OXFORD MEDICAL PUBLICATIONS

The Complete Recovery Room Book

Third Edition

THE COMPLETE RECOVERY ROOM BOOK

THIRD EDITION

ANTHEA HATFIELD

Armed Forces Hospital, Riyadh, Kingdom of Saudi Arabia

and

MICHAEL TRONSON

Box Hill Hospital, Melbourne, Australia

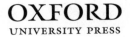

OXFORD
UNIVERSITY PRESS

OXFORD

UNIVERSITY PRESS

Great Clarendon Street, Oxford OX2 6DP

Oxford University Press is a department of the University of Oxford.
It furthers the University's objective of excellence in research, scholarship,
and education by publishing worldwide in

Oxford New York

Athens Auckland Bangkok Bogotá Buenos Aires Calcutta
Cape Town Chennai Dar es Salaam Delhi Florence Hong Kong Istanbul
Karachi Kuala Lumpur Madrid Melbourne Mexico City Mumbai
Nairobi Paris São Paulo Singapore Taipei Tokyo Toronto Warsaw
and associated companies in
Berlin Ibadan

Oxford is a registered trade mark of Oxford University Press
in the UK and in certain other countries

Published in the United States
by Oxford University Press Inc., New York

© Oxford University Press, 2001

First edition first published 1992
Second edition first published 1996
Reprinted 1998 (twice), 1999, 2000
Third edition first published 2001

A catalogue record for this title is available from the British Library

Library of Congress Cataloging in Publication Data
(Data available)

1 3 5 7 9 10 8 6 4 2

ISBN 0 19 263218 3 (Pbk)

Printed in Great Britain on acid free paper by
Biddles Ltd,
Guildford & King's Lynn

PREFACE

Many marvellous, and some disturbing, things have happened since we completed the second edition five years ago. Changes in anaesthetic, and surgical techniques allow many patients to have their operation and be discharged, either on same day, or the day after their surgery. In the 1950s patients stayed in hospital 21 days after a hysterectomy, but now the average stay is 2 – 3 nights. Most joint replacements previously stayed up to a month in hospital, and are now discharged to a rehabilitation centre in 4 – 7 days. Wound healing is much improved with the reduction of the stress response to surgery.[1]

Short acting anaesthetic agents allow patients to regain consciousness more quickly, but some now wake so abruptly that they become disorientated and upset. Research into pain mechanisms, and a better understanding of analgesics means more effective pain control. Despite initial hopes, patient controlled analgesia has not reduced hospital stay.

In an effort to reduce costs hospitals are increasingly efficient. While in most cases this has improved patient care; in others we look back through misted rose coloured glasses at the 'good old days' with their continuity of care. Patients are now on a standardized production line, the *clinical pathway*. In some centres surgeons do not even meet their patients until they see them on the operating table, and rely on someone else's assessment!

Preassessment clinics have reduced the incidence of unfit patients presenting for surgery, and this brings fewer unexpected problems to the recovery room. Anaesthetists and recovery room nurses have extended their care into the postoperative period resulting in better pain control, fluid balance and metabolic care. Patients receive preoperative education from medical, nursing and physiotherapy staff. Clinical pathways plan each step of the patient's progress through the hospital. Some big busy hospitals are practising *hot bedding* where patients for elective surgery are admitted and discharged throughout the day as beds become available. Occasionally this just-in-time philosophy means a patient will be held in recovery room until a bed becomes available.

The recovery room remains the most important room in the hospital for it is here that the patient is at most risk from inadvertent harm. Problems can evolve into critical situations extremely rapidly, and many of these are avoidable. Postoperative chest infections still frequently occur, but the big postoperative killers are now pulmonary emboli and myocardial infarction. Pulmonary embolism kills more people each year than breast cancer.[2] Deep vein thromboses almost certainly seed during the metabolic turmoil at the end of surgery, and the first half an hour in the recovery room. It is increasingly obvious that postoperative myocardial infarction trumpets its coming in the recovery room even though it may not finally appear until a few days later.[3]

Patients are increasingly seeking help outside mainstream medicine. Many patients are taking untested drugs (herbal remedies) with sometimes unpredictable, and occasionally tragic consequences particularly bleeding, disordered liver function, kidney damage, asthma and cardiac arrhythmias

The introduction of low molecular weight heparins have affected the use of spinal and epidural anaesthesia, and recent outbreak of spinal haematomas is worrying.

Recovery rooms are now a more hazardous environments to work in . Strict adherence to *universal precautions* is needed to prevent transmission of nasty diseases such as HIV or hepatitis. Latex allergy, almost unknown for the 80 years that latex gloves have routinely been worn, has suddenly emerged as a huge problem.[4]

At long last hypothermia has been recognised as a major cause of much postoperative morbidity and there are excellent devices now available for preventing perioperative heat loss.

Some problems remain with us. The most worrying is that clinical physiology of hypoxia is still not well understood by either medical or nursing staff, particularly the implications of oxygen saturation measured by the pulse oximeter. The danger and incidence of episodic postoperative hypoxaemia, especially at night, in elderly patients undergoing major joint replacements is still not generally recognized. This danger lasts for up to a week following surgery, and is particularly likely if the patient is receiving opioids.[5] Hypoxia quickly maims or kills, and oxygen is cheap and accessible.

Anaesthetists and surgeons are slowly becoming aware of the implications of the vigorous immunosuppression caused by homologous blood transfusion.[6]

So much research has been done into the effects of anaesthetic agents that the death and morbidity rates associated with anaesthetics in theatre has fallen dramatically. But we remain astounded at the continuing lack of worthwhile clinical research into the first few hours after surgery. Little has been done to describe or find the answers to some big clinical problems. How to prevent deep vein thrombosis in recovery room? How to prevent postoperative nausea and vomiting? How to predict and prevent postoperative myocardial ischaemia? How common is minor aspiration in the recovery room, and what part does this play in postoperative chest infections? And despite the knowledge collected over more than 120 years the physiology and destructive consequences of postoperative hypoxia remains poorly taught.

Recovery room staff are far better trained than in the past; and specialist perioperative nursing courses are common. Anaesthetists too, are extending their expertise to become perioperative physicians. It will not be long before recovery room becomes as much a specialty as intensive care is now.

Melbourne   A.H.
August 2000   M.T.

1. Chumbley GM, Hall GM. Editorial (1997) *British Journal of Anaesthesia* 78: 392-4
2. Hirsch J. Hoak M. (1998) *American Heart Association Scientific Statement.*
3. Personal communication September 1999, Prof. H. Salem (Haematologist) at Box Hill Hospital.
4. Ferguson SJ, Kam PCA, Thompson JF. (1998) *Australian Anaesthesia.*
5. Witt S. (1999) US Dept Labor Occupational Safety and Administration Technical Bulletin http://www.netcom.com/~nam1/tib.html
6. Dyson A. Henderson AM *et al* (1988) *Anaesthesia and Intensive Care* 16:405-10

PREFACE TO THE SECOND EDITION

This is a book for staff who, when alone and confronted with a problem in an isolated hospital, need practical advice on what to do. Its aim is to help you save lives. Saving lives includes preventing complications that may at worst permanently maim the patient, for example, brain damage; or less seriously, delay their discharge from hospital.

It is a practical book for those who are neither fully trained anaesthetists, nor specialist trained recovery room nursing staff. While the text is purposefully dogmatic and direct, the regimes described are effective under most circumstances. This book is not a substitute for personal instruction from an expert, nor an alternative for practical experience. It does not compare theories, or argue different points of view.

In the best of circumstances, in properly staffed teaching hospitals, the safety of about 30 per cent of patients is in jeopardy during the first postoperative hour, and up to 50 per cent of all postoperative deaths occur during this time.[1,2] The outcome of major complications is better if they occur during anaesthesia; than if they occur in the recovery period.[3] Our experience suggests that the death rate in the recovery room of an isolated hospital is higher than that at a major teaching hospital. Urban hospitals also have periods of isolation, for instance after-hours, at weekends, during holiday periods, and at night. At these times fully trained recovery staff may be unavailable, their places taken by part-time staff who are unfamiliar with routine procedures.

Recovery rooms are specialized intensive care units, where patients need frequent and careful observation. It is our opinion that the recovery room is the most important room in a hospital. It is here that a patient is at greatest risk, and it is here the staff need to give immediate and skilled attention to save lives.

Only a paradigm shift in the minds of anaesthetists, clinical staff, and administrators will further reduce perioperative mortality and morbidity. There have been astounding advances in anaesthesia in the past 25 years, the intraoperative death rate has fallen perhaps twenty-fold, and it is rare for a patient to suffer harm from the anaesthetic. The time has come to turn attention to the neglected first few hours after surgery. Clinical impressions, although statistically useless, are a good starting place to design trials. Clinical audit is essential, but impressions are needed to help guide what to audit. We believe that clinical research should now aim at identifying factors that predict the outcome of events in the recovery room For instance our own clinical impressions suggest that life-threatening events take place during the physiological and biochemical, turmoil of the first few hours after emergence from anaesthesia. It is at this time that events such as deep vein thrombosis, postoperative hypoxaemia, pneumonia, and cardiac problems begin. We believe that it is possible to achieve a further reduction in postoperative morbidity and mortality, but to achieve this, facts are needed; and as we have discovered, facts about the recovery room are hard to find.

Melbourne   A.H.
March 1996   M.T.

1. Zelcer J., Wells D. G. (1987). *Anaesthesia and Intensive Care*, 15: 168-173
2. *Report on Deaths Associated with Anaesthesia in Australia* 1988-1990; National Health and Medical Research Council Document.
3. Tirets L., Desmont J. M. (1986). *Canadian Anaesthetists' Society Journal*, 33: 336-44

DEDICATION

To Dr Michael Davies for his foresight and ingenuity at planning a recovery room of the 'future' in a climate of budget restraints, and to Carol Anders and the nurses in her team at the St Vincent's Hospital, Melbourne; and to the recovery room staff at Box Hill Hospital who devote their efforts so conscientiously in the pursuit of excellence in patient care.

THE ISOLATED HOSPITAL AND DEDICATION TO THE SECOND EDITION

The difficulties encountered by an isolated hospital are different from those of large, busy urban hospitals. The staff of isolated hospitals have often spent years without contact with people of similar interests and with no chance to exchange ideas and experiences. New techniques are slow to arrive, and drugs and other essential items are scarce. Equipment fails, and no one knows how to repair it. These problems are exacerbated by local health authorities, who seem to neither understand the problems, nor care. The grind of constant work, and the battle for limited resources, exhausts enthusiasm and depresses the spirit. The result is intellectual burn out; the standard of care imperceptibly drops, and untoward incidents occur. Morale falls and a feeling of helplessness begins to seep into the soul of the staff. The difficulties soon come to be regarded as inevitable. This is made worse by visitors who tactlessly point out what is wrong, without having any idea of the cause, or of the constant struggle required to maintain standards.

We dedicate this second edition of The Complete Recovery Room Book to all the doctors and nurses who, each day, strive to maintain standards despite overwhelming difficulties, and especially those we have met in the hospitals of the South West Pacific.

FIRST EDITION DEDICATED TO

Pamela Deighton, Palega Vaeau, and Grant Scarf
- the first recovery room team to Samoa

CONTENTS

INTRODUCTION

Eternal vigilance is the price of safety.

It is a common belief that patients are asleep during their operation. They are not asleep. They are in a drug induced coma, and to metabolize and excrete these drugs takes time. During this time they gradually recover consciousness, but remain unable to care for themselves. They are at risk from a range of disasters as they emerge from the protection of the anaesthetic. Suddenly, they are exposed to extreme physiological disturbances, caused by pain, hypothermia, hypoxia and shifts in blood volume. Not only do the recovery room staff have to be adept at the management of a comatose, and physiologically unstable patient; but also, in the care of a surgical patient with drains, drips and dressings.

Before recovery rooms were routinely available, almost half the deaths in the immediate postoperative period such as airway obstruction or aspiration of stomach contents were preventable.

The recovery room provides a way of smoothing the transition of patient care from the operating theatre to the wards. Its function is to safeguard the patient in the immediate postoperative period when he is least able to look after himself. It relieves the ward of the necessity to dedicate one nurse to one patient, and removes the need to duplicate equipment. It also enables staff with special training to be concentrated in one area so they can maintain their skills and train more junior staff.

Recovery rooms improve patient safety, save money,
and allow the wards to work more efficiently.

How to use this book
Use this book like an encyclopaedia to provide information quickly about an unfamiliar clinical problem, operative procedure, or an emergency. It is not intended to be read in one sitting. There are many cross references, and

at times deliberate repetition of material to help you find answers to your questions easily and quickly.

Terminology

In recent years the term *post anaesthetic care unit* (with its acronym *PACU*) has become popular. Recovery room, is still the most common term in the hospitals we work in. The word recovery emphasizes the function of this room; to safeguard patients recovering from the insults of surgery and anaesthesia; and for this reason we have retained it.

In the United Kingdom it has become customary to measure pressures in kilopascals (kPa); however most other countries continue to measure pressures, especially blood pressures, in millimetres of mercury (mmHg). We have decided to stay with common usage in our region, so blood pressures are recorded in millimetres of mercury, with kilopascals quoted for blood gases. Haemoglobin is now measured in gms/L and not gms%.

In our region (and in our book) medically qualified anaesthesiologists are called *anaesthetists*. In the USA anaesthetists usually are not medically qualified, whereas anaesthesiologists are.

Grammar

Most medical textbooks and journal articles are written in the past passive tense. This form is an academic convention and is sometimes ambiguous. It is also boring, and difficult to understand, for those who do not speak English as their first language. With these readers in mind, we have tried to keep our writing as simple, and as graphic, as possible. We have deliberately written much of this text in direct active speech, a "do this", "do that" form, which we hope will link educational goals with service needs.

Drug names

In the workplace, drug trade names are often more recognizable than generic names. Although this is theoretically undesirable, it is a fact, and for this reason the trade names of drugs are usually quoted after the generic names, for instance propofol (Diprivan®). It is not feasible to quote all the trade names, so where relevant we have used the trade name of the company that first developed the drug. The appendix on drugs will help you convert generic names to trade names.

Aphorisms
We make no apology for these simple, direct and obvious catch phrases scattered throughout the book. They are there to jog the memory. Staff may not remember the physiological reasons for something, but they do remember the phrase.

Tables
Some of the tables and lists are designed to be photocopied as wall charts.

Gender
For the sake of simplicity in the text, nurses and paramedical staff are referred to as she, and doctors and patients as he. This is still the commonest configuration in most parts of the world and no offence is intended.

Abbreviations
The number and variety of abbreviations used in medicine is increasing at a bewildering rate. We have made up a list of the ones we have collected over the years, but it is far from complete.

Drugs
Drug schedules are continually revised, new side effects and hazards recognized and formulations changed. For this reason every reader is urged to consult the drug company's printed instructions before administering any of the drugs recommended in this book.

Our opinions
Medical knowledge is advancing rapidly. New ideas come, and concepts that have been worshiped as dogma for years are dropped. In an attempt to keep this edition simple, and practical; and the cost down, we have pruned and simplified the text. We have decided not to attempt to describe every disorder, but to devote most of the space usefully, to commonly encountered problems. We have therefore excluded cardiac surgery and specialized neurosurgery. This book is written forthrightly, and the opinions expressed are our own. We appreciate that there are many different points of view on what is, and what is not, the correct treatment of a particular clinical problem. This book tells the way we do it, and not everyone may agree. This book is a guide, not a rule book. It offers suggestions, not instructions. It is impossible to cover every clinical situation, and sometimes you will need common-sense to modify treatment

to fit the circumstances. Safety is our prime concern; if you have any doubts about what you are doing, we urge you to consult a colleague.

In medicine there are rarely absolutes, events and outcomes may, or may not happen. Things may be possible, or probable. If an outcome is almost inevitable we have tried to avoid qualifiers such as may or probable. We have written this book to teach, and to be successful in this aim we have been purposely dogmatic. It is easier to remember that hypoxia is harmful, than hypoxia may be harmful under certain circumstances.

There are certain to be omissions of fact, and we would be grateful for suggestions on ways to improve this manual for a future edition.

Acknowledgements
We acknowledge thankfully all the people who have helped us, wittingly or unwittingly. Over the years we have accumulated notes, listened to presentations at conferences, read journals and texts, and absorbed large amounts of anecdotal data in operating theatre tea-rooms. Many of the sources of this information are lost, but to these our unknown teachers and advisers, we express our most grateful thanks.

Acknowledgements to the third edition
Sydney Jacobs and David Anders for editorial comments and corrections, Carol Anders, Ruth Crampton, Gretta Chandler, Luke Hickey, Hoang Vien and Vicki Woodruff for reading and commenting on the chapters: Design, Monitoring, Staffing, Equipment and Purchasing Equipment, and Drains. Claude Calandra for reading, commenting and contributing to Mothers and Babies. Eileen Halliday for reading and commenting on Paediatrics, Peter Hatfield for reading and commenting on the Intravenous Fluids and Renal chapter. Ian Cobble for the information on fire safety.

Book Design
Inhouse Design Group Ltd, 62 Ponsonby Rd, Auckland, New Zealand.

Illustrations
Arch MacDonnell, 94 Lincoln St, Auckland, New Zealand.

THE 20 GOLDEN RULES OF RECOVERY ROOM

1. The confused, restless or agitated patient is hypoxic until proven otherwise.

2. Your patient may be hypoxic even if the oximeter reads 98% saturated.

3. Never turn your back on your patient.

4. The blood pressure does not necessarily fall in haemorrhagic shock.

5. Never ignore a tachycardia or bradycardia, find the cause.

6. Postoperative hypertension is dangerous.

7. Never, ever, use a painful stimulus to rouse your patient.

8. Noisy breathing is obstructed breathing, however not all obstructed breathing is noisy.

9. Nurse your patient on his side in the recovery position.

10. Allow the patient to remove his own airway.

11. If your patient is slow to wake up, consider hypothermia.

12. Cuddle crying children.

13. The opioids do not cause hypotension in stable patients.

14. When giving drugs to the elderly, start by giving half as much, twice as slowly.

15. If you don't know all the actions of a drug, then do not use it until you do.

16. Treat the patient, not the monitor.

17. A patient with cold hands is haemodynamically unstable.

18. Pain prevention is better than pain relief.

19. Do not discharge a patient until he can maintain a 15 second head-lift.

20. If confused - read rule #1.

1. ROUTINE RECOVERY ROOM PROCEDURES

This chapter follows the patient from the operating theatre, discusses his care in the recovery room, and describes his discharge and transport to the ward.

PREPARATION BEFORE THE PATIENT'S ADMISSION

Before receiving a patient make it a routine to check all your equipment. Fatalities can happen for lack of something simple, like inadequate suction, or because of a disconnected oxygen line.

Everything must be ready
before the patient comes from theatre.

At the beginning of each shift check that:
- the resuscitation trolley has been checked. Enter this fact in the trolley's maintenance book or daily diary;
- the drug cupboard is restocked;
- disposable items have been replaced;
- sharps and rubbish containers are emptied and cleaned;
- suction bottles and tubing are clean and working;
- oxygen and suction supplies are adequate;
- a good supply of warm blankets, clean gowns and gloves are available;
- alarm bells are working.

Before each patient arrives check:
- a clean high capacity sucker is switched on and working;
- oxygen mask is connected and ready;
- if oxygen cylinders are being used then check there is sufficient oxygen in them;
- some means of assisting the patient's breathing, such as a Mapleson's C circuit, or an Ambu®, or Laerdal bag®, with properly fitting mask is available;
- pulse oximeter is switched on and working;
- Non invasive blood pressure (NBP) machine is working and cuffs of each size are available;
- intravenous drip hangers are ready.

Transport to the Recovery Room

Moving the patient from the operating table to the special recovery room trolley requires skill and care. Lines, drains and monitors easily become disconnected at this stage. Never leave the patient alone for any reason. Keep the trolley sides up at all times.

Many hands make light work.

The anaesthetist, and a nurse must accompany the patient from the operating theatre to the recovery room.

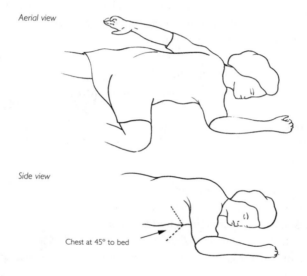

Aerial view

Side view

Chest at 45° to bed

fig 1.1 Typical recovery position

Wheel the patient from the operating theatre feet first. The anaesthetist walks forwards (never backwards) maintaining an airway. Generally the patient will lie in the left lateral, or recovery position.

Admission to the Recovery Room

This is a most important procedure where the immediate care of the patient is being handed from the medical staff to the recovery room nursing staff. Both the anaesthetist and the nurse need to hand over independently, to a competent member of the recovery room staff.

Anaesthetic handover should include:

- age of the patient;
- significant medical conditions;
- procedure (this may differ from the scheduled operation);
- details of vital signs: blood pressure, pulse, respiratory rate;
- untoward incidents during or before surgery;
- analgesia given and anticipated analgesic needs;
- blood loss;
- fluids given and expected future needs;
- antibiotics given, and when the next dose is due;
- urine output during the procedure, and expected output for the next few hours;
- the patient's anxiety level and pre-operative psychological problems;
- monitoring required in the recovery room;
- investigations required.

Before the anaesthetist leaves the recovery room the patient must have an adequate airway, good oxygen saturation and a satisfactory blood pressure. He should also tell the nursing staff where he will be so that they may contact him quickly if the need arises. The anaesthetist should not be far away while the patient is still in the recovery room.

Maintain the patient's airway
during the handover.

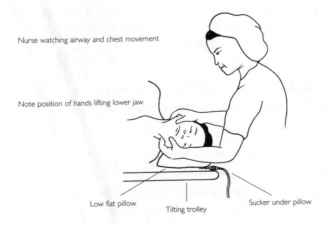

Nurse watching airway and chest movement

Note position of hands lifting lower jaw

Low flat pillow

Tilting trolley

Sucker under pillow

fig 1.2 Attention to the patient's airway

Nursing staff handover includes:

- Checking the name of the patient against their notes and identity bracelet;
- care and placement of drains;
- precautions about dressings;
- special nursing requirements, such as the position of the patient;
- nursing problems, such as pressure areas, and psychological status;
- organization of the patient's notes;
- ensuring the correct charts and x-rays accompany the patient;
- personal belongings, such as dentures and hearing aids.

PERCEPTIONS OF THE RECOVERY ROOM

Staff perception of a patient's recovery

If the patient is comatose his airway will need support, and his pharynx and mouth kept clear of secretions. At this stage the patient may not respond to any stimuli. Plantar reflexes may not react, or if the patient is emerging will show an upgoing response. The pupils may not react to light As the patient responds, his gaze becomes divergent and the pupils constrict in reaction to light. A few moments before awakening pupils dilate and the patient starts to move his limbs and perhaps shiver or shake. His pulse and blood pressure often rise. He then usually takes a big breath; or sighs just before opening his eyes. Although awake the patient may have clouded consciousness for 5 to 10 minutes. He probably will have no memory of this stage.

Occasionally the patient is confused, restless, disoriented and possibly fearful. You will not be able to reason with him. This period of delirium, is called an *acute brain syndrome* (see page 437).

Exclude hypoxia and hypoglycaemia
as the cause of postoperative restlessness.

Patient's perception of their own recovery

Hearing is the first sense to return. Voices are very loud, distorted and sometimes frightening. Even the sound of a telephone ringing can be alarming. Lights seem unduly bright hurting the eyes. Vision is blurred. Arms and legs feel heavy. Pain may be unbelievable and is often described as the worst the patient has ever experienced. Finally sense of locality and memory return. The patient feels disoriented and giddy, and often asks "Where am I?"

Visitors

Apart from mothers of children it is probably unwise to allow visitors to see patients who are recovering from anaesthesia. Visitors can become distressed if they see a loved one disoriented, vomiting, or in pain.

INITIAL ASSESSMENT

On admission to the recovery room, immediately after applying an oxygen mask to the patient's face, check in the following order the A,B,C,D and E:

A Airway

- Make sure the patient has a clear airway, is breathing and the air is moving freely and quietly in and out of the chest.
- If necessary gently suck out the patient's mouth and pharynx. If he is still unconscious make sure an oral airway is properly located between his teeth and tongue and lips are in no danger of being bitten.
- Administer oxygen with a mask. Begin with a flow rate of 6 litres of oxygen per minute. Attach a pulse oximeter.

B Breathing

- Check his chest is moving and you can feel air flowing in and out of his mouth.
- Look for any sign of cyanosis and note the reading on the pulse oximeter. If it is reading less than 96 per cent, search for the reason. (See hypoxia page 295). Do not allow the patient to snore, noisy breathing is obstructed breathing.

C Circulation

- Only then measure the blood pressure, pulse rate and rhythm and record these observations on the chart.
- Note his *perfusion status* (see page 255) and record this in the notes.

D Drugs, Drips and Drains and Dressings

- Note drugs given in theatre, particularly analgesics, that may affect the patient's breathing. Check whether the patient has any allergies, and what drugs he will require while in the recovery room.
- Note intravenous fluids in progress, how much fluid and what type have been given during the operation. Check that the drip is running freely, and is well sited. Make sure that no pieces of tape

encircle the arm, replace these if necessary. Tape encircling the arm can cause distal ischaemia if the arm swells for any reason. Splint the infusion site if the cannula lies across the wrist or elbow joint.

- Note drain tubes; with what, and how fast they are draining. Make sure the urinary catheter is not obstructed, note the contents of the collecting bag.

E   Extras

- Measure the patient's temperature. This is essential for all babies and any patient who has had major surgery (see page 146).
- If the patient is a diabetic measure his blood glucose or urinary sugars.
- Check the patient's history to see whether there are any risk factors that predispose to hypoglycaemia;
- Plaster checks;
- Pulses following arterial surgery;
- Circulation of graft sites.

CONTINUING CARE IN RECOVERY ROOM

Phases in recovery[1]

PHASE 1: The patient returns to consciousness with intact protective reflexes. (If this takes longer than 10 minutes then see page 441). He should be able to sustain a head lift for 5 seconds, deep breathe, and cough effectively.

PHASE 2: During this phase the patient recovers the ability to think clearly and movement returns. At the end of this phase the patient can return to the ward.

PHASE 3: At the end of this phase all the effects of the anaesthetic should be gone. This can take 48 hours or more.

Oxygen, why is it so important to give it?

If the patient does not receive supplemental oxygen after general anaesthesia he is at risk of hypoxia because:

- nitrous oxide washing back into the patient's lungs displaces air containing oxygen. This process is called *diffusion hypoxia*;
- shallow breathing may cause carbon dioxide to build up in his lungs, displacing air containing oxygen. This process is called *hypoventilation*;
- opioids, such as fentanyl, morphine or pethidine, given during the

anaesthetic depress the respiratory centre's stimulatory response to rising carbon dioxide levels in the blood. This causes shallow breathing.

- Volatile anaesthetic agents, such as isoflurane, sevoflurane, enflurane, depress both the peripheral chemoreceptors in the carotid body, and the chemical receptors stimulatory response to a falling oxygen tension in the blood.

- Hypothermic patients may shiver which increases the skeletal muscles oxygen requirements more than seven-fold. In response the heart must greatly increase its cardiac output, and this may not be possible.

Even the patients who have had spinals or epidurals need additional oxygen because:

- they have vasodilated extremities and the heart has to work harder (using extra oxygen) to pump the blood through these dilated vessels;

- they are susceptible to low blood pressures.

Continue to give oxygen
while the patient is in recovery room.

MONITORING AFTER ADMISSION

Monitors alert you to life threatening situations, and allow you to more easily follow trends in the patient's physiological variables, such as blood pressure, pulse, and oxygenation.

Treat the patient not the monitor.

Blood pressure

Take the blood pressure on admission, then at 5 minute intervals for 15 minutes, (or follow your hospital protocol) and then every ten minutes thereafter. If a patient has had intravenous analgesia or other drugs in recovery room measure the blood pressure more frequently. A non-invasive blood pressure (NBP) monitor is useful for patients with cardiovascular instability, following major blood or fluid loss, and in head injured patients. The NBP monitor is subject to errors, and is especially inaccurate if the pulse is irregular. Always check the first one or two readings with a manual blood pressure machine. If the pressure is extremely high or extremely low, check it manually as well (see page 29).

Pulse

Record the pulse rate, rhythm and volume. If the pulse rate is irregular, suspect an arrhythmia and apply an ECG. The most common cause of an irregular pulse is sinus arrhythmia, a normal variation in young people where the pulse rises and falls with respiration. More insidious are atrial fibrillation or ventricular premature beats (see page 266).

If you detect an irregular pulse
monitor with an ECG.

Respiratory rate

Causes for a rising respiratory rate include sputum retention, developing heart failure, rising temperature, or a change in intracranial pressure. The commonest reason for a decreasing respiratory rate is opioid overdose.

Temperature

Measure the patient's temperature when they first arrive in recovery room. The normal range of core temperature 36.5 and 37.2°C. Patients are often cold so have extra blankets nearby. If their temperature is below 36°C consider warming them with a forced air convection heater such as Bair Hugger™. If their temperature is raised, advise the surgical team. Read more about temperature on page 145.

Pulse oximeter

All patients need access to this facility. In some isolated hospitals you may only have one pulse oximeter — share it between patients.

If you detect an irregular pulse,
monitor with an ECG.

ECG

Monitor with an ECG, any patient who is at risk of cardiac arrhythmias, or ischaemic heart disease. There is a list of major risk factors on page 276. Also read more about ECG on page 245.

INJECTIONS

Give deep intramuscular injections only into the upper (outer) lateral quadrant of the thigh. Adults of normal weight and muscle mass can tolerate a maximum of 5 ml of injection. Patients less than 45 kg can tolerate no more that 2 ml injectioned into their muscles. Make sure the needle is long enough to deposit the drug into the muscle, and not into the fat covering it. Fat is poorly perfused and the drug absorption will be delayed. Wait until the preparation fluid is dry. Grasp the injection site firmly, and insert the needle at 90°. Dart the needle in, and press the plunger slowly to avoid sudden painful distension of the muscle. Do not massage the injection site, but encourage the patient to move his leg around.

Intramuscular injections should never be given into the buttocks of children. Sometimes drugs have been accidentally injected into the sciatic nerve, permanently damaging it, and causing the leg to become paralysed.

In children, and thin adults avoid injections into the deltoid muscle as this can injure the circumflex nerve. The upper outer lateral aspect of the thigh is the only safe intramuscular injection site in children.

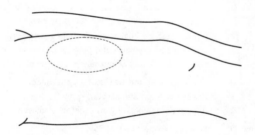

*fig 1.3 Safe area for intramuscular injections in children
on the upper outer lateral quadrant of the thigh*

SUGGESTED NEEDLE SIZES		
PATIENT SIZE	NEEDLE SIZE (inches)	NEEDLE SIZE (mm)
Obese adult	21 G x 1.50	0.80 x 38
Average adult	23 G x 1.25	0.63 x 32
Thin or emaciated adult	25 G x 1.25	0.50 x 25
Child	25 G x 1.00	0.50 x 22

Recovery Room Scoring Systems

The recovery room records are a continuation of the anaesthetic record. It is better to keep them on the same chart, with the anaesthetic record on the left of the chart, and the recovery room record on the right side.

Many recovery rooms have a scoring system for assessing, and monitoring their patients to ensure they are safe and comfortable for discharge.

PATIENT ADMISSION ASSESSMENT

SAFETY CRITERIA

Respiration	0	Needs assisted ventilation.
	1	Laboured or > 20 or < 10 breaths/minute.
	2	Normal rate 12 – 15 breaths/minute. Can take deep breaths and cough.
Perfusion	0	Cyanotic or dusky colour.
	1	Pale with cold hands.
	2	Warm and pink.
Power	0	Unable to lift head or move limbs on command.
	1	Moves limbs but unable to sustain head lift.
	2	Sustains head lift for full 5 seconds.
Circulation	0	Blood pressure increased or decreased by 50% of preoperative level; or pulse >150 or <45.
	1	Blood pressure 20% above or below preoperative level.
	2	Stable blood pressure and pulse with no significant changes for 3 sets of quarter hourly readings.
Sedation	0	Does not respond to shaking by shoulder.
	1	Rouses only on stimulation.
	2	Awake communicating and seldom drowses.
Temperature	0	Axillary temperature < 35°C.
	1	Axillary temperature 35 – 36°C.
	2	Axillary temperature > 36°C.

Score out of 12

COMFORT CRITERIA

Nausea	0	Nauseated and vomiting.
	1	Nauseated only.
	2	Neither nauseated nor vomiting.
Pain	0	Severe distressing pain.
	1	Uncomfortable.
	2	Pain free.

Score out of 4

For analysis data can be entered on a standard spread sheet computer program, and presented every month at the recovery room meeting. There have been many different proposed scoring systems, however the one shown here is useful. With some score systems the patient can be hypertensive, hypoxic and at risk of myocardial infarction or ischaemia, yet scored as fit for discharge from the recovery room.

In using these scores consider two separate issues. Firstly, is the patient safe to discharge from the recovery room, and secondly is he comfortable?

These scores are simple to use and they provide objective evidence on which to base quality assessment and educational programs. They enable statistics to be gathered, workloads assessed, and staff deployed for maximum efficiency. A scoring system gives them feedback on specific areas of their work, and makes potential problems more easily defined. For instance, any patient who does not score at least 10 out of 12 within the first 30 minutes should be reported to the anaesthetist.

PROCEDURES

Exercises for the emerging patient

STIR-UP EXERCISES: Once the patient is awake encourage him to do a number of simple exercises to reduce the chance of postoperative pneumonia and deep vein thrombosis. The exercises are sometimes referred to as *stir-up exercises.*

Most deep vein thrombosis starts in the recovery room.

DEEP BREATHING EXERCISES: The aim is to inflate segments of lung that inevitably collapse during general anaesthesia. Encourage the patient to take 2 - 3 very deep breaths every 5 minutes.

COUGHING EXERCISES: These clear the airways of mucus and dried secretions. Sit the patient up if possible. If he has an abdominal wound then show him how to hold it when he coughs. Coughing exercises must not be done after open eye, middle ear, intracranial, facial or plastic surgery.

LEG EXERCISES: These prevent a deep vein thrombosis forming. Get the patient to move their feet up and down, and to bend their legs at the knees. In patients at risk from thromboembolism anti-embolic graded elastic stockings should be fitted before the patient goes to theatre. They are effective in preventing deep vein thrombosis.

Pressure care

Check the patient's body for pressure areas. Make sure the patient is lying on a soft smooth surface. If areas of redness are still present when the patient is ready to leave recovery room, then point them out to the ward staff. Do not rub red areas; they are already traumatized enough, just pad them, and remove the weight from the area.

Beware of red areas in elderly, thin and malnourished patients.

Suction

PHARYNGEAL SUCTION: Keep a high flow, high capacity suction under each patient's pillow. Unconscious patients are unable to cope with their secretions and need to be nursed in the standard recovery position.

Patients are much safer on their sides,
try to keep them from lying on their back.

If necessary clear the mouth and pharynx with a dental sucker. Do not force the sucker between the teeth or you may damage the delicate mucosal lining of the mouth and pharynx, dislodge restorative dental caps or loose teeth. If the sucker touches the posterior pharyngeal wall of the soft palate, it can make the patient gag or vomit. Patients recovering from an anaesthetic, where a volatile agent has been used, sometimes clench their teeth tightly making it difficult to pass the sucker into their mouth. In these cases pass a soft 16 G plastic Y-suction catheter down along the floor of their nose into their pharynx. Remember the floor of the nose runs straight back, and not upwards. Frequently the patient will respond by tossing his head from side to side, and opening his mouth enabling you to insert an oropharyngeal airway

TRACHEOBRONCHIAL SUCTION[2] (*sucking out*): Occasionally patients are intubated or have a tracheostomy when they return to the recovery room. Their endotracheal tubes need to be aspirated at intervals to clear the accumulating sputum. Smokers produce more sputum than a normal patient, and need more nursing care.

Excessive mucus in the airways can be heard as a harsh rattling sound during breathing. This is a sign the patient requires sucking out. Palpation of the chest will reveal a coarse vibration as air gurgles past the mucus in the trachea or major bronchi.

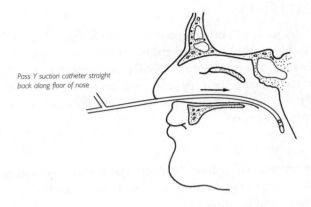

Pass Y suction catheter straight
back along floor of nose

fig 1.4 Transnasal suction of nasopharynx

Suction is not necessary in every patient.

Be careful with tracheobronchial suction. It is distressing and painful for an awake patient, similar to having a lump of food 'go down the wrong way'. Vigorous coughing sharply raises the blood pressure, intracranial pressure, and intraocular pressure, and causes venous congestion in the head and neck. Hypoxia is a constant risk; reflex bradycardia or tachycardia can occur. Take care to use a catheter that is less than half the diameter of the lumen of the endotracheal tube.[3] A dangerous, and sometimes fatal, decrease in intrathoracic pressure can rupture lung tissue if too large a suction catheter is used.

Many patients who have heart disease, with unstable circulations, are at risk from arrhythmias and hypoxia. To prevent endotracheal suction causing a sharp rise in blood pressure, with the risk of aggravating bleeding, or causing other complications, instill lignocaine 1 mg/kg down the endotracheal tube. Similarly use lignocaine in patients with the following risk factors:

- head injury;
- eye surgery;
- ear surgery;
- neurosurgery;
- plastic surgery on the head or neck;
- hypertension;
- ischaemic heart disease.

INTUBATED PATIENTS

Occasionally the anaesthetist will bring a patient to the recovery room still intubated. Reasons for this include, a prolonged operation, poor respiratory function, elderly patients, sicker patients, difficulty reversing the muscle relaxants, hypothermia. Usually these patients will be extubated in the recovery room before they are returned to the ward. They may or may not need ventilating during this period.

Extubation[4]

About 5 per cent of patients will require extubation in the recovery room. Before this can be safely performed the patient must fulfil three criteria.

1. They must be able to breathe adequately.
2. They must not be unduly depressed by narcotic drugs.
3. They must be able to protect their own airway against accidental aspiration of material in the pharynx.

1. CAN THE PATIENT BREATHE ADEQUATELY?

It is probably safe to extubate:
- If the patient has normal lungs and can take deep breaths on command through the endotracheal tube;
- If you are uncertain whether the tidal volume is adequate, measure it for one minute with a Dragermeter®, or Wright's Respirometer®. Before extubation the patient's tidal volume needs to be 5 - 7 ml/kg with a respiratory rate greater than 10 breaths/minute;
- If you do not have either of these instruments, then prime an anaesthetic machine with oxygen and attach the patient. When the

USEFUL TIPS

- To obtund the violent responses and patient distress to this unpleasant procedure use 1% lignocaine 0.1 ml/kg down the tracheal tube, and repeat after one minute;
- Explain to the patient what is to happen;
- For unstable patients get an assistant to help you;
- Pre-oxygenate on 100% oxygen for at least a minute;
- It is a sterile procedure, so wear sterile gloves;
- Hold your own breath while you a sucking the patient out to remind you how long the patient is holding his breath;
- Gently and slowly withdraw the catheter, watching for secretions;
- If the sputum is tenacious, try instilling 2 – 3 ml of 0.9% saline down the tube;
- Turning the head to one side often allows the sucker to go down the opposite bronchus.

patient takes a deep breath the black reservoir bag should deflate by 800 ml or more. To gauge the volume it is useful to remember the volume of a normal adult clenched fist is about 350 - 400 ml.

2. IS THE PATIENT UNDULY DEPRESSED BY NARCOTIC DRUGS OR ARE THEIR LUNGS AFFECTED IN OTHER WAYS?

- Attach the patient to a 'T-piece' and observe their ventilatory rate. If it is less than 8 breaths per minute do not attempt extubation. If it is less than 5 breaths a minute, then assist the patient's breathing and assume that his respiration is depressed by narcotics. Unless the patient is distressed, delay extubation if the arterial PCO_2 is greater than 50 mmHg (6.6 kPa) or the arterial PO_2 is less than 100 mmHg (13 kPa) while breathing 35% oxygen.
- The oxygen saturation meter can help you make a decision about whether the PaO_2 is high enough to extubate the patient. (See the table on page 28).

TEN STEPS IN EXTUBATION

1. Put the patient on high inspired concentration of oxygen for 3 minutes before proceeding. Bring the resuscitation trolley to the bedside. Attach a pulse oximeter and an ECG.
2. Check the pharynx with a laryngoscope making sure there is no foreign material, such as a throat pack present, if so remove it.
3. Under direct vision suck out the pharynx to remove all secretions and blood. Remember to check the nasopharynx behind and above the soft palate for blood clot, secretions and foreign material. A clot forming in the nasopharynx cannot be seen by merely looking in the pharynx. In the past these clots have fallen into the larynx, or have been aspirated into the trachea obstructing it suddenly. It may be the coroner who finds this on post mortem, hence its name.
4. Lay the patient on his left side.
5. Remove the ties and tapes securing the endotracheal tube, and deflate the cuff slowly with a 20 ml syringe.
6. Disconnect the catheter mount. If the patient has audible secretions in their chest pass a soft suction catheter down the endotracheal tube. While applying suction ask the patient to take a big breath in. At the end of inspiration with one smooth movement withdraw the tube together with the suction catheter. The patient will now have a lung full of air and will cough.
7. Put the patient on an oxygen mask with a 6 litre per minute flow.
8. Encourage a few deep breaths and coughs to reassure both the patient and yourself.
9. Watch the oximeter to check the patient's saturation remains good.
10. Watch for signs of postoperative hypoxia or hypercarbia. Encourage the patient to deep breathe and cough.

3. CAN THE PATIENT PROTECT HIS OWN AIRWAY?
- Unless the patient is fully conscious it is unwise to extubate the patient if there is a suspicion that he may have a full stomach.
- Delay extubation until the patient is conscious if the intubation was difficult, or the patient has an abnormal upper airway.
- Do not extubate a patient, unless on command, he can sustain a 5 second head lift from the pillow; and touch the tip of his nose with his finger.
- If a restless patient is co-ordinated enough to reach up and grab his own endotracheal tube, he will be conscious enough to look guard his airway.

If the patient takes out his own airway,
then he is safe without it.

DISCHARGE AND TRANSPORT

Length of stay in the recovery room

ADULTS: Ideally patients stay in the recovery room for at least an hour after general anaesthesia and half an hour after local anaesthesia. Each hospital has its own protocols, but the following guidelines are widely accepted. Patients with regional anaesthetic blocks, such as spinal and epidural anaesthesia stay at least an hour after the blood pressure becomes stable. Patients stay 30 minutes after an intramuscular dose of opioid.

CHILDREN: Observe healthy children for at least 30 minutes if they have received inhalational anaesthesia by mask or laryngeal mask. Observe healthy children who have been intubated for at least an hour, because laryngeal oedema may take this long to become obvious. Following tonsillectomy, adenoidectomy, cleft palate repair, pharyngeal or other major intra-oral procedures observe the patient for 90 minutes. Infants less than 12 months of age, and those who have received naloxone are best observed for a minimum of two hours. Premature babies must stay longer if less than 18 months old.

The anaesthetist, or a member of the medical staff, must review the patient's status before discharge, and make an appropriate note on the patient's chart. The anaesthetist must be certain that the patient is safe to leave his immediate care, and that some other member of the medical staff is available, and properly instructed, to take over responsibility for the patient's welfare.

Discharge to the ward

1. Minimum criteria for discharge to the ward are:
   - the patient has a stable pulse rate, rhythm and blood pressure;
   - the patient is conscious and able to lift head clear of the pillow on demand;

PROTOCOL
CARE OF THE PATIENT AFTER SPINAL ANAESTHESIA

OBSERVATIONS
Standard post-anaesthetic observations.
Sensation should return within 4 hours. If after 4 hours the patient remains numb, and there is no 'pins-and-needles' sensation, notify the anaesthetist.

ANALGESIA
Severe pain may return suddenly once the spinal block has worn off. Give analgesia at the first complaint of pain.

FASTING
Fasting is not necessary unless it is a surgical requirement, such as after abdominal operations.

POSTURE
It is not necessary to lie the patient flat for 24 hours. The patient should be allowed to sit up as soon as the analgesia has worn off.

AMBULATION
If not surgically contraindicated the patient may get out of bed 2 hours after the return of normal sensation, but only with assistance. Before getting the patient out of bed sit him up slowly, and check his blood pressure. If the systolic blood pressure falls more than 20 mmHg, or if the patient feels faint, dizzy or nauseated, then lie the patient down, and notify the anaesthetist.

POTENTIAL COMPLICATIONS

POSTURAL HYPOTENSION
Lie the patient in bed, and notify the anaesthetic registrar on duty who will increase the fluid intake, or will order vasopressors.

URINARY RETENTION
Encourage the patient to void when sensation returns. If the patient has not voided within 4 hours, or his bladder can be palpated, he will require a catheter.

Please report any abnormalities
or concerns to the anaesthetist immediately.

   - the patient is able to take a deep breath on command;
   - the patient is able to touch tip of his nose with his forefinger;

- pain has been relieved;
- there is no excessive loss from drains or bleeding from wound sites;
- observation charts are completed;
- patient is clean, dry, warm and comfortable.

2. Remove all unnecessary intravenous lines.

3. Remove ECG dots, and check the diathermy pad is not still attached.

4. Check that the medical and nursing staff have completed all the charts and notes and send them back to the ward with the patient.

5. Ensure the patients recovery room record is clear and concise. The ward staff will need an accurate record to quickly identify any deterioration.

6. Allow thirty minute to elapse between the last dose of analgesia and the patient's discharge from the recovery room.

Handover to ward staff

The recovery room staff must be certain that the ward nurse understands the patient's problems, and is willing and competent to accept responsibility for the patient's care. This fact should be noted on the patient's chart.

If the patient has received blood or blood products in theatre inform the ward nurse about this as part of your handover. If she is to give further blood discuss this too. Blood is a living tissue and will deteriorate if not looked after properly. If the additional transfusion is to be given immediately she should take the blood, with the patient, to the ward. If it is to be given later then it should go back to the blood bank and be reissued from there when required.

Always send all unused blood and blood products back to the blood bank as soon as the patient leaves theatre.

Transport patients facing forward and semi-sitting.

Transport

A nurse and an orderly should always accompany the patient when they return to the ward. Every trolley needs to carry portable oxygen and suction. Good combination units are commercially available. Keep an emergency box containing a self-inflating resuscitation bag, airways and a range of masks on the trolley.

Discharge to the intensive care unit (ICU)

If the patient is going to the intensive care unit send for the bed, and check it has the following equipment with it:

- a full cylinder of oxygen with flow meter. Remember to turn the cylinder flow on to at least 6l/min (less than this gives a lower inspired oxygen than room air);
- a portable battery powered ECG monitor and defibrillator;
- a pulse oximeter;
- suction;
- emergency drugs, syringes, and needles in a closed sealed carrying box;
- an anaesthetist, or member of the medical staff, should accompany patients returning to the intensive care unit.

If recovery rooms are properly staffed and equipped sick patients can be held overnight instead of discharging them to intensive care. This may be an economical option.

Patients who need admission to intensive care postoperatively include:

- those who are already in ICU but are having an operative procedure, such as a tracheostomy;
- those patients having uncomplicated surgery, but with severe intercurrent medical conditions, such as diabetes, myasthenia gravis or unstable angina;
- those patients having a big operation, such as oesophagogastrectomy, liver or pancreatic surgery or prolonged plastic surgery;
- those patients where it may be reasonably anticipated that complications will arise, such as the head injured multiple trauma patient who is unable to protect his airway.

It is better to plan an elective admission to the intensive care unit, than to attempt an operation and find that the patient is too unstable to transfer back to the ordinary surgical ward. This is largely a matter of common sense, and a properly run audit will identify potential problems.

1. Adams AP. (1994). *Recent Advances in Anaesthesia and Analgesia*, 18:123-43. published; Churchill Livingstone, London, England.
2. Voss TJ. (1994). *Australian Anaesthesia*, pp 115-25, published by Australian and New Zealand College of Anaesthetists, Melbourne, Australia.
3. Rosen M, Hillard EK. (1960). *British Journal of Anaesthesia*, 32:486-504
4. Hartley H, Vaughan RS. (1993). *British Journal of Anaesthesia*, 71:561-8.

2. MONITORING

When your patient arrives in recovery room make a quick overall visual check. Monitors will warn you of approaching problems, but they are not a substitute for carefully observing the patient. On emerging from anaesthesia, and for some time afterwards, the patient is in an unstable physiological state. Monitoring is first and foremost careful observation by the nurses and doctors in recovery room

The most useful electronic monitor in the recovery room is the pulse oximeter. This, with blood pressure monitoring, is all you require for most healthy patients having straightforward surgery. For an infant, a debilitated, sick, hypothermic, or elderly patient, you will need an ECG.

Much modern equipment is complex, and can confuse even the most competent staff. All personnel in the recovery room need to know how to use the monitoring equipment, and especially, how to understand what can go wrong with it. This requires a continuing education program, both for newcomers, and to refresh the memory of more experienced staff. If you are worried about the readings from a monitor, (and before assuming the monitor is faulty) go to the patient, and check the colour, pulse, breathing, blood pressure (manually) and the temperature.

If a patient arrives with a central venous pressure (CVP) or arterial line take the opportunity to study these forms of monitoring. When they are essential, as in post transplant patients, or after major bowel surgery, you will be quick and confident.

PULSE OXIMETERS [1] (SEE PAGE 486)

Pulse oximeters are the most important monitors we have and should be available in every recovery room. Providing a patient is well perfused the measurements are accurate. Use a pulse oximeter on all patients until their protective reflexes return, and they have oxygen saturations greater than 96 per cent when breathing room air.

Causes of erroneous readings: [2]
- long fingernails and nail polish;
- poor peripheral perfusion with hypothermia, shock or vasoconstrictor drugs;

- ambient light (particularly infrared lamps used to warm infants) entering a poorly fitting probe;
- bilirubin in heavily jaundiced patients;
- movement;
- iodine containing skin preparation;
- carboxyhaemoglobin gives a false high reading;
- methaemoglobin caused by prilocaine or nitroglycerine causes a trend toward 80 per cent saturation irrespective of the true haemoglobin saturation;
- dyes such as methylene blue give a false low reading.

Some pulse oximeters run on rechargeable batteries which last about 10 hours. Remember to charge them every night for use the next day.

A useful way to protect the delicate sensory probe, is to encase it in plastic foam. This also excludes ambient light, which is a cause of erroneous readings.

THE SATURATION METER AND ITS CORRELATION WITH PaO_2

Oxygen saturation	PaO_2 at pH 7.25	PaO_2 at pH 7.40	PaO_2 at pH 7.55
60	36 < critical level	31	24
70	44	37 < critical level	28
80	53	45	34
81	55	46	35
82	56	48	36 < critical level
83	58	49	37
84	59	50	38
85	61 < danger level	52	39
86	63	53	40
87	65	55	41
88	67	57	43
89	69	59	45
90	72	61 < danger level	47
91	75	64	49
92	79	67	51
93	83	70	54
94	88	75	57
95	94	80	61 < danger level
96	102	87	66
97	113	96	73
98	129	109	83
99	157	134	101
100	241	204	155

Figures are calculated from Kelman modification of the Hill Equation for the oxygen dissociation curve.[3]

The saturation of haemoglobin can be used to calculate the patient's arterial PaO_2. The relationship between haemoglobin saturation and PaO_2 is described by the oxygen saturation curve (see page 304).

Pitfalls occur in use of the oximeter, because there is a false belief that a saturation is greater than 90 per cent means the patient is not hypoxic. As the table below shows this depends on the pH of the blood.

In summary, once the saturation falls to 90 per cent the symptoms of hypoxia accelerate. A PaO_2 less than 60 mmHg (7.9 kPa) is dangerous, and a PaO_2 less than 35 mmHg (4.6 kPa) is potentially lethal even in an otherwise well patient.

Treat the patient, not the monitor.

BLOOD PRESSURE
Manual blood pressure
First:
- Explain to the patient what is about to happen;
- Check that the pulse is regular;
- Quickly inflate the cuff to above the expected arterial pressure;
- Estimate the blood pressure by feeling the return of the pulse with your finger on the radial artery;
- Quickly re-inflate the cuff to 30 mmHg above the arterial pressure;
- With the stethoscope over the brachial artery in the cubital fossa, let the cuff deflate no faster than 5 mmHg per second. To be accurate some authorities maintain this should be 2 mmHg per second,[4] however this is most uncomfortable for the patient;
- Listen for the point where the first sound is heard, this is the systolic blood pressure. The diastolic pressure is taken at the point where the sounds disappear completely; not the point at which the sounds become muffled.

Also make sure to:
- use the correct sized cuff, the standard adult cuff should be 12.5 cm wide. If you are making your own cloth blood pressure cuff covers, then the bladder length should be at least 80 per cent, and the width at least 40 per cent of the circumference of the upper arm.
- keep the mercury manometer at eye level to prevent parallax errors;
- check the blood pressure in both arms, if the patient has vascular disease or diabetes;

• do not allow the mercury column to fall too swiftly as you may pass the correct blood pressure between beats.

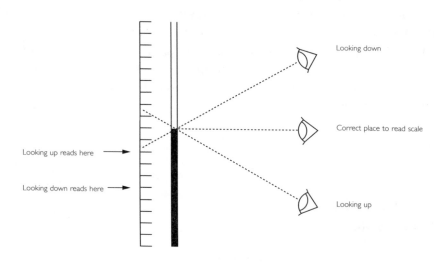

How you position a mercury blood pressure machine may cause errors in the readings.

fig 2.1 Diagram of parallax effect

False readings occur because:
• cuff is the wrong size for the limb;
• cuff deflation is either too slow, or too fast;
• the mercury manometer is not at eye level;
• air leaks give spuriously low readings.

In elderly patients, *pseudo-hypertension* may deceive you. The cuff cannot compress the rigid calcified arterial walls to occlude the blood flow, so you can still feel the pulse even though the cuff pressure is above the real systolic pressure. Many arteriosclerotic patients have different blood pressures in each arm. Continue to check both sides manually especially if this varies from the non-invasive blood pressure (NBP) reading by more than 20 mm Hg.

Non-invasive blood pressure (NBP)

Non-invasive blood pressure devices use an oscillotometric technique which underestimates at high pressures and overestimates at low pressures and doesn't work very well at all in patients with arrhythmias. The most accurate pressure with these devices is the mean pressure. Cuff width is also important. Narrow cuffs tend to overestimate pressure. Complications from cuffs of the incorrect size include limb oedema, bruising and blisters.

If the blood pressure is low the NBPs are slow to read and constantly re-cycle. They cause other problems including distal ischaemia or vessel damage. If you suspect this, measure the blood pressure on the opposite side.

Invasive-blood pressure

Invasive-blood pressure uses an intra-arterial cannula attached to a transducer. These devices are commonly thought to be an absolutely accurate measure of continuous blood pressure. However, if the fluid dynamics of the system are not correct, errors of 70 per cent or more, can occur. The catheters must be matched to the transducer and must not be too stiff, too pliant, or too long; so use reputable makes. Check the first few readings with a manual blood pressure machine. As with non-invasive pressure the mean pressures tend to be more accurate. Other problems that may occur are loss of power supply, incorrect calibration, broken or faulty transducers, failure to correctly level the transducer to the isophlebotic line on the patient.

Do not disturb the dressings around the arterial cannula. If the cannula is accidentally disconnected, put a syringe on the cannula and prepare to set up a new sterile line. If the cannula falls out, immediately apply pressure to the site with your gloved hand. If you cannot control the bleeding then inflate a pressure cuff on the arm to 250 mmHg to act as a tourniquet until help arrives. If the arterial line crosses the wrist or elbow joint, splint the arm to prevent the cannula kinking.

The incidence of radial artery thrombosis is 2 - 25 per cent. Factors increasing the risk are:
- emboli arising in the heart;
- large or long catheters;
- the length of time the cannula is left in the artery;
- prolonged hypotension;
- the use of vasoactive agents;
- accidental injection of drugs into an arterial line (see page 444).

Temperature Monitoring

Check the temperature of all patients entering recovery room and is essential for all babies. The normal temperature range is from 36.5° - 37.2°C.

Infra-red tympanic thermometers[5] are the best and easiest way to accurately measure a patient's core temperature. They respond rapidly, and measure the core temperature, because the tympanic membrane shares the same blood supply as the hypothalamus. This is where the body's thermoregulatory control centre is located. Be gentle when using this device, the ear is easily damaged. If they are not aimed properly at the tympanic membrane they read lower than the true core temperature. Do not use a glass clinical thermometer, because these do not measure low temperatures. Never put a glass thermometer into the mouth of an unconscious or semiconscious patient. In ill patients, or patients recovering from anaesthesia, the oral temperature poorly reflects pulmonary artery temperature, while the axillary temperature is absolutely useless.

Hyperthermia
Should the patient's temperature rise above normal, consider malignant hyperthermia. It has high mortality unless quickly treated (see page 149). Other causes include thyroid crises, blood transfusion reactions and pre-existing febrile states.

Hypothermia
This is defined as a core temperature of 35°C or less (see page 145). About 60 per cent of patients arrive in recovery room with temperatures less than 36.5°C[6]. About 75 per cent of patients, who have had either their chest or abdomens open, become hypothermic. If you suspect hypothermia feel the skin temperature on the patient's chest with the palm, not the back, of your hand.

Urine Output

Urine output is a useful guide to cardiac output as the kidney receives 25 per cent of this. Adequate output in postoperative patients should exceed 1 ml/kg/hr. Diuretics will abolish the usefulness of this monitor. Make sure you have the correct measuring bag or urinometer.

Glucose

Check the blood sugar of all diabetic patients, alcoholics and neonates with a gluconometer. Read more about diabetes on page 416.

Electrocardiography (ALSO SEE PAGE 245)

About half the arrhythmias detected in the recovery room are 'human detected' and the other half are 'monitor detected'. The ECG does not detect serious physiological changes such as hypoxia, hypercarbia, and hypotension. Indeed a normal ECG in a dangerous situation may lead to unwarranted complacency.[7]

Arrhythmias detected in the recovery room
can forewarn of serious postoperative cardiac problems.

A normal resting ECG does not exclude coronary artery disease, but it is reassuring. Adverse cardiac events occur in only 2 per cent of patients with a normal preoperative ECG; compared with 23 per cent if the pre-operative ECG is abnormal.[8]

Studies have found that myocardial ischaemia and cardiac arrhythmias are common in the recovery room particularly if the patient has pre-existing risk factors.[9] A good rule is to monitor any patient with risk factors for ischaemic heart disease.

Guidelines to select those at risk
1. Patient factors:
   - known or suspected cardiac disease;
   - patient on drugs affecting the heart such as digoxin;
   - hypertension, or systolic blood pressures greater than 160 mmHg;
   - age over 50 years;
   - peripheral vascular disease;
   - major intercurrent medical illness such as diabetes;
   - pulse greater 100 beats per minute or less than 60 beats per minute;
   - smokers over the age of 35 years;
   - lung disease;
   - oximeter reading arterial saturation of 95 per cent or less;
   - abnormal perfusion status;
   - anaemia;

- electrolyte imbalance;
- obese patients.

2. Surgical factors:
   - thoracic operations;
   - emergency major surgery;
   - head injuries and neurosurgery;
   - patients with burns.

3. Anaesthetic factors:
   - arrhythmias during the anaesthetic;
   - severe pain in patients over the age of 45 years;
   - hypothermia;
   - patients from intensive care unit;
   - large blood transfusion;
   - improperly reversed muscle relaxation.

To read more about arrythmias see page 266.

Hints

- Post a diagram on the notice board so that every one knows exactly where to place the sticky ECG electrodes (see illustration below). Take care to have the left arm electrode over the fifth intercostal space in the mid axillary line.
- If serious arrhythmias, or signs of ischaemia occur then do a 12 lead ECG so the trace can be kept and analyzed later.

The commonest reasons for a poor quality ECG trace are:
- the electrode has poor contact with skin. Shave and clean the skin with an alcohol swab. Re-apply an electrode;
- the patient is moving, or shivering;
- the leads are faulty;
- the leads are picking up interference; usually because they are lying across power cables, or other metal objects. This can be seen as 50 cycle AC hum making the trace blurred or smudged. If you look at the trace closely you will see a tight sine wave pattern. Solve the problem by moving the leads away from the source of interference. Coiling the lead may also help.

Make sure your screen and printouts are properly calibrated. On the vertical axis 1 cm = 1 millivolt; and on the horizontal axis 1 large square = 0.2 seconds.

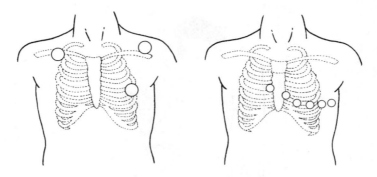

Modified CM5 position for the ECG electrodes   Position of ECG electrodes for a 12 lead trace

fig 2.2 Placement of electrodes

To detect ischaemic ST changes the modified CM5 lead is the most useful. Place the left arm electrode over the fifth left intercostal space in the mid axillary line, and turn the 'lead select' switch to Lead I.

Lead II is the best lead to detect changes in rhythm, and to view the P-wave.

CENTRAL VENOUS LINES

If the patient comes to you with a central venous line and you intend to use it, check the X-ray to make sure it is in the right vena cava. Blood should aspirate freely through the catheter and you should observe changes in pressure with respiration. In post operative patients it is useful to assess fluid deficits. Monitoring makes it safe to give fluid boluses to a patient with a low blood pressure.

If you do not have access to sophisticated equipment it is still possible to monitor Central Venous Pressure (CVP) using traditional methods. The normal value for (CVP) is 0 - 5 cm of water. Unlike blood pressure which is measured in millimetres of mercury (mmHg), the CVP is recorded in centimetres of water.

How to measure a CVP without a modern transducer
The principle involved is to balance the column of water in the manometer tubing with the pressure in the great veins. To achieve this there must be a continuous column of fluid between the great veins and the manometer.

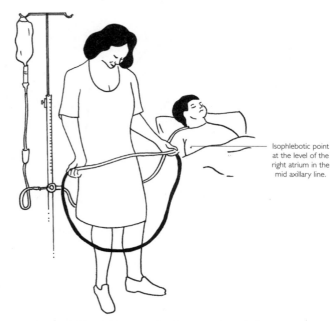

Isophlebotic point
at the level of the
right atrium in the
mid axillary line.

fig 2.3 How to measure central venous pressure with reference to the isphlebotic point

Fix the manometer to the central venous catheter and attach it to a drip stand. If you have positioned it correctly the fluid in the manometer should swing freely as the patient breathes. To get the zero point on the manometer level with the patient's isophlebotic line you can either use a carpenter's spirit level, or a closed loop U-tube filled with coloured fluid.

Three way taps can cause confusion:

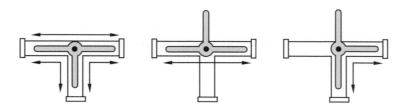

fig 2.4 Direction of flow with three-way taps

Management

1. If the CVP is inserted in recovery room first order a chest x-ray before using it to check position and ensure there is no pneumothorax.
2. Monitor blood pressure, pulse and respiratory rate.
3. Ensure the zero pressure reference point is at the specified place, usually the mid-axillary line (*isophlebotic line*). Frequently check the readings with a spirit level, or a loop of tubing partially filled with coloured fluid.
4. Keep the line free of air bubbles.
5. Have a continuous flowing infusion to ensure the line remains patent.
6. Lock all connections to prevent accidental disconnection.
7. Maintain strict aseptic care of ports and infusions. Clean the puncture wound with poviodine (Betadine®), dry and dress it with clear plastic dressing.
8. Before you take any reading make sure the fluid in the manometer is swinging normally with the patient's breathing. If it is not swinging, then the catheter is, either blocked, or in the wrong place. If there are large pressure swings, the catheter tip is probably in the right ventricle; so pull it back a bit.
9. Securely fasten the lines to the skin so that they are not accidentally pulled out.
10. Warn the patient to notify the nursing staff immediately if the line becomes disconnected.
11. Sometimes a wide bore 10 gauge sheath is inserted into a central vein, to give blood at a fast rate.

> *If you find a collapsed patient and a disconnected central line*
> *- treat for air embolism.*

Using a CVP in a bleeding patient

The CVP is a useful guide to fluid replacement in a bleeding, or traumatised patient. Normally about 3 litres of the blood volume are stored in the floppy walled great veins. There is a further one litre in the arteries, and another litre in the heart and lungs. When a patient bleeds, his blood volume falls. To start with, most of this blood comes from the veins, which gently contract to maintain the pressure inside them.

The first sign of a low blood volume is a gently falling central venous pressure. After a blood loss of about 500 mls the pulse rate starts to rise, and by the time 800 mls is lost the CVP will fall rapidly, this is followed later by a fall in the arterial blood pressure.

As the diagram below shows, the CVP does not change as much as the blood volume changes between 0 - 5 cm H_2O where the graph line is almost flat. In other words you cannot tell whether the veins are almost full or almost empty. So, in a bleeding patient, it is better to aim to raise the patient's CVP to 5 cm H_2O. You may be surprised by how much fluid is needed, but you are unlikely to give too much fluid provided the CVP does not go over 10 cm H_2O.

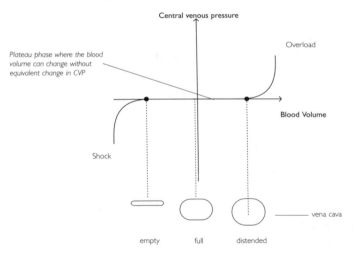

Cross-sectional shape of great veins as they follow the blood volume

fig 2.5 Diagram of how central venous pressure follows blood volume

A useful way to determine where on the curve a patient bleed volume lies is to do a *CVP stress test*. Give 200 mls of a colloid, such as blood or polygeline (Haemaccel®) and note how much the CVP rises. If it rises less than 5 cm H_2O (3 mm Hg) then you may safely give another bolus over the next 5 minutes. If the CVP rises more than 5 cm of water the patient's blood volume is probably adequate. It would be unwise to give further fluids.

Some drugs, especially inotropes require a central line for administration.

Complications of central line insertion

1. Pneumothorax occurs in 2 - 5 per cent of subclavian insertions, and in less than 1 per cent if the line is inserted through the internal jugular vein. If a chest x-ray shows that the lung has collapsed with greater than 3 cm between the lung and the chest wall, or the patient is short of breath, you will need to insert an underwater thoracic drain (see page 96).

2. If arterial puncture occurs press firmly on the site for 10 minutes. Monitor the patient's blood pressure, pulse and breathing. Watch for signs of continuing haemorrhage.

3. Air embolism occurs if the line become disconnected. The incidence is under 0.5 per cent, but can be fatal (see page 235).

If you find a collapsed patient
with a disconnected central venous catheter,
assume the patient has an air embolis.

4. Other problems are catheter sepsis, thromboembolism, brachial plexus injuries, damage to the thoracic duct, catheter kinking (or even knotting), pericardial tamponade, and cardiac arrhythmias.

CARDIOPULMONARY CATHETERS (SWAN-GANZ CATHETERS®) [10]

If the patient has lung or heart disease and you need to know about left heart function CVP monitoring will not be reliable, and further monitoring via a pulmonary artery catheter will be required. Studies in Europe and North America show that 50 per cent of users of the pulmonary artery catheter cannot correctly interpret the pulmonary artery occlusion pressure from a clear trace.[11]

Swan-Ganz® catheters are balloon tipped catheters used for measuring *pulmonary artery* (PAP), and *pulmonary artery wedge pressures* (PAWP). When the balloon is inflated, the tip floats forward and wedges in a small pulmonary artery blocking the flow of blood. The pressure in this still column of blood in the pulmonary capillaries can be measured. This gives valuable information about the filling pressures of the left atrium, and performance of the left heart. They are often used in specialized units in patients with cardiovascular disease, or those having open heart or vascular surgery. Some catheters have a heat detecting thermistor at the tip, which is connected to a computer. If cold saline is injected up stream, the speed at which this saline reaches the tip can be used to calculate the cardiac output.

NORMAL VALUES OF CARDIAC PRESSURES	
Central venous pressure	0 – 7 mmHg
Pulmonary artery pressures	14 – 32 mmHg systolic
	4 – 13 mmHg diastolic
	8 – 19 mmHg mean
Wedge pressure	6 – 12 mmHg
Cardiac output	70 – 100 ml/kg
Cardiac index	2.5 – 3.6 litres/min/m^2
Pulmonary vascular resistance	700 – 1500 dyne-sec/cm^5
	77 – 150 kPa-sec/cm^5
Systemic vascular resistance	20 – 120 dyne-sec/cm^5
	2 – 12 kPa-sec/cm^5
Oxygen consumption	3.5 ml/kg/min

Perfusion status reflects cardiac output. As people come in different sizes, cardiac output is often standardized by calculating the *cardiac index*.

$$\text{Cardiac index} = \frac{\text{cardiac output}}{\text{body surface area}} = \frac{5.0}{1.34} = 3.73 \text{ litre/m}^2$$

Most monitors that measure cardiac output will have the facility to calculate the body surface area from the patient's weight and height.

Pulmonary oedema is likely to occur in healthy lungs if the wedge pressure is greater than 20 - 25 mmHg. Pulmonary oedema can occur at normal, or lower pressures if the patient is septic, has adult respiratory distress syndrome (ARDS), or very severe hypoproteinaemia.

Problems that may arise during insertion of a Swan-Ganz® catheter and may appear in the recovery room are:
• carotid or sub clavian artery puncture and haematoma of the neck;
• pneumo- or haemo-thorax;

- catheter kinking, and occasionally intravascular knotting;
- balloon ruptures;
- rupture of pulmonary artery due to inappropriate inflation of the balloon;
- cardiac arrhythmias;
- valvular damage or incompetence.

BLOOD GASES

Arterial blood gases are best taken from an arterial cannula, or failing that the radial or femoral artery. You can use the brachial or dorsalis pedis arteries, but do not use them in diabetics or patients with peripheral vascular disease. Occlusion of these end-arteries can cause gangrene. Before sticking a needle into the radial artery, use a modified *Allen's test* to check patency of the collateral ulnar artery.

Reasonably cheap commercial kits are available for the collection of blood gases. If you do not have these, use a 23 gauge needle, and a 5 ml glass syringe which has the lining lubricated with heparin. Make sure no heparin drops are left in the syringe, and no air enters the syringe. Air bubbles cause errors in the estimations. Once taken, the blood should be stored in melting ice and quickly sent to the laboratory. The results will be unreliable if more than 10 minutes elapse between taking the blood and processing it. The laboratory will also need to know the patient's temperature, and his inspired oxygen concentration.

ALLEN'S TEST

Get an assistant to curl the patient's hand into a fist. Compress both the ulnar and radial arteries. Release the ulnar artery first, and note if the hand flushes. If there is adequate collateral flow, the hand will flush within 15 seconds. If there is inadequate flow the hand will remain pale. It is unwise to puncture or cannulate the radial artery if there is not enough flow in the ulnar artery to supply the hand.

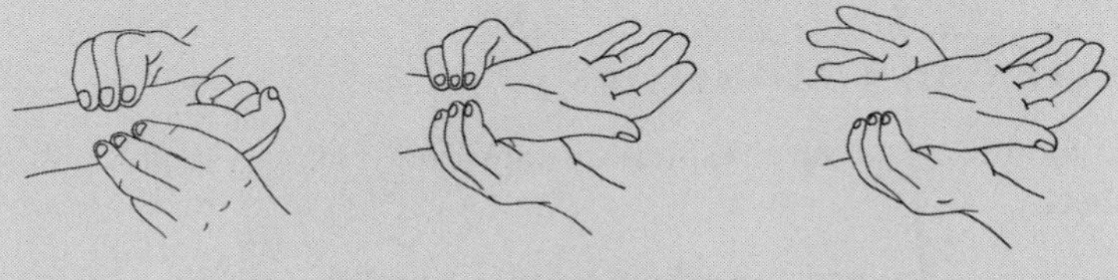

fig 2.6 Allen's test

To prevent painful haematomas, use a pad to press firmly on the puncture site. After a measured 3 minutes, remove the pad to check if bleeding has stopped. Re-apply the pressure if necessary. Do not just tape a cotton-wool swab over the site, because unobserved the artery may continue to bleed.

Assess and treat any abnormal result quickly.

QUICK GUIDE TO INTERPRETATION OF BLOOD GAS RESULTS				
	pH	PaO₂ mmHg (kPa)	PaCO₂ mmHg (kPa)	Standard HCO₃ mmol/l
Normal*	7.35 – 7.42	90 – 100 (11.8 – 13.2)	35 – 42 (4.6 – 5.5)	22 – 26
Danger	< 7.25	< 60 (< 7.9)	> 45 (> 5.9)	< 16
Critical (moribund)	< 7.12	< 35 (< 4.6)	> 60 (> 7.9)	< 12

Acid base balance in a hypothermic patient

Physiological pH and PCO_2 alter with the patient's temperature. Traditionally, arterial blood gases (ABGs) are measured in the laboratory at 37°C and then corrected back to the patient's temperature (*pH-stat*). Maintain the blood gases to achieve levels of pH 7.40 and a PCO_2 of 40 mmHg when the blood is at 37°C. If the hypothermic patient's ABGs are correct at 37°C, then they will be physiologically correct at whatever they might read in the hypothermic or hyperthermic patient. For instance, if the blood gases are normal at 37°C, and read pH 7.52 and a PCO_2 of 25 mmHg at 28°C, then this is the value at which the patient's physiology is optimal for that temperature; so do not attempt to correct it.

RESPIRATION MONITORS

Some monitors measure respiratory rate from changes in the voltages of the ECG.

There are sensory pads on which neonates and young children can lie to detect apnoeic periods. These should be used postoperatively, on any infant under the age of 12 months who was born prematurely (see page 392).

Capnography

Capnographs measure carbon dioxide concentration in the airways by shining infrared light through samples of expired air, and calculating how much light is absorbed. A microprocessor looks for the highest reading at the end of a breath. It is assumed that this is the concentration of carbon dioxide in the alveoli, hence the other name for these devices; end tidal CO_2 monitors. The commonest reason for malfunction is water entering the sampling line.

Although frequently used during anaesthesia, capnography is not routinely used on extubated patients because it is difficult to obtain an undiluted sample of expired air. Capnography swiftly detects some emergencies:
- disconnection from, or malfunction of, a ventilator;
- obstruction of an endotracheal tube;
- a rapid fall in expired PCO_2 due to a fall in cardiac output, or a pulmonary or an air embolism;
- a rapid rise in CO_2 production is often associated with malignant hyperthermia.

X-RAY

Portable X-ray may be needed for the following:
- respiratory distress;
- pneumothorax;
- following central venous line insertion;
- heart failure;
- suspected aspiration;
- following nephrectomy where there is a chance the pleural space has been entered;
- misplaced surgical Raytec® swab.

NEUROMUSCULAR BLOCKADE

Do not use a nerve stimulator on a conscious patient because it is painful. The best test of proper reversal of muscle relaxants is to ask the patient to lift their head from the pillow. Patients must be able to sustain a 15 second head lift before they are discharged from the recovery room. Other tests of muscle power are straight leg lift, coughing, and hand grip. To test hand grip offer only two of your fingers, otherwise you may be hurt.

If a patient is still unconscious and you suspect incomplete reversal of their muscle relaxing drugs. A nerve stimulator can be used to gauge residual neuromuscular blockade after the use of relaxant drugs such as vecuronium or suxamethonium.

Frequent use of a nerve stimulator during an operation may cause post-operative paraesthesia with a feeling of 'pins-and-needles' around the little finger and down the ulnar side of the hand. This resolves within a few hours.

HOW TO USE A NERVE STIMULATOR

Put two skin electrodes over the ulnar nerve near the wrist joint. Attach the negative electrode distally. Look for a twitch of the thumb as the nerve is stimulated. It should jerk toward the palm of the hand as flexor pollicis brevis is stimulated. Ignore movement in the other fingers because the current directly stimulates the muscles so they will curl even if the nerve itself is not stimulated.

Two stimuli are given, a *train-of-four* twitches or a *tetanic stimulus* with a whole run of stimuli close together.

Using a train-of-four in the unparalysed patient causes the thumb to twitch equally all four times. The ratio of the fourth response of a train-of-four to the first response is a measure of recovery from neuromuscular blockade. The fourth twitch disappears when there is about 75% neuromuscular blockade still present. The third when there is about 80%, the second when there is 90% paralysis. Absence of all four corresponds to complete paralysis. Neostigmine and atropine will not adequately reverse neuromuscular blockade if two twitches or less are seen in a train of four. Three or four twitches need to be seen before the patient is safe to be reversed with neostigmine and atropine.

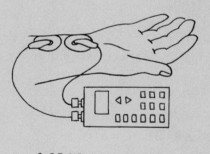

fig 2.7 *Where to place electrodes*

VENTILATORY VOLUMES

The patient's tidal air exchange can be measured by a respirometer, (sometimes called an anemometer). To prevent expired air escaping it needs a tightly fitting mask, laryngeal airway or endotracheal tube to get accurate results. The two types available are a Wright's Respirometer® and the Drager Volumeter®.

VOLUME METERS

WRIGHT'S RESPIROMETER®

In this device gas passes over a two-bladed rotor which spins to measure the flow passing through it. These instruments, are very accurate, but are also very fragile. Look down the inlet port and you will see the paper-thin metal aerofoil blades. These aerofoils are easily torn by a moderate blast of air. If someone blows hard into this type of respirometer, the blades will shear off and the tiny cogs will be stripped. They are very expensive to repair or replace. To test a Wright's respirometer, wave it through the air, the dial will indicate an airflow.

DRAGER VOLUMETER®

This device is much more robust, a bit more bulky, but not quite so accurate. Two lightweight meshing rotors measure the volume of air passing over them. It has a useful timing device which stops measurement after one minute has elapsed, making it easy to get consistent readings. If necessary this device may be autoclaved.

Both instruments tend to under read at low flow rates and over read at high flow rates.

1. Alexander CM, Teller LE, (1989). *Anaesthesia and Analgesia*, 68: 368-376.
2. Alexander CM, Teller LE, (1989). Anaesthesia and Analgesia, 68: 368-376.
3. Kenny GNC, (1979). British Journal of Anaesthesia, 51: 793.
4. 'The Management of Hypertension—A consensus statement' Medical Journal of Australia (1994) suppl. 160: S1-S16.
5. Edge G, Morgan M, (1993). *Anaesthesia,* 48: 604-7.
6. Vauhn MS, Vaughn RW, *et al.* (1981). *Anaesthesia and Analgesia* 60: 746-751.
7. Ludbrook GL, Russell WJ, *et al.* (1993). *Anaesthesia and Intensive Care*, 21: 558-64.
8. Carliner NH, Fisher ML, *et al.* (1985). *American Journal of Cardiology*, 56:51-8.
9. Hollenberg M, Managano DT, *et al.* (1992). *Journal of American Medical Association*, 268: 205-9.
10. Gnoegi A, *et al.* (1997). *Critical Care Medicine*, 25 (2): 213-20.
11. Gnoegi A, *et al.* (1997). *Critical Care Medicine*, 25 (2): 213-20.

3. DAY SURGERY

INTRODUCTION

With the growing confidence of medical and nursing staff, sicker patients are undergoing day surgery. The American Society of Anesthesiologists (ASA) physical status III (see page 409) is now regarded, in some units, as acceptable fitness for day surgery, provided the disease is medically stable, and the anaesthetist agrees the risks are acceptable.[1]

Day surgery is popular with hospital management, and the authorities who finance them. It is cheaper to treat day patients, than have them stay overnight, or longer in hospital.[2] Many patients prefer to go home, even if it means a certain amount of discomfort. Despite this enthusiasm up to 35 per cent of patients do not go to work the following day.[3]

About 25 per cent of day cases suffer from nausea, headache and excessive drowsiness after their discharge from the hospital.[4]

Problems likely to be encountered in recovery room after day case surgery include:

- pre-existing disease, lack of proper preoperative evaluation, and explanation about the procedure to the patient;
- it cannot be assumed that the patient is reliably fasted:
- it is difficult to explain postoperative instructions;
- if the patient's condition deteriorates following his return home, he will be relying on family and friends to get the medical attention he needs. The 'carer' who comes to take him home might not be capable of this responsibility;
- drugs that the patient may already be taking, such as diazepam, can prolong the effect of anaesthesia, or have untoward effects once he arrives home.

ADVANCES IN ANAESTHESIA

Day surgery, is to a large extent possible because of the advances in the pharmacology of anaesthetic drugs. Ten years ago, patients would have been too debilitated by their anaesthetic to leave hospital with 24 hours of their operation. Modern drugs used for day surgery anaesthesia have fewer side effects.

DRUGS USED IN DAY ANAESTHESIA

PROPOFOL (DIPRIVAN®)

Propofol is a rapidly metabolized intravenous agent used for induction of anaesthesia and sedation for regional procedures. Patients emerging from propofol anaesthesia are clear headed and sometimes mildly euphoric. The actions of the drug are terminated, as it is diluted, by the extracellular fluids, and later it is broken down in the liver. Propofol has been reported to cause convulsions, but is also a most effective anticonvulscent. Of concern is a report of a day case patient who fitted after discharge and sustained a mild head injury.[5] In view of the current uncertainty about the association of propofol with convulsions it would be wise to be cautious about early discharge if any abnormal muscle movement occurs during induction. Special equipment (such as the Diprofusor™) has been developed to titrate suitable doses of propofol for *total intravenous anaesthetic* (TIVA), however there are concerns about intraoperative awareness.

MIDAZOLAM (HYPNOVEL®)

Midazolam is a water soluble short acting benzodiazepine which is rapidly metabolized by the liver. It is used for sedation during endoscopic procedures such as gastroscopy and colonoscopy. Midazolam is cleared by the liver ten times faster than diazepam. In some cases there have been concerns about antegrade amnesia. It impairs the patient's memory of both the procedure, and things you tell him before and afterwards. We recall a case where a 35 year old man was discharged home after a day case gastroscopy. He later denied ever having had the procedure, and had no recollection of his stay in the day centre. Although the sedative effects of midazolam are reversed by flumazenil (Anexate®), which works for about 30 minutes, the amnesia can persist. We do not recommend using flumazenil to hasten recovery in day surgery patients; it is better to wait until the sedative effects of midazolam or diazepam wear off in their own time.

ATRACURIUM (TRACIUM®)

Atracurium, a short acting muscle relaxant, breaks down spontaneously (Hoffman degradation) into inactive products and its elimination from the body is independent of the liver and kidney.

ALFENTANIL AND SUFENTANIL

These two opioid analgesics have very short action and are only used in the operating theatre. They are both profound respiratory depressants, but this will have worn off by the time the patient reaches the recovery room.

SEVOFLURANE

Sevoflurane is a volatile anaesthetic agent. Its short action makes it suitable for day cases. Gaseous induction with sevoflurane is smooth and rapid in both children and adults, and therefore useful for those with a phobia of needles, or those with difficult venous access. Children are often restless and disoriented on emergence from sevoflurane.[6] Adults who have received sevoflurane for more than about 20 minutes may also feel agitated and jittery on emergence.

DESFLURANE

Desflurane has a pungent odour and requires a special vaporizer. Desflurane causes sympathetic stimulation and a tachycardia. Fentanyl will block this effect. Awakening from desflurane anaesthesia is rapid, but there are problems with emergence delirium.

Plan of Day Surgery Recovery Room

Recovery from anaesthesia must be as well supervised as in-patient surgery. Plan for the day surgery recovery room to be close to the operating theatre. You will need full recovery room facilities with the same equipment, monitoring, supervision and management as a normal recovery room. There should be an area set aside, where a patient, having recovered consciousness, can sit and comfortably complete his recovery. This area is this step down bay. No patient should leave this area unless he is in the company of a responsible adult.

Organization

Some points to consider:

1. It is better to have operations under general anaesthesia only in the mornings. Afternoon surgery should be done under local anaesthesia.
2. If the patient does not speak English keep an interpreter or, less optimally, the relative close by until you are quite certain the surgeon and anaesthetist will not require help with translation.
3. Obtain a contact phone number before the relative, who brings the patient, leaves. This is important if the case is cancelled and the collection time alters.
4. Surgeons and anaesthetists like all the patients on the list to be present before the list starts. This can be a problem with space. Consider staggering the patients' arrival times but make sure they are ready well in advance of their scheduled operation time.
5. It is useful to employ a community liaison sister. (*Hospital in the home*) who visits the patients in their homes. Ideally she will see them within a few hours of discharge. Her duties include monitoring and treating postoperative pain, nausea, vomiting and headaches. Also tending to changes of dressings and removal of sutures.
6. About 0.2 - 3 per cent of the patients are unfit to go home, and need admission to hospital overnight. The most common causes for admission are nausea and vomiting, haemorrhage and uncontrolled pain.
7. Recovery room staff duties are similar to a normal recovery room but the requirement for a receptionist-secretary is greater.

Written protocols should cover:
- admission and discharge;
- routines for checking equipment and drugs;
- the duties of all medical, nursing and paramedical staff;
- problems and how to handle them;
- lines of communication.

Responsibilities
Work these protocols out carefully, and write them down so everyone is clear about what their duties are. Many units use the following criteria.

Responsibilities of the anaesthetist are:
- supervising the recovery period;
- authorizing the patient's discharge;
- accompanying the patient to the recovery room;
- proper hand over to the nursing staff;
- providing written and verbal instructions to the recovery room staff;
- prescriptions for analgesics and antiemetics;
- specifying the requirements for oxygen supplements;
- remaining close by until the patient is safe to leave in the care of the nursing staff.

Responsibilities of the surgeon are:
- authorizing the discharge of a patient from the recovery room when this depends on a surgical decision;
- being available to consult with the anaesthetist and recovery room staff about the patient's welfare.

Clinical aspects
As with all postoperative patients watch them closely until they have:
- regained consciousness;
- a stable arterial blood pressure;
- are in control of their airway;
- breathing adequately.

Once awake, the patient will appear to be lucid and able to carry on an intelligent co-ordinated conversation. However instructions given, or conversations held at this point are usually forgotten, and the patient may have no recall what-so-ever of the conversation. Occasionally after returning home, a patient will deny that he has even had a procedure. This profound amnesia occurs more frequently if midazolam has been used during the procedure.

Step down procedure
Recovery in day patients is usually a two step procedure.

STEP 1: The patient recovers on the trolley, lying in the coma position until he is awake. After about fifteen minutes, providing his blood pressure is stable, the patient can be moved into a sitting position. If the patient has been intubated he should remain, for at least a full hour, in the recovery room before being discharged to the step down area.

Criteria for leaving the recovery room for the step down area:

- awake;
- minimal pain;
- no active bleeding;
- vital signs stable;
- no drug intervention likely;
- minimal nausea;
- no crying or anxiety;
- no vomiting;
- if relaxant drugs were part of the anaesthetic can he lift his head for 5 seconds;
- oxygen saturation above 96% on air.

STEP 2: After an hour or more, the patient is encouraged to get up, and walk to an arm chair. During this stage, providing nausea is not a problem, he can be offered fluids, and something light to eat.

Pain relief

Analgesia for day surgery has its own requirements.[7] Simple oral analgesics, such as paracetamol or paracetamol-codeine compounds are usually sufficient to control pain. If a nerve block has been used, give the patient oral analgesia before it wears off. Opioids used, either during, or after the procedure increase nausea and vomiting, they are nevertheless the best form of pain relief and should be given if appropriate.

Nausea and vomiting

From the patient's point of view, nausea and vomiting is a disaster; but over 50 per cent of day patients will suffer from it when they get home. In adults it is more likely after ear surgery, laparoscopy, eye surgery and orthopaedic surgery. In children operations for orchidopexy, squints, and tonsillectomy have a high incidence of postoperative nausea and vomiting. Check the notes, a history of motion sickness, or vomiting after previous anaesthetics will alert you. (For treatment of nausea and vomiting see page 227.) If this problem persists make enquiries about admitting the patient. Do not leave the organisation of this until the end of the session.

DISCHARGE PRECAUTIONS

It is difficult to tell how well a patient has recovered following anaesthesia. No single test can demonstrate that a patient is free from the effects of the anaesthetic, and is safe to leave the hospital. There is no substitute for clinical evaluation by the anaesthetist before a patient is discharged.

Have a permanent bed availability arrangement for patients who are not ready to leave when you want to close down the facility for the night.

All patients must be 'street fit'
before discharge.

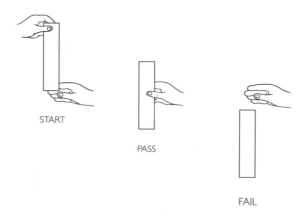

fig 3.1 Ruler test

Ruler test

A simple test we have found useful to determine street fitness is to sit the patient on a chair, and rest the wrist of his dominant hand over the edge of a table. Suspend a 30 cm ruler between his fore-finger and thumb. Tell him to grab it as it falls. If the distance the ruler falls is one third more than the pre-anaesthetic value his reflexes are still impaired and he should remain another half an hour for observation.

Street fitness

Street fitness is a useful, but not a well defined concept. The criteria for street fitness include:

• the patient is awake and fully oriented in time and place;
• there are no active surgical complications;
• the dressings have been checked and there is no bleeding;
• there are no anaesthetic complications such as nausea or giddiness;
• able to dress themselves with no unsteadiness when standing;
• able to walk unassisted to the bathroom, to void without feeling faint;
• stable vital signs for 60 minutes;
• has preferably eaten, and had a drink without feeling nauseated;
• pain is controlled;
• absence of breathing problems.

INSTRUCTIONS FOR THE PATIENT AND HIS RELATIVES

Appendix VI on page 559 has a sheet of questions, answers and instructions for the patients. You might wish to photocopy this and give it to them.

In some hospitals, patients for day case surgery go home from the recovery room. If this is so, make sure they have written orders describing in detail, the medication they are to take, what the effects of the procedure are likely to be, and what to do if any problems arise. Have the responsible adult, who is to care for the patient, present while you tell them the instructions. Give them both written instructions. If you just tell the patient, most will forget what you have said.

Make sure that:
• he will be escorted by a competent adult;
• he has access to a telephone at home, and the phone numbers of the doctor, the hospital, and other support staff;
• he has a follow up appointment.

Immediately before discharge:
• check the blood pressure and pulse rate while sitting and then standing;
• stand him up and ask him to close his eyes to check that he is steady on his feet. Be prepared to steady him if necessary;
• check the dressings for ooze or haemorrhage;
• ask about pain;
• ask about nausea;

- make sure the patient has his medication;
- make sure he has all his belongings.

What to expect for 24 hours:
- a mildly sore throat, especially if he was intubated;
- perhaps some nausea and vomiting especially after the car journey home;
- mild headache for 12 hours which will be relieved by simple analgesia;
- possibly some muscular aches;
- mild to moderate pain;
- a blood stained weepy ooze from wound.

For the first 48 hours following general anaesthesia patients must be formally warned:
- not to drive a motor vehicle;
- not to use machinery that requires judgement or skill;
- not to drink alcohol;
- not to cook (because of the risk of burns);
- not to take medication unless prescribed by a doctor;
- not to sign any legal documents;
- not to make major financial decisions;
- not to be the only person in charge of children, or other dependent individuals.

In 1992 the Royal College of Surgeons of England issued a policy statement that the time limit for these precautions should be extended from 24 to 48 hours.[8] One survey showed that nearly 10 per cent of patients drove themselves home after day surgery, and 30 per cent of these had driven within 12 hours of their anaesthetic.[9]

1. Parness SM, (1990). *Anesthesiology Clinics of North America*, Vol 8. No. 2 pages 399-421.
2 . Kitz DS, Lecky JH, *et al.* (1987). *Anaesthesia and Analgesia*, 66: 97.
3. Carroll NV, Miederhoff P, Cox FM, *et al.* (1995) 'Postoperative Nausea and Vomiting After Discharge from Outpatient Surgery Centers', *Anaesthesia and Analgesia*, 80: 903-909.
4 .Watcha MF, White PF, (1992). 'Postoperative Nausea and Vomiting: Its Etiology, Treatment, and Prevention', *Anaesthesiology*, 77: 162-184.
5. *Reported to the Victorian Consultative Council on Anaesthetic Mortality and Morbidity.* Information Bulletin No. 3 February (1994).
6. Davis PJ, (1999). *Anaesthesia and Analgesia*, 88: 34-8.
7. Baker AB, (1992). *Medical Journal of Anaesthesia*, 156: 274-280.
8. 'Guidelines for Day Surgery Cases' (1992). Royal College of Surgeons of England, London.
9. Ogg TW. (1985). *Anaesthesia Rounds*, No. 18 Imperial Chemical Industries (Pharmaceutical Division) Macclesfield, England.

4. Surgical Operations

Abdominal Surgery

Abdominal surgery is sometimes associated with postoperative hypoxaemia, because pain inhibits deep breathing and coughing; and general anaesthesia compromises lung function. Intercostal blocks or a thoracic epidural will help with most, but not all, of the pain. Encourage deep breathing, and coughing while supporting the wound. After major surgery on the lower abdomen, such as a total hysterectomy, or abdominoperineal resection, patients will need a urinary catheter to prevent retention. Make sure this is attached to a urinometer for an accurate assesment of output. If the patient has a central venous line (CVP) attach a manometer (see page 36). Record your measurement on a fluid balance chart. Some patients require a large amount of fluid postoperatively. It is safer to monitor this with CVP measurements. Ideally, the CVP reading should be maintained between +2 and +10 cm H_2O.

Abdominal Lipectomy

Abdominal lipectomy (*apronectomy*) is a traumatic operation. The incision traverses the abdomen, and is closed under tension. Blood loss can be considerable. Many of the problems are similar to those of the obese patient (see page 426). Transfer the patient to her bed as soon as possible.

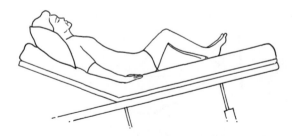

fig 4.1 Banana position for recovering after abdominal lipectomy
(cot sides would normally be in place)

Keep her knees bent, and upper body leaning forward, to prevent traction on the wound. Check that there is no swelling or wound ooze before giving analgesia. Pain is often the first sign of a developing haematoma. If she wishes to sit up, raise the head and the foot of the bed into the *banana position*.

AORTIC SURGERY (SEE VASCULAR SURGERY PAGE 85)

BREAST SURGERY

After a mastectomy nurse patients on their back with their heads turned to one side in case they vomit. If they are obese, sit them up as soon as they are fully conscious. As the dressings are sometimes bulky and tight, check that the patient can breathe properly.

Elevate her arm on the operative side on two pillows. If the surgery has involved the axilla, the venous drainage of the area may be impeded, causing the arm to become congested. If the arm is blue, or otherwise discoloured notify the surgeon. If the patient is uncomfortable help her to change her position, so that she does not hurt her arm, or put tension on the sutures. Before discharging the patient to the ward, check the drainage bottles for excessive bleeding.

Postoperatively breast binders are still occasionally used in an optimistic attempt to reduce postoperative bruising. They seriously impede deep breathing and coughing.

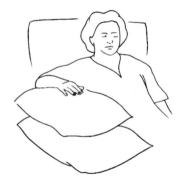

fig 4.2 Patient after right sided breast surgery

Mammoplasty

AUGMENTATION MAMMOPLASTY: A developing haematoma is usually painful. Check for swelling before prescribing analgesia.

REDUCTION MAMMOPLASTY: With large breasts more than 1500 mls of blood can be lost during the operation. Check the patient's perfusion status, and be prepared to replace the losses.

BRONCHOSCOPY

Patients often cough uncontrollably after a bronchoscopy. The anaesthetist will have probably sprayed the throat, and larynx with lignocaine before the patient comes to the recovery room; but despite this, they may cough violently, becoming hypoxic and distressed. Sit the patient up, and support him on two or three pillows. This will make him more comfortable. If coughing is excessive, then give lignocaine 1.5 mg/kg intravenously.[1] Take care that nothing the patient coughs up touches any part of your body. Wear gown, gloves and goggles while attending him.

BURNS

Patients with burns are haemodynamically unstable after surgery, so assign your most experienced staff to look after them. A ketamine infusion (see below) is helpful to dissociate them from thinking about their fearful experience. Secure intravenous lines are essential. These patients have a high fluid requirement.

Airway obstruction
Patients with facial burns will have airway burns, and probably smoke damage to bronchi and lung tissue too. The airway becomes progressively oedematous and swollen. Wheezing, or noisy breathing will warn you of impending airway obstruction. Watch for agitation, or restlessness heralding hypoxia.

If the lips and tongue swell to close the airway, you may need to gently insert a soft nasopharyngeal airway as a temporary measure. Lubricate it well with 2% lignocaine gel. These airways are well tolerated, even in a conscious patient. Avoid rigid plastic tubes that can damage tissues, rupture nasal cartilages, and introduce infection into the paranasal sinuses.

Monitoring
It can be difficult to find somewhere to put the ECG dots, or blood pressure cuff. The ECG dots can go anywhere on the limbs, and they can even be put on the head if necessary. All you need to do, is place them, so they form

the corners of triangle around the heart. If the arms are burnt, use a large blood pressure cuff on the thigh or calf to measure blood pressure.

Pain

In full thickness burns to the skin the nerve endings are destroyed, and the burn is painless. After debridement, burns, especially of the hands and feet, are very painful. Donor sites are more painful than the grafted area. Regional blocks are impractical if the debrided areas are extensive.

The pain of burns has a strong psychological component. Understandably the patient dreads the disfigurement, and in the recovery room may become distressed by the pain. If high doses of opioids are ineffective, or only give short periods of pain relief, try ketamine. Use a loading dose of ketamine 0.1 mg/kg followed by an infusion of 1 - 4 mg/kg/hr. Use the larger dose in a young person, and smaller in the elderly. To reduce the chance of hallucinations, keep the environment quiet, and do not disturb the patient. Use a small dose of diazepam or diazamuls to reduce the chance of hallucinations; midazolam is too short acting to be useful.

Hypothermia

Hypothermia is a serious problem,[2] especially in the operating theatre where the ambient temperature is low and the evaporative losses are high. Burnt patients are invariably hypothermic after their operations. To minimise further heat loss, increase the air temperature in the recovery room to above 30°C. Cover the patient with a warm air blanket, space blanket and warm towels. Warm all intravenous, or dialysate fluids. Heat and humidify the inspired air if possible. Monitor the patient's core temperature with a rectal thermistor probe, or tympanic membrane sensor.

Fluid balance

Monitor central venous pressure and urinary output. It is well known that patients with burns lose a lot of fluid, there are risks of renal failure, and shock if fluid replacement is not adequate. There is also a risk of over enthusiastic resuscitation causing pulmonary oedema. Maintain the central venous pressure 9 - 12 cm of water above the level of the right atrium. Use a dopamine infusion of 3 - 5 microgram/kg/minute to preserve renal function, and try to keep the urine output greater than 60 ml an hour. If possible avoid diuretics, because the hourly urine output is a useful guide to volume replacement in the early stages of burns resuscitation.

Burns oedema and limb ischaemia

About 18 hours after a burn the patient will become oedematous. Circumferential burns on a limb act like a nonflexible tourniquet as the oedema develops. Regularly check peripheral capillary return. If a limb becomes congested or white, an *escharotomy* is urgently needed. This involves cutting the tight band of dead tissue strangling the limb. It is a relatively painless procedure and does not require an anaesthetic, but it may bleed vigorously so be prepared to give a rapid transfusion.

Bleeding

Grafted, and donor sites can bleed extensively. Watch the bandages carefully for signs of further blood or fluid loss. Monitor the patient for signs of impending hypovolaemia: tachycardia, a urine output less than 30 ml/hour, and poor peripheral circulation.

Septicaemia

All burns are potentially infected, and may release septicaemic showers during manipulation. If this happens the patient will become sweaty and hypotensive. Use large bore intravenous cannulae for all fluids, so you can resuscitate him quickly if necessary.

*If a burnt patient
becomes sweaty and hypotensive
consider either septicemia, or hypovolaemia.*

CAROTID SURGERY (SEE VASCULAR SURGERY PAGE 85)

CLEFT PALATE

A tongue suture enables the tongue to be pulled forward to clear the airway. Leave the suture in place for 36 hours until the risk of swelling in the mouth subsides. Keep the face clean, and watch for oozing from the nose or mouth. Notify the surgeon if this ooze does not slow and stop.

Splint the arms of children so that they cannot suck their fingers. To minimise distress, give analgesia early. Monitor the child's oxygenation with a pulse oximeter. Never turn your back on children, because respiratory obstruction occurs quickly, and without warning. You will find it easier to measure a child's pulse rate by feeling his apex beat, or brachial artery, rather than the radial or carotid pulse. (Read more about looking after children in chapter 20).

Never turn your back on a child.

DENTAL SURGERY

Many of the problems are similar to those of tonsillectomy. Recover the patient in the 'recovery position', without a pillow under his head, until he is conscious. Hypoxaemia is a risk in these patients.[3] All should receive oxygen until they are able to sit up and breathe deeply. Dental patients are sometimes patients with mental impairment, who have not looked after their teeth. Despite their emphatic denial they may have had food or drink before the procedure, so keep a watch out for regurgitation or vomiting. Never leave the patient unattended until he is able to lift his head, cough, and spit out blood and secretions on command. Pain may be severe and cause restlessness. Once conscious he will be more comfortable sitting up.

EAR SURGERY

Giddiness, vomiting, and nausea are common after operations on the ear. Anti-emetics such as either ondansetron (Zofran®) or prochlorperazine (Stemetil®) are usually given by the anaesthetist before the patient leaves the operating theatre. If the patient is still nauseated, give an antiemetic from a different group to the one they have already received. A second dose of the same drug within 6 - 8 hours is not usually effective and can cause side effects (see page 234). Do not let the patient lie on his affected side. Patients are given deep anaesthesia for ear surgery and are slow to wake. Pain may raise his blood pressure and pulse rate. If possible transfer the patient directly from the operating table to his bed. Remember to ask the orderly, in ample time, to fetch the bed from the ward. Following ear surgery coughing, or straining may disrupt the surgery especially if the tympanic membrane has been opened or grafted. For the management of coughing (see page 318).

Eye Surgery

Nausea and vomiting is a difficult and persistent problem following opthalimic surgery. Tell the patient to warn the nursing staff if he feels nauseated, so that antiemetics can be given before vomiting becomes a problem. These patients are often more comfortable sitting up once they are awake. (See chapter 13 for control of nausea and vomiting). Try to prevent coughing, if it persists give 1.5 mg/kg lignocaine intravenously.

There have been reports about transient multiple cranial nerve palsies complicating retrobulbar blocks, this may extend to involve the brain stem causing apnoea and loss of conciousness, occasionally also hypotension and paralysis.[4]

Cataract

Cataract surgery is usually done under local anaesthetic. General anaesthesia is avoided in the elderly because of the risk of chest infections and postoperative confusion. Diabetes is commonly associated with cataracts so check the blood glucose level with a gluconometer. It is better to send them back to the ward to a warm sweet drink, than give them intravenous solutions.[5]

These patients must not cough vigorously, as their iris may prolapse through the wound. Use a bolus dose of lignocaine 1 mg/kg intravenously to alleviate coughing if it becomes a problem. Give the patient oxygen, especially if they have had sedation as well as the eye block. Try to discourage the use of anxiolytic drugs in addition to blocks. Elderly people are not normally anxious, and these drugs can cause disorientation.

Squints

These operations are usually done on young children, commonly as day surgery. Postoperative and nausea can be reduced by keeping the child well hydrated. The incidents of nausea and vomiting is as high as 80 per cent.

Facial Surgery

Following *blephoroplasty*, or *meloplasty* (face lift) sit the patient up. The eyes are usually covered with tight bandages. If the patient complains of pain, it may mean a haematoma is developing beneath the dressings, so inform the surgeon.

Iced, water soaked, gauze pads will help reduce the swelling after blephoroplasty. Do not encourage these patients to cough. Let them recover quietly. Before discharging the patient from the recovery room check that there is no double vision, which is another sign of a developing haematoma.

This surgery is often performed under very light anaesthesia such as *total intravenous anaesthesia* (TIVA). This means they will be completely awake, and very sensitive to comments about their face lift made in their presence.

Facio-maxillary procedures and jaw fractures
The operations are frequently long, and the patient may still be intubated on admission to the recovery room. These patients have had a deep anaesthetic, and take some time to wake up. The anaesthetist will not extubate them until they are sufficiently awake to look after their own airway. Rubber bands are normally used to stabilize the jaws, because these are easy to remove in an emergency. Modern bone plates allow stabilization of the jaw without mouth closure. Keep the patients in the recovery position until you are really sure that they will not vomit.

Malar fracture
Malar fractures, even after surgical reduction, are unstable. To prevent the pillow displacing the fracture, lie the patient with their fractured side uppermost. Mark the affected cheek with an ink cross, so that everyone knows it is an unstable fracture. Before the patient is discharged to the ward, check he does not have double vision, indicating that the fracture has become displaced.

Tongue sutures
When the patient comes to the recovery room there may be tongue suture protruding from his mouth. This allows the staff to pull his tongue forward if it swells to obstruct his pharynx and airway.

GYNAECOLOGY

Patients sometimes have psychosocial problems, becoming distressed and tearful especially after the termination of pregnancy. For a short time after wakening they may become disinhibited, and talk or swear in an embarrassing way. Do your best to preserve their dignity.

Analgesia

Although lower abdominal operations are less painful than upper abdominal operations, patients still need good analgesia, and there will be a number of patients who require opioids.

Initially try to manage pain in day patients without opioids. The NSAIDs, particularly mefenamic acid, and tenoxicam are effective for uterine cramps following curettage.[5] The onset of pain relief with NSAIDs may take 1 - 2 hours. Panadol suppositories are useful (see page 208).

Vaginal surgery

Vaginal surgery is performed with the legs in lithotomy position. Check for pressure areas, and numbness or tingling in the feet. Hip pain or back pain can be caused by over extension of the legs during the operation. If this occurs, note it in the record, and inform the surgeon. Patients who have been in lithotomy position with their legs up in stirrups during the operation may be hypotensive when they come to the recovery room. Nurse them with their legs elevated on pillows for the first hour following surgery. Check their pads for continuing vaginal bleeding. Some patients need urinary catheters to prevent postoperative urine retention. Check with the surgeon if a catheter is necessary, before sending the patient to the ward. Encourage leg movements to prevent deep vein thrombosis.

Laparoscopy

Laparoscopy is less painful than open surgery. NSAIDs, especially as supositories given preoperatively, help with postoperative pain relief. In spite of this, opioids may still be required to control the pain; especially if the fallopian tubes have been cauterized. Some surgeons drip 0.5% bupivacaine 5 mls with 1:200 000 adrenaline onto the cut end of the fallopian tubes at the end of the procedure.[6] This provides excellent pain relief for the first postoperative hour. Shoulder tip pain is a common complaint, and is probably due to gas accumulating under the diaphragm. It resolves quickly, but can be distressing while it lasts; sitting the patient up helps. Many of these patients want to go home on the same day as their surgery, but occasionally they are detained because of uncontrollable pain or postoperative nausea and vomiting.

Hysteroscopy

Irrigation fluid causes the same problem as TURP syndrome (see page 81).

HAND SURGERY

Much hand surgery is done under regional blockade. The appropriate drug to use is lignocaine. If you see that bupivicaine has been given, explain to the patient that the numbness can last for a very long time. Since the arm is both numb and paralyzed, warn the patient not to try to move his arm, because it can fly about uncontrollably. Patients have hit themselves in the face while attempting to investigate their new plaster, risking black eyes or even fractured noses. Following hand surgery the arm is usually splinted with at least a plaster back slab. Elevate the arm in a box sling to reduce the swelling, and make sure it is comfortably positioned. Report to the surgeon, any problems with perfusion of the arm.

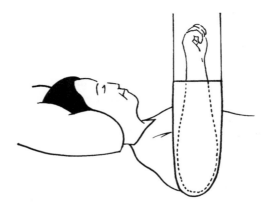

fig 4.3 Position of the arm after hand surgery

HYPOPHYSECTOMY (SEE NEUROSURGERY PAGE 66)

LIPOSUCTION

Liposuction is a procedure for removing unwanted fat. It is frequently performed as day surgery, often under local anaesthesia. Large volumes of fluid containing local anaesthetic are injected into the fat and a lot of fluid is absorbed resulting in a diuresis. Check the patient's bladder as soon as she reaches recovery room. The combined effect of hypothermia, and the adrenaline used in the subcutaneous fluid can cause the patients to shake and shiver after the procedure. Many suffer from headaches[7], which can be controlled with paracetamol. Toxicity from the absorption of the local anaesthetic does not appear to be a common problem.

MEDIASTINOSCOPY

Patients come to the recovery room with a small wound and no drainage tubes. Major complications can occur during the procedure, such as, bleeding, or tearing of the lungs or airways. Pneumothorax is the main complication. Watch for signs of airway obstruction, deviation of the trachea, and progressive dyspnoea. Consider a chest X-ray if there is any deterioration in the patient's condition. On the chest film look for widening of the mediastinum, pneumothorax, and pneumomediastinum. Air can track into the neck, so feel for *crepitus* (crackling under the skin), especially at the sternal notch. If you feel the crepitus, or the patient is distressed, give high flow oxygen, and send for the surgeon. Prepare to insert a chest drain (see page 96). The patient may need to return to theatre if the complications do not resolve.

NASAL SURGERY

Following nasal surgery the nose is usually packed with stuffed glove fingers, gauze or silk. A partially conscious patient finds it difficult to breathe through his mouth, is distressed at having his airway blocked, and may become restless and thrash about. A large number of these patients are also young and fit and have never had an anaesthetic before. Have a strong orderly at your side and ask the anaesthetist to remain with the patient until he is fully conscious. Sit him up as soon as possible. This helps reduce venous bleeding into the soft tissues around the eyes, and prevents postoperative facial swelling.

Pain relief

Opioids are best given intraoperatively for nasal surgery and NSAIDS postoperatively. Many surgeons inject local anaesthetic so pain is not usually a problem.

Blood clots

Sometimes a piece of tissue, or blood clot will fall on to the vocal cords causing laryngospasm, coughing or a hoarse voice. If you suspect this has happened check the larynx, and pharynx with a laryngoscope.

A large blood clot can easily be hidden in the nasal pharynx where it cannot be seen. This *coroner's clot* can be aspirated without warning into the trachea, to totally block the airway (see page 329). After surgery on the upper airway gently use a dental sucker to explore the nasopharynx.

An excessively dry throat may make the patient restless. Once he is fully conscious, give him a piece of wet gauze to suck or little sips of water.

Eye irritation

Sometimes small bits of plaster get into the eyes and irritate them. If this happens, notify the surgeon, and record the fact in the history. Irrigate the eyes with sterile normal saline. Check the eyes are not red before discharging the patient to the ward. Cold wet swabs to their eyes are comforting, and help prevent peri-orbital bruising.

Neurosurgery

Postoperative care after intracranial surgery requires close monitoring of the conscious state. Record the patient's pupils, state of consciousness, respiratory rate, and best reactions to stimuli on a *head injury* chart.

Usually the *Glasgow coma scale* (GCS) is used to record the depth of coma. The lower the score the more deeply unconscious is the patient. With a score less than 8 the patient will be comatose, and need his airway protected.

GLASGOW COMA SCALE		
	RESPONSE	**SCORE**
Eyes open	Spontaneously	4
	To command	3
	To pain	2
	No response	1
Best motor response	Obeys	6
to command	Localizes	5
to pain	Flexion: non-localizing	4
	Flexion; decorticate	3
	Extension: decerebrate	2
	No response	1
Best verbal response	Oriented and converses	5
	Disoriented and converses	4
	Inappropriate words	3
	Incomprehensible sounds	2
	No response	1
	Score 3 – 15	

Take care to administer the intravenous fluids exactly as prescribed. Carefully record the intake and output.

Never do anything to cause pain to a comatose neurosurgical patient, because this will raise his intracranial pressure. Minimize activity around the trolley. Those who have just had intracranial operations, must be moved carefully, and not jolted, or handled roughly. If possible have the patient's bed available so that he does not have to spend time on a trolley, and be moved again later.

Signs of rising intracranial pressure are:
- deterioration of conscious state, and changes in respiratory rate or breathing pattern;
- decreased movement, and muscle power on one side of the body;
- a dilated, or oval pupil indicating transtentorial herniation of brain.

If any of these occur notify the neurosurgeon, and the anaesthetist immediately.

Beware of the unilateral dilating pupil.
Report it straight away - don't delay!

Most neurosurgical patients are extubated before returning to the recovery room. If the patient is still intubated sedate him with lignocaine 1 mg/kg intravenously before aspirating the trachea.

The requirement for pain relief is minimal in these patients, if they do need analgesia, dihydrocodeine is the drug of choice. Dihydrocodeine cannot be given intravenously.

Hypotension
A fall in mean blood pressure will decrease cerebral blood flow, and can lead to hypoxia and fitting. Likely causes include:
- decreased blood volume;
- intraoperative diuretics;
- drug reactions, or interactions;
- adrenal cortical failure;
- decreased cardiac contractility.

Hypertension
A rise in blood pressure increases intracranial pressure, increases the risk of haemorrhage at the operation site, and aggravates oedema formation. If the blood volume has been kept up during surgery, the blood pressure will rise once vascular tone returns. Hypertension may be a protective reflex to maintain cerebral blood flow. Eliminate hypoxia and hypercarbia as a cause. Aim to decrease the blood pressure slowly, watching carefully for signs of deteriorating conscious state.

Head injuries

Head injured patients are likely to progressively develop cerebral oedema for the first 48 hours. Cerebral oedema can cause brainstem compression. An early sign of brainstem compression is a change in respiratory rate. It first rises then falls. A change of as little as 3 breaths a minute may be significant, so it is important to measure the respiratory rate for a full minute, noting rate, depth, and rhythm. Put your hand on the patient's chest when monitoring breathing so you can feel the rise and fall.

A change in respiratory pattern, or rate
indicates a change in conscious state.
Get help!

As cerebral oedema develops, intracranial pressure will rise. This can disrupt blood supply to cause irreversible brain damage. It is important to keep the intracranial pressure low. If the patient is being ventilated, give morphine 0.01 mg/kg. Hyperventilate to acutely reduce intracranial pressure. Start an infusion of 1 gm/kg of 20% mannitol over 10 minutes, and notify the neurosurgeon. A late sign of raised intracranial pressure with brain stem ischaemia is the dilation of one or both pupils. Unfortunately, by the time this has occurred, the brain will be damaged.

Cerebral aneurysm clipping.

Vasospasm is a problem after neurosurgery for clipping of the intracranial aneurysms. This slows intracerebral blood flow, and predispose to strokes. Aim to keep the PaO_2 greater than 150 mmHg (19.7 kPa) and the mean blood pressure greater than 100 mmHg. Give at least 35% oxygen by mask. You may need a dopamine, or noradrenaline infusion to maintain the blood pressure. To dilate the cerebral arteries, and override vasospasm a nimodipine infusion is often used. Nimodipine is a calcium channel blocking drug used for the management of cerebral vasospasm after intracranial surgery. The initial dose is 15 microgram/kg/hr for 2 hours then 30 microgram/kg/hr if the blood pressure remains stable. Its side effects are hypotension and bradycardia and a decrease in renal blood flow.

Hypophysectomy

Surgical ablation of the pituitary gland is performed through the nose. Therefore the patient has had both a nasal, and an intracranial operation. Monitor the patient in the same way as one who has had a craniotomy.

Occasionally bleeding occurs around the base of the brain triggering excessive sympathetic nerve activity. This will cause hypertension, and cardiac arrhythmias, and aggravate further bleeding.

If massive polyuria occurs and persists for more than an hour, commence fluids with 0.45% saline (1/2 N saline), and 5 mmol potassium per litre to replace urinary losses. Measure urinary electrolytes, and replace deficits accordingly. Give desmopressin (DDAVP®), 2 microgram as a slow intravenous infusion to control the polyuria. The syndrome usually resolves in 2 - 3 days.

Brainstem surgery

Occasionally patients who have had brainstem surgery get lower cranial nerve dysfunction, with vocal cord paralysis, difficulty in swallowing, and partial airway obstruction. Make sure they fulfil the criteria (on page 20) before extubating them. Watch them closely for obstruction, and for loss of gag reflex. If this happens, reintubate the patient.

Spinal cord surgery

If the cord is intact, spinal cord surgery is painful. If the surgeon agrees to place an epidural catheter during the procedure, then a thoracic epidural is the best way to control this pain. Otherwise use high doses of morphine, but watch for respiratory depression. High spinal cord injury can cause *Ondine's Curse* where the patient appears to forget to breathe. It may be necessary to re-intubate, and ventilate these patients. The problem usually resolves after 2 - 3 days. High spinal cord injury or surgery can disrupt sympathetic outflow tracts causing hypotension and bradycardia. Vasopressors may be needed to support the blood pressure. Tracheal suction gives these patients a bradycardia. Use atropine 0.6 mg intravenously to prevent this. They are often cold after surgery. If their sympathetic nervous system has been damaged they have no mechanism for preventing heat loss. Note of their temperature and use warm blankets, a space blanket, or hot air from a Bair Hugger™.

OESOPHAGECTOMY[8]

Oesophagectomy is a traumatic operation performed for cancer of the oesophagus. Bowel is pulled up through the mediastinum, and a piece, with its blood supply intact, is used to replace the oesophagus. This operation is a major physiological insult that predisposes the patient to cardiac arrhythmias, especially atrial fibrillation, and major respiratory complications.[9] Be prepared to treat the arrhythmia (see page 273). These patients are frequently hypomagnesaemic which contributes to the cardiac arrhythmias sometimes seen in recovery room. The patient may still be intubated on admission to the recovery room, and will have all the problems associated with a long operation. If the carcinoma has involved the larynx he will have a tracheostomy and be unable to speak.

Nasogastric tube

This is needed to prevent the stomach distending. Make sure the nasogastric tube is well secured, because it crosses the anastomosis, and moving it puts stress on the stitches holding the anastomosis together. If the nasogastric tube comes out it can be a disaster. It cannot be easily replaced, and the distending gut may tear the anastomosis apart.

ORTHOPAEDICS

Operations on bones are painful. Young patients especially, need more than the average amount of opioid to control their pain. It is best to start pain relief before they leave the operating theatre so that they have already received a loading dose on reaching the recovery room. Major orthopaedic operations are sometimes performed with spinal anaesthesia, or regional blockade.

Arthroscopy

Arthroscopy is a painful procedure. Many surgeons instil a long acting local anaesthetic such as bupivacaine into the joint to help control the pain. Adding morphine to this injection improves the duration of analgesia. The patient is more comfortable after knee operations if the legs are elevated on pillows.

Tourniquets

Operations performed under tourniquet, such as total knee replacements, may bleed vigorously in the recovery room, so watch the drain bottles for losses. It is not unusual for a knee replacement to lose a litre of blood in the first few hours after surgery. Check that blood is cross-matched, and available.

Hip surgery

During hip replacements and femoral neck fractures, several litres of blood can be lost. Blood spilled on the floor, and drapes make it difficult to estimate the blood loss during surgery, and the patient may come to the recovery room either hypovolaemic, or having had too much fluid. Try and estimate the fluid balance, how much has been given and how much has been lost and make a note of this. Often patients continue to bleed after coming to the recovery room, and if this is not detected the patient may become shocked later after returning to the ward. Up to a litre of blood can be lost into the thigh before it starts to swell noticeably. Occasionally a patient will neglect to tell the medical staff he has been taking aspirin in one of its many guises, or a herbal remedy, such as St John's Wort or Gingko balboa which may explain excessive postoperative ooze.

It is usually the elderly, with all their other medical problems, who have hip surgery. These patients commonly become hypoxic in the recovery room, especially if they have had a general anaesthetic. Periodic hypoxaemia occurs for up to five days after surgery.[10] If a patient has fractured her neck of femur, she will probably be already hypoxic before coming to the operating theatre; and the hypoxia will be worse postoperatively.[11] Hypoxia, together with fat emboli are the main reasons for postoperative confusion that is so common in these patients.[12] The problem is aggravated if opioids are used for postoperative pain control, and severe hypoxia occurs when the patient is asleep.[13] If the patient has been taking antidepressants the postoperative confusion is even worse.

Patients having hip surgery often have other arthritic joints. Take care especially of their necks when you move them.

Hypoxia is a constant threat
to elderly patients
having orthopaedic operations.

Abduction pillow

After hip replacement an *abduction pillow* (Charnley pillow) is used to keep the legs apart, and strapped in the extended position. This pillow is often put on by staff in recovery room. Before you put on the pillow, check the skin on the legs thoroughly for signs of break down or abnormality, and check the perfusion of the limbs. Put the wide end between the ankles. Apply the straps in such a way that you can easily slip your finger between the strap and the skin. Be careful not to compress the peroneal nerve with the straps. Check the pedal pulses, and the perfusion of the feet before the patient leaves recovery room.

Routine orthopaedic observations

Additional special orthopaedic observations should include:

1. Check the drain bottles every 15 minutes; and record their patency, the amount of drainage, its colour, and its character.

2. Check neurovascular status every 15 minutes. This includes; peripheral pulses, limb colour, limb temperature, capillary refilling, presence of numbness, or tingling, swelling, and if possible movement.

3. Check the position. Keep the limb in the correct position, set by the surgeon. Initially the bed should be flat. While the patient is lying flat have a sucker ready, because they are at risk of aspirating if they vomit.

4. Check for signs of fat emboli (see page 337).

Plaster checks

These include:

- warmth, colour, and capillary refilling;
- movement of fingers or toes;
- sensation and presence of pain, numbness or tingling;
- pulses;
- state of plaster.

To help prevent a plastered limb from swelling elevate it on a pillow. Do a plaster check every 15 minutes, and record your findings. The main danger is that the limb will swell inside the tight plaster, and cut off the distal circulation. If this occurs the patient will complain of 'pins-and-needles', followed by pain and then numbness. These important symptoms may be absent if a local, or regional anaesthetic has been used. Feel the character of the pulse, and compare it with the pulse in the unplastered limb; they should be the same. Look carefully to see that the extremity is not changing colour, and that the skin capillaries are not congested and blue. Check capillary return by pressing on a nail bed, and note how fast the capillaries fill when you let it go. This should be about one second, but if the limb is congested it will be faster. If the limb is ischaemic, the capillaries will fail to fill. It will be necessary to split the plaster if the limb perfusion is impaired. Occasionally muscles go into spasm inside the plaster and this is best treated with valium 0.1 mg/kg either intravenously or as a suppository. Small suppositories are available for babies.

Check that blood is not seeping through the plaster. If it is, then mark out the boundaries with a felt tipped pen so its progress can be followed. The surgeon should review the plaster before the patient returns to the ward.

Fat emboli

Orthopaedic and trauma cases are at risk from fat embolism (see page 327).

Deep vein thrombosis (DVT) [14]

Patients with hip fractures and pelvic fractures are at risk of deep vein thrombosis. Up to 50 per cent have evidence of deep vein thrombosis. Up to 2 per cent die from pulmonary embolism with elective surgery and up to 7 per cent from emergency surgery. Epidural and spinal anaesthesia decrease the risk slightly; probably by increasing blood flow to the limbs during the operation. How to prevent deep vein thrombosis, and pulmonary embolism remains a controversial issue. [15]

Risk factors include:
• emergency surgery;
• increasing age;
• previous history of thrombosis, or embolism;
• obesity;
• malignancy;
• prolonged immobilisation;
• oral contraceptives containing oestrogen ;
• cardiac failure.

Prophylaxis in the recovery room include:
• encouraging active leg, and foot exercises;
• low dose heparin, or low molecular weight heparins used preoperatively, and sometimes given again in the recovery room. Low molecular weight heparins are more effective than standard heparin.
• less effectively, intra-, and postoperative infusions of dextran 70; use 10 ml/kg;
• graduated compressive pressure stockings;
• where possible raise the patient's legs to prevent pressure on the calf muscles.

Pulmonary embolism (PE)

Pulmonary embolism uncommonly occurs in the recovery room, and is more likely to occur in the ward 2 - 14 days postoperatively. Consider pulmonary embolism if a patient becomes abruptly short of breath, has pleuritic chest pain; or collapses. Patients with an acute pulmonary embolis are apprehensive, fearful and panicky. A chest X-ray, or ECG in recovery room usually reveals nothing at this early stage. A wheeze can be sometimes heard over the affected lung. Treatment is difficult in the first few days after an operation, because thrombolysis with streptokinase will dissolve all clots, precipitating postoperative bleeding. Heparin can be commenced cautiously.

PERINEAL OPERATIONS

Operations on the perineum are painful. The anaesthetist sometimes puts in a caudal block to control the pain. Warn the patient he may have a numb bottom for some hours, but as soon as the anaesthetic starts to wear off to ask the ward staff for pain relief. Caudal analgesia tends to wear off abruptly.

PLASTIC SURGERY

Do not let patients become restless after plastic surgery operations. If patients thrash about they are likely to disrupt the surgery. This applies especially to skin grafts, vascular flaps, and nerve and tendon repairs. Diazamul, or diazepam, 1 - 5 mg intravenously is suitable sedation. Give it slowly in 1 mg increments, and supplement it with oxygen by mask.

Check the perfusion of pedicle grafts. Signs of poor perfusion are pallor, coolness, blue discolouration, and poor capillary return.

Plastic surgery is frequently performed under deep anaesthesia. To avoid emergence delirium let the patients wake up slowly, and quietly.

Epidural analgesia will provide continuing regional anaesthesia for operations on the abdomen, or lower limbs; and additionally will keep the operation site well perfused.

Tissue grafts

Following microsurgery for free vascularized tissue grafts, put patients on supplemental oxygen, and keep the surgical site warm. A good blood supply is essential for a successful graft. Good analgesia will help prevent cutaneous vasoconstriction that might jeopardise the viability of the graft. Do not let the patient become hypotensive or hypovolaemic. Monitor his oxygenation with a pulse oximeter. If the grafted tissue appears pale or white, suspect problems with its arterial blood supply. If it appears dark, or blue the venous drainage is impaired. Inform the surgeon.

Hypotensive anaesthesia

Some plastic procedure operations are performed under hypotensive anaesthesia to reduce bleeding, and make it easier for the surgeon to see what he is doing. When the blood pressure is returned to normal the surgical site may bleed. Be prepared for this. Do not discharge the patient to the ward until his blood pressure has been stable at preoperative levels for an hour.

If a patient is confused, restless, slow to awaken, or complains of a headache after hypotensive anaesthesia inform the anaesthetist. This may be a sign of intraoperative cerebral hypoxia.

THORACOTOMY

Analgesia is best achieved with either a thoracic epidural, or intercostal blocks. Some surgeons use a cryoprobe on the intercostal nerves as they are closing up. It takes some weeks for the nerves to regain function. In the recovery room the patients are nursed in the sitting position. Check the underwater drains to ensure they are draining and swinging. The drain tubes must never be tied to the bed linen or the cot side. As the patient moves the drains can be accidentally pulled out. Under some circumstances it is dangerous to clamp thoracic drain tubes, particularly if the drain tubes are bubbling into the bottle. Clamping a bubbling drain will cause a pneumothorax, because the air cannot escape from the chest. (see pneumothorax, page 333). Never clamp drain tubes if the patient is receiving positive pressure ventilation.

Do not lift the drain bottles higher than the base of the bed, because fluid may run from the bottle back into the patient's wound. Moving these patients from trolley to bed requires many hands.

Never *milk* thoracic drain tubes with one of those old fashioned roller drain tube milkers. These milkers grasp the tubing between two stainless steel rollers, they generate enormous suction pressures that can make the lungs bleed.

A complication of thoracotomy is cardiac tamponade.

THYMECTOMY

This operation is performed to relieve the symptoms of myasthenia gravis. The patient will normally be taking neostigmine, or physostigmine to counteract muscle weakness. These drugs are usually omitted on the morning of surgery, and recommenced in the recovery room. Their side effects are bradycardia, weakness, and excessive oral and bronchial secretions.

The Tensilon® test

The Tensilon® test is used to find the optimal postoperative dose of neostigmine. Edrophonium (Tensilon®)is a short acting anticholinesterase. If a dose of edrophonium causes an increase in muscle power then increase the dose of neostigmine.

Do not extubate the patient until he has achieved maximum strength. Following extubation the patient must be watched for weakness in the facial, and neck muscles, and for any difficult in swallowing secretions.

As after any mediastinal operation, watch for the signs of concealed haemorrhage, respiratory distress or subcutaneous emphysema indicating the patient has developed a pneumothorax.

THYROIDECTOMY

Sit these patients up as soon as they regain consciousness. Their bandages will need to be checked and resecured. The patients are frequently nauseated, because of surgical traction on, and around the vagus nerve. They may have been given an antiemetic as part of the anaesthetic. Check which they have received. Use either metoclopramide 5 mg IV, or prochlorperazine 6.25 mg I/M or ondansetron 4 - 8 mg I/M.

Stridor

Concealed bleeding from below the deep fascia in the neck can cause airway obstruction. If the patient develops noisy breathing, or stridor in the recovery room immediately notify the anaesthetist, or the surgeon. Do not attempt to reintubate these patients unless you are skilled; because the laryngeal opening, and even the pharynx, will be obscured by oedema. Intubation requires an inhalational induction.

If you cannot find someone to help, relieve the obstruction yourself.

Stridor is a medical emergency.

Thyroid storm (see page 153)

PARATHYROIDECTOMY

Nausea and vomiting is a problem in these patients. Check whether they have received an intraoperative antiemetic and give a different one in recovery room. They can also become hypocalcaemic, suspect this if you observe muscle twitching, especially around the mouth or cheek.

MANAGEMENT OF STRIDOR AFTER THYROID OPERATIONS

Step 1. Put the patient on high inspired oxygen, and sit him up.

Step 2. Take out the skin clips or sutures. The wound will fall open.

Step 3. Using sterile instruments take out the sutures running transversely in a straight line in the bottom of the wound. The tissues will fall open, and allow the blood to drain out. No harm can be done by this procedure, and it may save the patient's life.

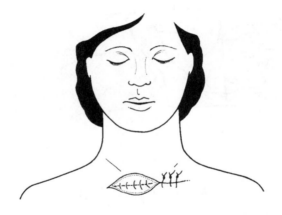

fig 4.4 Removal of sutures after a thyroidectomy

TONSILLECTOMY

Following tonsillectomy concealed bleeding into the pharynx is a danger. Nurse these patients in the *recovery position* without a pillow until they are conscious. For patients weighing less than 50 kg, put a pillow under their hips, and tilt them head down to let the blood drain from their mouths.

Tonsillectomy is painful, but there are problems if the patient is deeply sedated after this operation, so check with the surgeon, and anaesthetist before giving further opioids. This precaution applies especially to patients who have a history of sleep apnoea. These patients are at risk of obstructing their airways, and with an opioid depressing their respiratory centre, silently become apnoeic. Have a working sucker under their pillows. Do not use metal suckers, but rather soft plastic suction catheters that are less likely to damage the friable surgical site. Most tonsillectomy patients need intravenous fluids for 24 hours after surgery. Give adults metoclopramide (Maxolon®) before they return to the ward, because they tend to swallow a lot of blood and feel nauseated. Read more about the care of children in chapter 20.

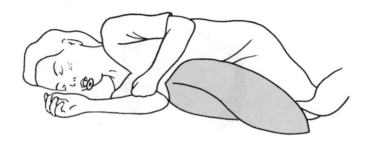

fig 4.5 Tonsillectomy position

The bleeding tonsil

This is a major recovery room emergency. Establish a free running intravenous line after tonsil surgery. If it does not run well, or is pulled out, replace it immediately. If you are sucking blood from the pharynx every few minutes advise the surgeon. Very gently look with a laryngoscope. Remember a small child is seriously compromised once he loses 10 per cent of his blood volume. This can easily be overlooked.

TRACHEOSTOMY

This may be performed as part of a laryngectomy, or on patients who have been intubated for a period in the intensive care unit.

Keep the airway clear. Use soft plastic Y-catheters to suck out blood and secretions. Thoroughly pre-oxygenate the patient before carrying out this procedure. While suctioning the patient hold your own breath and mentally count to 10. Never suck longer than this without stopping to give the patient a rest, and some more oxygen. Suctioning is a sterile procedure; use sterile gloves, and a non-touch technique (see page 18). Be very careful that none of the patient's secretions contaminate you. If you are splashed, clean the area thoroughly and immediately.

Change the dressings before the patient returns to the ward. Check to make sure the tracheostomy tube has been formally and firmly stitched in place, rather than just tied in with tape. Warn the ward staff if it has just been tied in place. If the tracheostomy tube falls out in the next 3 - 4 days it is almost impossible to replace, because a clear tract will not yet have formed through the oedematous tissue. Send sterile dressing scissors, tracheostomy dilators, and a spare tracheostomy tube back to the ward with the patient. These instruments will be needed urgently if the tracheostomy falls out. Keep them in a sterile plastic bag on the head of the bed until the stoma hardens in 4 - 6 days.

Humidification

Start humidification with a heated humidifier as soon as possible. Spontaneously breathing patients can be humidified, and oxygenated using a T-piece (see page 483). Do not use a condenser humidifier unless it has been specially designed for tracheostomies. Jamming a normal condenser humidifier (eg. Humidvent®) on to the tracheostomy tube can suffocate the patient if he coughs up a glob of phlegm which blocks the paper filter.

UROLOGICAL SURGERY

Patients undergoing urological surgery are often elderly and have other intercurrent illnesses. They frequently develop problems that show up in the recovery room. Keep a patient who has had urological surgery in the recovery room until you are sure that he is not going to have trouble, 60 - 90 minutes is appropriate. If the patient has had a spinal anaesthetic he will be awake, and awake patients tend to receive less close attention from recovery room staff. There is a protocol on page 23 for the routine care of patients after spinal anaesthesia.

Urological patients who have spinal anaesthesia are especially vulnerable to complications, because they have been exposed to large volumes of fluid, they get cold and they have had their legs raised for long periods of time. Take extra care of these patients, Give them all supplemental oxygen, monitor their blood pressures and oximeter readings, and report to the anaesthetist if the saturation falls below 93 per cent.

Urological operations include:
• transurethral resection of the prostate (TURP);
• percutaneous nephrolithotomy (PCNL);
• transurethral bladder tumour resection (TURBT);
• nephrectomy.

Problems include:
• complications of spinal anaesthesia;
• TURP syndrome;
• hypothermia;
• hypotension;
• plasma volume overload;
• pain;
• clot retention;
• ruptured bladder;
• sepsis;
• blood loss;
• clot retention;
• pneumothorax (after nephrectomy).

Spinal anaesthesia

Spinal anaesthesia is used routinely during prostate surgery because it allows early detection of the TURP syndrome, promotes vasodilation and reduces the risk of volume overload and blood loss. It also provides postoperative analgesia and helps the patient tolerate the urinary catheter. There is also a reduced incidence in postoperative myocardial infarction in this elderly age group, when compared with those who have general anaesthesia.

Other significant problems with spinal anaesthesia include:
• hypotension;
• post dural (spinal) headache;
• backache;
• neurological complications;

SPINAL HEADACHES. These are not common in older patients but they still occur. Good hydration helps prevent spinal headache. Advise the ward to keep his drip running for the first 24 hours, even if the patient is eating and drinking.

The best treatment for a post-spinal headache is a blood patch (see page 216). Although customary to lie patients flat for some hours after spinal anaesthesia, this is not necessary, and will not reduce the incidence of post-spinal headache.

BACKACHE is common after spinal or epidural anaesthesia. It is usually attributed to periosteal damage done by the tiny needles. This is unlikely, a far more likely cause is that the patient has lost the tone of the muscles normally supporting the arch of his lumbar spine. If he has not been properly positioned on the table he may have lain in an uncomfortable position for some hours. Considering these factors it is surprising that backache is not more common. Support the patient's back with a folded towel and be very slow and gentle when moving a patient's limp lower body.

DANGER OF DAMAGE TO A NUMB LIMB. The patient will normally be fully conscious but unable to feel the lower half of their body. This total analgesia persists for 1 - 4 hours depending on the type of the local anaesthetic agent used. The patient may be injured if a numb leg falls off the trolley, or the patient is knocked while being transferred from the trolley to his bed.

TURP syndrome

Most recovery room problems for urology patients follow transurethral resection of the prostate (TURP). The TURP syndrome is a serious complication. It occurs if irrigation fluid used to flush the blood away during surgery is absorbed into the blood stream causing and hyponatraemia vascular volume overload, confusion and even convulsions. This complication can also occur following percutaneous nephrolithotomy (PCNL).

A confused urological patient?
Consider hypoxia, and water intoxication.

Irrigation solutions used during TURPs or PCNLs are isotonic, non-toxic and will not conduct the electric current used to cut and coagulate tissues. Commonly used solutions include: 1.5% glycine, and 3% mannitol. Distilled water is no longer used because if it is absorbed it will cause haemolysis, shock and renal damage. If the patient has received more than 15 litres of irrigation solution, or has been on the operating table for more than one hour you should check their sodium and haemoglobin, and report these results to the surgeon and the anaesthetist.

GLYCINE TOXICITY

When glycine enters the circulation in large amounts it is toxic to the heart and the retina causing transient blindness with or without cardiac failure. The signs of glycine toxicity are nausea, vomiting, convulsions, slow respiratory rate, spells of apnoea, hypotension, cyanosis, and anuria. This problem can be counteracted by adding the amino acid arginine to the irrigating glycine solution. Transfer the patient to ICU for supportive treatment.

BLINDNESS ASSOCIATED WITH GLYCINE TOXICITY

The patient complains of blurred vision and and see halos around bright objects. The pupils become dilated and unresponsive. This frightening event resolves spontaneously after 8 - 48 hours. In contrast to cortical blindness the patient can still see light and his blink reflex is not impaired.

AMMONIA TOXICITY

Ammonia is a by-product of glycine metabolism. Ammonia toxicity occurs within one hour of surgery, with signs of nausea, vomiting and then deteriorating conscious state that quickly becomes a coma. Blood levels of ammonia may exceed 500 micromol/litre (normal level 10 - 35 micromol/litre). The patient will remain in coma for 10 - 12 hours, emerging only when the blood ammonia level falls below 150 micromol/litre. Ammonia toxicity may be due to arginine deficiency. Transfer the patient to ICU for management.

Hypothermia

A falling core temperature is a problem in elderly urological patients, who may have received many litres of cool bladder irrigation fluid. Check their temperature as soon as possible. Use a Bain Hugger™,or blankets and Mylar® sheeting.

Hypotension

Hypotension in recovery room could be an effect of the spinal anaesthesia. Nausea is a sign of hypotension in patients after spinal or epidural anaesthesia but you must exclude other causes. These include:

1. Bleeding. Look for blood in the urine bag. If you can't see light through the urine bag then tell the surgeon and anaesthetist.
2. TURP syndrome.
3. Heart failure. Signs may include shortness of breath, cough or wheeze. The patient's oxygen saturation may fall below 95 per cent.
3. Myocardial ischemia may cause ST segment changes on the ECG or Arrhythmias such as vetricular premature beats.

4. Sometimes frusemide (Lasix®) is given to patients to encourage a urine output, and flush away clots. The combination of a spinal anaesthetic, a diuretic, and an elderly patient with poor cardiac function is a potent recipe for hypotension.

If the blood pressure falls establish the cause. Replace blood loss with either blood or colloid. Use 100 ml aliquots until either the blood pressure or jugular venous pressure rises. If the patient has warm hands and a normal pulse rate consider using ephedrine in 3 - 5 mg doses slowly intravenously. Repeat this at 5 minute intervals up to a limit of 0.75 mg/kg. If the problem persists use dopamine infusion to support the blood pressure (see page 520). Heart failure may be a problem. If the JVP rises, and the blood pressure remains low, suspect heart failure (see page 281).

After a spinal anaesthetic, if the patient sits up abruptly, the blood pressure will fall. Sit him up slowly, and measure his blood pressure frequently. If he becomes hypotensive, lie him flat.

Beware of hypotension in the urological patient
Measure the blood pressure frequently.

Plasma volume overload

During the early stages of spinal anaesthesia the patient is often given large amounts of intravenous fluid. He can absorb this as his circulation is dilated. As the anaesthetic wears off the fluid is recirculated and could put a susceptable patient, with cardiovascular or arterial disease, into left ventricular failure and pulmonary oedema. Suspect this if the patient becomes breathless or begins to wheeze. Listen to his chest for crepitations. If he is accumulating fluid in his lungs give frusemide. Start with 5 mg intravenously and if necessary give up to 40 - 80 mg. Be cautious if the patient has received gentamicin during the procedure as the combination of frusemide and gentamicin can be nephrotoxic.

Ruptured or perforated bladder

After a spinal anaesthetic signs of a ruptured bladder, very severe pain, are masked. Suspect this complication if the patient has nausea and shoulder tip pain. Check the fluid balance very carefully and alert the surgeon.

Sepsis

The prostate may harbour a variety of bacteria. If the prostatic venous sinuses are opened during surgery, irrigation can push bacteria into the blood stream. These patients may develop a short episode of hypotension, severe chills, fever, and capillary dilatation. The symptoms only last a few hours, and then the patient recovers spontaneously. This event is probably due to bacterial endotoxins entering the circulation. Gentamicin is the antibiotic of choice. Use an initial loading dose of 2 mg/kg IV.

Blood loss

Patients should stop taking apirin or NSAIDs at least one week before surgery. If they have not done so suspect this as a cause of postoperative bleeding. Blood loss is difficult to estimate during transurethral surgery (one old man went back to the ward and proudly told his friends "They took two buckets of blood out of me !") It certainly looks like that but most of it is irrigating fluid. Some of this irrigating fluid is also absorbed, contributing to overhydration and masking the usual signs of blood loss, hypotension and tachycardia. Check the patient's haemoglobin in recovery room. This should have been checked preoperatively and during the procedure, changes will indicate a trend. Discuss the result of this investigation with the surgeon. He is the only one who really has an impression of the amount of blood lost.

Dilutional thrombocytopaenia occasionally occurs, so check their platelet count if bleeding persists. Sometimes particles of prostate gland, rich in tissue thromboplastin, enter the circulation and trigger *disseminated intravascular coagulopathy* (see page 346). Urokinase, released from the prostate during surgery may prevent clots forming, or dissolve those that do form. This is called *primary fibrinolysis* and the treatment is tranexamic acid, or epsilon-amino-caproic acid (EACA).

Confusion

Post-operative confusion occurs in about 6 - 10 per cent of patients undergoing transurethral resection of the prostate. The confused patients pull on their catheters causing trauma to the raw urethral surface.

> *A confused urological patient?*
> *Consider hypoxia, and water intoxication.*

If a patient remains confused or aggressive after prostatic surgery, transfer him to a high dependency nursing area for further management. These patients can disturb a normal ward.

Pain

TURP surgery is not usually very painful. If there is severe pain, suspect a complication such as clot retention or ruptured bladder. Percutaneous nephrolithotomies (PCNL) and nephrectomies are painful. Pain after nephrectomy is best controlled with thoracic epidural blockade, intercostal blocks are a less optimal alternative. PCNLs usually require NSAID suppositories as well as patient controlled analgesia (PCA).

Drug toxicity (see also box on page 139).

Some urological surgeons use prophylactic gentamicin to prevent infection. Keep in mind that the combination of gentamicin and frusemide is both nephrotoxic and ototoxic in a saline depleted patient. Ringing in the ears is an early sign, and may first occur in recovery room. Unfortunately the damage is irreversible, and deafness is a risk.

Catheters - see page 98.

Drains - see page 91.

Vascular Surgery

Angiographic procedures

Problems presenting in the recovery room include intimal dissection at the puncture site, haematoma, embolism of debris or clot to the limb causing ischaemia or infarction, and hypersensitivity to the contrast dye. The radiocontrast dye can induce an osmotic diuresis that may present with urinary retention, or hypotension, secondary to an osmotic diuresis.

Perfusion

It is most important to be alert to the risk of the graft blocking in the first few hours postoperatively. The risk is higher in the recovery room, because of the coagulation and blood flow changes that occur during emergence. The graft is more likely to block after general anaesthesia than regional anaesthesia.[16] Check the perfusion of the limbs below the surgical site. Record the warmth, colour, pulses and perfusion of the limb on the recovery room chart.

Myocardial ischaemia

About 60 per cent of patients with peripheral vascular disease have ischaemic heart disease and many suffer from silent ischaemia. They have a high risk of myocardial infarction in the first postoperative week. Frequently the first signs of ischaemia develop in the recovery room so monitor the patient with a pulse oximeter and ECG, and look for signs of myocardial *ischaemia* (ST elevation or depression). Keep the patient on oxygen all the time he is in recovery room, and send him back to the ward with oxygen as well. If the patient returns to the ward with unrecognised ischaemia there is a high risk that he will have a myocardial infarct, or cardiac arrhythmia and die. The risks rise to a maximum on the first and second postoperative day. Many anaesthetists will prescribe prophylactic beta blockers; nitroglycerine paste is also frequently used.

Hypertension, and tachycardia
may precipitate cardiac ischaemia.

Analgesia
Vascular patients need good analgesia. Ideally this should be provided with an epidural infusion. Opioids help reduce the added stress of postoperative pain.

Hypothermia
Patients undergoing aortic surgery frequently become hypothermic. Do not attempt to extubate vascular patients until their temperature is at least 36.5°C. Hypothermia delays metabolism, and excretion of drugs, and there is a danger of persistent residual effects of opioids, and muscle relaxants. To overcome this risk, the patient may need ventilating, monitoring, and ionotropic support in recovery room for a few hours. After prolonged vascular surgery patients are often moderately acidotic, but providing the cardiovascular system remains stable and responding to ionotropes, this does not need correction, and will rapidly resolve as the patient warms.

Renal function
Up to 25 per cent of aortic surgery patients develop deterioration in renal function postoperatively.[17] A renal dose of dopamine (an infusion of 3 - 5 microgram/kg /min) will help improve renal blood flow, urine output, drug excretion and renal function. This is usually started in theatre, transferred to recovery room, and continued in the ward for at least 24 hours. Aim to maintain a urine output of greater than 60 ml/hr. Resist the urge to use frusemide to maintain a urine output unless it is less than 20 ml/hr.

Before giving frusemide 40 mg IV, check that the patient:
• is not volume deplete;
• has warm hands and feet, indication good perfusion;
• and a CVP of between + 2 cm and + 9 cm above the isophlebotic line, in the mid axilla;
• has a patent urinary catheter.

The commonest cause of low urine output
after vascular surgery is hypovolaemia.

Major aortic surgery

These patients appear haemodynamically stable on the operating table at the end of the procedure, but as soon as they are moved on to their bed or trolley for transport, they usually drop their blood pressure and central venous pressure. If the patient arrives in the recovery room hypotensive, raise his legs on pillows. Tipping a patient head down will alter the blood flow through his lungs worsening his oxygenation.

Check the surgical blood loss. Has it been adequately replaced? Check his central venous pressure. Rapidly infuse 5 ml/kg boluses of blood, polygeline (Haemaccel®), hetastarch or plasma. If the central venous pressure rises, then falls again quite rapidly keep repeating the boluses until the central venouspressure is sustained above 5 cm. The pulse will slow and the urine output increase when the patient has an adequate fluid load. You may need to infuse a litre or more to achieve this. After each bolus, listen to the chest for fine crepitations indicating left ventricular failure. Check the respiratory rate, and monitor the oxygen saturation with a pulse oximeter. If the respiration rate is rising and crepitations are heard, or the oxygen saturation falls, slow the fluid rate. X-ray the chest to check for pulmonary oedema. If the central venous pressure rises and the urine output drops below 30 ml/hr, consider starting a dopamine infusion of 3 - 5 microgram/kg/min through a central venous catheter.

The general stress response to the surgery, the haemodynamic consequenses of the cross-clamping and unclamping the aorta, the fluid shifts, the altered coagulation,the changes in pulmonary physiology all cause a reduction in the oxygenation of the heart. Closely monitor the ECG and watch at all times for ischaemic changes. Keep the patients warm and give high flow oxygen. (See page 461 for treatment of shock.)

Carotid endarterecomy[18]

Patients undergoing carotid endarterectomy have had their operation primarily as prophylaxis against stroke. It is devastating, therefore, if a stroke should occur because there is a lapse in postoperative monitoring of the patients' physical signs. Keep these patients in recovery room for at least 2 hours. They must be close to theatre in case they deteriorate and further urgent surgery is required.

There is a high incidence of coronary artery disease in these patients, so watch carefully for postoperative ischaemia. Look for ST changes (either elevation or depression) on the ECG monitor. Arterial pressure monitoring is most appropriate for the management of their blood pressure.

The operation removes the thick plaque lining the artery to improve cerebral blood flow. In the first few postoperative hours haemorrhage into the neck can occur. It may not always present with external swelling, but occasionally distend into the pharyngeal mucosa causing airway obstruction. This can happen suddenly, it is usually preceded by difficulty in swallowing saliva, noisy breathing, and then stridor. If this occurs call the anaesthetist and the surgeon. If blood does not come out of the drain tube suspect this complication

A major postoperative problem is a blood clot forming on the raw lining of the carotid artery. This occurs in 1 - 7 per cent of patients, usually in the first 2 hours after operation, and will cause a stroke. If the artery is surgically unblocked within 30 minutes the stroke may resolve. Watch for changes in conscious state, and diminished power in the limbs. Check that the patient can lift each leg off the bed, and has a firm hand grip. Check his co-ordination by asking him to touch the tip of his nose with each forefinger. Watch for any slurring of speech, difficulty in swallowing, facial drooping, or changes in the size, or reactivity of the pupils. Report to the surgeon immediately if any of these signs occur.

Hypertension is a systolic blood pressure greater than 160 mmHg, or 20 mmHg above preoperative levels, or a diastolic greater than 100 mmHg. Hypertension may be the first sign of impending deterioration of neurological function.[19] Up to 65 per cent of patients get reflex hypertension, particularly if the patient has previously been hypertensive. This is because the surgery disturbs the baroreceptors located at the bifurcation of the common carotid, and internal carotid arteries. Usually there are no symptoms, but cardiac ischaemia may be revealed by the ECG monitor. You will need good minute-to-minute control of the blood pressure to maintain flow (*pressure dependent perfusion*) and reduce the risk of clots and strokes. Treat hypertension with short acting agents such as nitroglycerine. This can be given sublingually initially and then followed by an infusion 0.3 - 2 microgram/kg/minute. Avoid giving hypotensive agents, such as hydralazine which have a slower onset of action and longer duration.

Up to 45 per cent of patients will become hypotensive in the recovery room, or within 2 - 3 hours of returning to the ward. The patient may show evidence of cerebral hypoxia, such as confusion, agitation, or disorientation. Hypotension often leads to cardiac ischaemia. Watch for nausea and vomiting as a sign of developing hypotension. Initially treat the hypotension with a small dose of ephedrine 5 - 10 mg, and give colloid such as Gelofusin® to restore the patient's blood volume. Treat persistent hypotension with a dopamine infusion.

Hyperperfusion syndrome, with loss of autoregulation of cerebral blood flow, sometimes causes unilateral migraines. Transient postoperative dysfunction of adjacent cranial nerves and recurrent laryngeal nerve dysfunction can also occur. If the patient has had his surgery with a cervical plexus nerve block his phrenic nerve can be temporarily paralysed. This will not affect a healthy patient but it will cause an increase in $PaCO_2$ which could be a problem for someone with COAD.

It is preferable that these patients spend 2 - 3 hours in recovery room rather than immediate transfer to ICU. Their complications, develop quickly and often require surgical attention. Once the first few postoperative hours are past the patients are normally out of danger and can go to an ordinary ward.

1 Jakobsen CJ, Alburg P, et al. (1991). Acta Anaesthesia Scandinavia, 35:238-41.
2 Shiozaki T, Kishikawa M, et al. (1993). American Journal of Surgery 165:326-30.
3 Lanigan CJ. (1992). British Journal of Anaesthesia, 68:142-5.
4 Jackson K, Vote D, (1998) Anaesthesia and Intensive Care, 26:662-4.
5 Magos AL, Baumann R, et al. (1989). Lancet, 2:925-6.
6 Wheatley SA, Miller JM. (1994). British Journal of Obstetrics and Gynaecology, 101:443-6.
7 Benvenuti D. (1993). Plastic Reconstructive Surgery 92:1423.
8 Blyth PL, Mullens AJ. (1991). Australian Clinical Review, 11:45-50.
9 Nagawa H, Kobori O, et al. (1994). British Journal of Surgery 81:860-2.
10 Dyson A, Henderson AM. et al. (1988). Anaesthesia and Intensive Care, 16:405-10.
11 Fugere F, Owen H, et al. (1994). Anaesthesia and Intensive Care, 22:724-8.
12 Gustafson Y, Berggren D. (1988). Journal of the American Geriatric Society, 36:525-30.
13 Catley DM, Thornton C, et al. (1985). Anesthesiology, 63:30-28.
14 Dehring DJ, Areus JF. (1990). Anesthesiology, 73:146-64.
15 Gooucke CR. (1989). Anaesthesia and Intensive Care, 17:458-65.
16 Rosenfeld BA, Beattie C. et al. (1993). Anesthesiology, 79:435-43.
17 Martin LF, Atnip PA. (1994). American Journal of Surgery, 60:163-8.
18 Garrorich MA, Fitch W. (1993). British Journal of Anaesthesia, 71:569-79.
19 Garrorich MA, Fitch W. (1993). British Journal of Anaesthesia, 71:569-79.

5. DRAINS AND CATHETERS

DRAINS

Surgical drains allow body secretions and tissue debris to flow away from the surgical site, where, if they accumulated, they could:
- become contaminated with bacteria and be a source of infection;
- distend hollow cavities and tear the sutures;
- allow secretions, such as pancreatic juice, to accumulate and delay healing;
- exert undesirable pressure, for example in the pericardial sac, pleura, or inside the skull.

Principles of care
- Fluids drain with gravity, so keep the collecting containers below the level of the patient at all times;
- do not apply high pressure suction to any drain, not even for a moment.

A routine drain check includes patency of the tubing, the amount of drainage, the colour of the drainage, and its character, as well as checking the insertion site.

TYPES OF DRAINS

1. Simple drains that open to the dressings.
2. Sump drains.
3. Closed drains that flow into a container.
4. Pleural or thoracic drains.

Simple drains
Examples of the open type are: Yates, Penrose, corrugated rubber, wicks, and ribbon drains. Simple drains are usually covered by a pad. Once the pad becomes soaked, replace it. If the loss becomes excessive tell the surgeon. Keep the outside of the pad dry to prevent bacterial contamination .

Sump drains
A *sump drain* is sometimes used in bowel surgery. It consists of two tubes one used to flush the wound, and one to remove fluid, clots and debris.

Low pressure continuous suction can be applied to drains from special suction devices. Do not attach them to high pressure suction inlets on the wall suction, because serious tissue damage can occur.

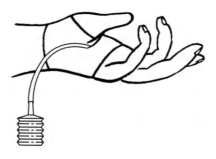

fig 5.1 Concertina drain

Closed drains

Examples of the closed type are free drainage tubes and vacuum suction tubes. Commercially available ones include 'Redivac®', 'Manovac®' or 'Haemovac®'. Vacuum drains must have their *concertinas* collapsed to function correctly.

Pleural drains [1]

Pleural or thoracic drains remove fluid, and air from the pleural space, and allow low pressure, low flow suction to be applied to aid re-expansion of the lung; but special safeguards have to be used to avoid accidental damage to the lungs, or to prevent a pneumothorax occurring. Following cardiothoracic surgery two chest tubes are often used. One is placed high and anteriorly within the thoracic cavity to drain air, and the other low and posteriorly to drain fluid. Do not use Y-connector tubes when fluid is being drained from two or more tubes, because it makes it difficult to account for, and localize, excessive drainage. You can use a Y-connector if one of the drains is primarily for air and the other for fluid. This minimizes the number of bottles around the bedside.

Sometimes, pleural drains have to be inserted as an urgent procedure. Keep a sterile thoracic drainage tray set up ready.

There are three forms of closed chest drainage:
- water seal (one bottle) drainage;
- water seal (two bottle) drainage;
- suction (three bottle) drainage.

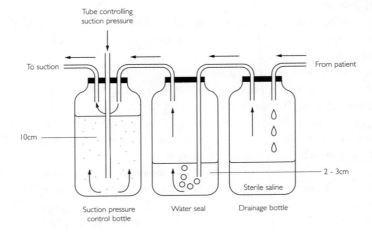

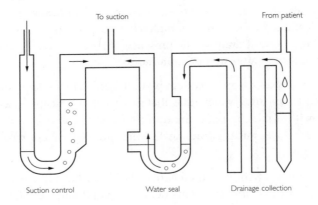

fig 5.2 Set up for continuous three bottle low pressure drainage of the thoracic cavity. Notice how the prinicple of the three bottle drainage is incorporated into a modern plastic drainage system moulded to form three chambers.

While these glass bottle systems are a bit cumbersome they are effective, and it is easy to see how they work. Once you understand the principles, you can apply them to set up any of the commercially available disposable plastic systems. They all work on the principle of either, water seal, or suction drainage.

Water seal drainage
Principals and hints:
- underwater seals act as a one-way valve allowing air to be expelled from the pleural space and preventing it from re-entering during the next inspiration;
- the system must be kept air tight;
- always keep the collection chambers below the level of the patient to prevent fluid siphoning back into the patient;
- if possible keep the collection chambers at least 100 centrimetres below the level of the chest because suction pressures of minus 80 cm H_20 can occur if breathing becomes obstructed;
- frothing in the chamber makes measurement of the volume drained difficult. Reduce frothing by using saline in the bottles instead of sterile water;
- never turn off wall mounted suction units, because there will be no outlet for the drain;
- if there is no respiratory swing (*oscillation*) of fluid in the glass 'straws', this means : the drain tube is obstructed by clots or kinks, or the airtight seal is leaking, or the lung is completely re-expanded;
- clamping a pleural drain in the presence of a continuing air leak invites the formation of a tension pneumothorax.

One bottle acts as a trap to collect pleural fluid. This is kept sterile. It is connected to an underwater tube that allows air to escape whenever the pressure within the chest and the trap rises above one or two centimetres of water pressure, but prevents air leaking into the system whenever the pressure falls.

Keep the stoppers tightly secured in their bottles. Check the tips of the long glass tubes (*straws*) are 2 - 3 cms below the fluid surface. Make sure the short glass straw is not obstructed, and is serving properly as an air vent.

Suction drainage
Suction drainage exerts a continuous negative pressure. It is the most common form of drainage used. The first bottle acts as a trap for pleural fluids. If the tube entering it from the pleural space is just below the fluid level in the trap it will detect any air leak. The first bottle serves as a water seal, in case the system is disconnected from the source of suction.

The centre bottle acts as a break in the system. It allows air to enter if the suction pressure exceeds a set limit. This pressure limit is determined by depth the tip of the centre straw extends below the surface of the liquid. The third bottle serves as a fluid trap.

THORACIC DRAIN TRAY

one medium stainless steel tray	one suture scissors
one small kidney dish	one needle holder
two small gallipots	one scalpel blade size 10
one scalpel handle No 3	three drapes
one toothed dissecting forceps	five cotton wool swabs
two pair artery forceps	one $1/10$ atraumatic silk suture
five medium gauze swabs	

ADD

local anaesthetic

disposable syringes and needles

Povidone (Betadine R) skin preparation

Size 28 drain tube and trochar (Argyle R or similar)

smaller trochar sizes for children

Make sure the level of water in the tube swings with respiration. It may bubble at first, but once the air is removed from the pleural space, and the lung is fully expanded the bubbling will stop. The glass tube in the suction control bottle is usually 10 cm below the fluid level, but it may be increased to 20 cm or more should the surgeon require stronger suction. If the patient is moved, clamp the tubes first. Do not leave the tubes clamped. Do not lift the bottles above the level of the bed without first clamping the tubing, or fluid will run back into the chest. Do not clamp the drains if the patient is being ventilated, because of the risk of a tension pneumothorax. Two rubber tipped clamps should accompany the patient to the ward; this precaution is taken in case the water seals become disconnected during transport.

Never *milk* pleural drains with a roller clamp. These archaic devices generate enormous pressures, and can damage lung tissue. Avoid dependent loops in the tubes, because fluid will collect in the loops and interfere with the drainage.

EMERGENCY INSERTION OF A PLEURAL DRAIN

The commonest reason to insert a pleural drain in the recovery room is to drain a pneumothorax. Drain a pneumothorax if it exceeds twenty per cent of the pleural volume, or if the patient becomes dyspnoeic.

If the patient is not in danger, get an erect chest X-ray before proceeding. Keep the film where you can see it as you insert the catheter.

Distrust anything other than an erect chest X-ray,
when assessing a pneumo- or haemothorax.

Check the side is correct, and that there are no underlying abnormalities. Use intercostal catheters (Argyle®) size 20 G, 22 G, for draining gas, and 32 G for draining fluid or blood. Use the size 16 G in prepubertal children.

Have the erect chest X-ray on view
when inserting intercostal catheters.

THE AXILLARY APPROACH

This is preferable for draining fluid collections. Using pillows or towels to lie the patient comfortably in a supine position, but slightly on their side. The catheter is inserted in the 4th or 5th intercostal space, just posterior to the midaxillary line.

THE ANTERIOR APPROACH

Here the catheter is inserted in the second intercostal space just lateral to the midclavicular line. This site is most suitable for removing air. Have the patient sitting comfortably in bed propped up at 45° on three or four pillows. Use ample local anaesthetic.

Use blunt dissection
when inserting intercostal catheters

CAUTIONS:

Never insert an axillary catheter, unless you have previously detected fluid with a small 19 G aspirating needle.

* To avoid damaging the heart, never angle the catheter anteromedially when inserting it on the left side;
* never insert a catheter anterior to the mid-axillary line;
* always check the size and site of the heart shadow;
* to avoid damage to the liver or spleen, never go below the level of 6th intercostal space in the mid axillary line;
* use your finger or stout curved forceps to penetrate the thoracic wall. Never push hard. If you are pushing hard then your technique is wrong. Use gentle blunt dissection to find your way.

Secure the tubing to the bed, leaving plenty of slack, to prevent it being accidentally pulled out. A large rubber band attached to a strong safety pin is useful for this purpose. Whenever the patient is moved check the security of the tubing, and make sure the patient is not lying on it. To stop the tube kinking as it comes out of the drain bottle tape a small tongue depressor to the point where it goes through the rubber stopper.

Chest drains are painful when the patient deep breathes or coughs. Give effective analgesia, preferably with intercostal or paravertebral blocks, or a thoracic epidural. Intrapleural analgesia does not work as well as might be expected.

NASOGASTRIC TUBES

Nasogastric tubes stop the stomach from distending with gas or fluid. They are used after bowel surgery, or whenever it is thought the patient might develop a paralytic ileus. Take care not to displace them. In some operations, such as after an oesphagectomy or gastrectomy, the nasogastric tube lies across the surgical suture lines. This is to prevent distension of the bowel that would tear the stitches. If the nasogastric tube is accidentally pulled out, it is impossible to reinsert it safely. Some anaesthetists suture them into the frenulum of the nose so that they cannot be accidentally pulled out. In any case nasogastric tubes should be guarded well, and firmly taped into position.

Check with the surgeon, whether to clamp the nasogastric drain or leave it on free drainage.

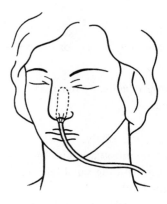

fig 5.3 Fastening of nasogastric tubes

Aspirate nasogastric tubes gently. Do not suck hard with a syringe, because the soft mucosal folds of the stomach will wrap around the tip of the tube. If nothing comes back after gentle suction on the tube, blow 10 - 20 mls of air down it to free the tip from the folds of the fragile gastric mucosa, and attempt to aspirate gently again. If there is still no aspirate then the stomach is probably empty. Do not kink off the tube to prevent air going down to the stomach. Air will not rush down the tube to fill up the stomach.

Never aspirate nasogastric tubes using the unmodified suction from the wall suction point, because it will severely damage the delicate mucosa making it bleed.

Before the patient leaves the recovery room, check inside his mouth to make sure the nasogastric tube is not coiled up there, or in his pharynx. Check the position of the nasogastric tube by injecting 10 - 20 ml of air into the tube and listening with a stethescope over the stomach. There should be a gurgling sound as air enters the stomach. Check there are written orders for the nursing staff in the ward about the care of the tube.

Urinary Catheters

Because of the problems with allergy, latex and silastic catheters are being replaced in most units by Hydrogel® catheters. They are suitable for both short term and long term use up to 3 months.

If the patient already has a urinary catheter in when he arrives in the recovery room then check that:
• urine flows freely;
• the bladder is not distended;
• the male foreskin is covering the tip of the penis; and record the urine output.

Urinary catheters are prophylactically inserted:
• after surgery or trauma;
• before pelvic surgery;
• to measure urine output accurately;
• to distinguish between retention and anuria;
• to manage shock, and impending renal failure;
• to provide access to the bladder;
• in patients who have epidural catheters for pain relief;
• in patients who have spinal anaesthesia.

HINTS FOR INSERTION OF URINARY CATHETERS

1. Use plenty of lignocaine lubricating gel.
2. Small catheters sometimes buckle in the urethra, try a larger one.
3. Do not try to force the insertion of a urinary catheter, the urethra is easily damaged. If you have difficulty call for expert help.

Males
Insert the catheter all the way to the Y-junction before inflating the balloon, then pull back gently. The catheter will have the volume needed to inflate the balloon printed on it. Replace the foreskin over the tip of the penis, otherwise it may form a constrictive band (*paraphimosis*) around the penis. This causes pain, and can be difficult to pull down at a later time.

Females
Check the catheter actually enters the urethra, and not the vagina.

Catheterization is a sterile procedure.

Catheter care
- Connect the catheter to a closed sterile collecting system;
- strap the catheter over (not under) the patient's thigh to minimise the risk of faecal soiling;
- do not strap the catheter to the bed or the bed linen.

If urine will not flow:
- try pressing gently on the suprapubic area;
- the catheter may not be in far enough or be wrongly positioned;
- the catheter may be blocked. Irrigate it gently with saline using a 50 ml syringe;
- check the bladder is empty by palpating above the pubic symphysis. If it is empty, irrigate the catheter with 50 ml of sterile saline; all this saline should come back again. If the saline goes in, but does not return, the catheter is either blocked, or not in the bladder.

Blocked catheters
Patients who have had bladder surgery will pass clots through the catheter. Gently milk the tube from time to time to ensure free flow. If the catheter seems to be blocked by clots, take a 60 ml syringe, and using a sterile

technique wash it out with water or saline. Gently instil 30 ml then ask the patient if he is in pain. Pain is a sign of an over filled bladder. Aspirate, if this is successful instil 30 ml quickly and aspirate again. Repeat this several times to break up the clots. If you are unsuccessful in relieving the obstruction call the surgeon.

Continuous irrigation

This is a technique for washing out the bladder, to stop clots forming. Make sure fluid is continuously draining out, and the bladder is not distended. If the outlet is blocked with clots, and fluid is continues to go in, there is danger of rupturing the bladder or disrupting the surgery.

Suprapubic catheterization

It may be necessary to insert a suprapubic catheter if urethral catheterisation is unsuccessful; or is contraindicated. Use an Argyle® or Ingram® 12 - 16 F trocar catheter, or an equivalent. A suprapubic catheter is safer for the patient if there is any suggestion of urethral stricture.

Contraindications to suprapubic catheters are:
• a bladder that is not easy to define by palpation or percussion;
• a lower midline abdominal scar warning of the danger of puncturing adherent bowel.

1 Kam AC, O'Brien M, et al. (1993) Anaesthesia, 48: 154-61.

6. INFECTION CONTROL

Transmission of infectious diseases between patients and staff is preventable. If you do not adhere to strict protocols you place everyone at risk. Universal precautions assume that every patient is an actual source of infection, and not just a possible source of infection. Take time to train new staff in your recovery room's infection control procedures. Do not assume that all staff either know what to do, or do it properly until they prove it to you. Test their knowledge of hospital protocols, and observe how they deal with spillage, take blood, and dispose of contaminated material. Do they understand the terms, clean, disinfected, and sterile? Are they aware of the terrible consequences of catching diseases such as hepatitis, tuberculosis or HIV/AIDS?

INFECTIONS AND YOU

Staff working in recovery room are at risk of catching infections from the patients, and this risk is rising continuously. You are exposed to aerosols from cough and sneezes, blood, saliva, urine and faeces in your daily contact with patients, and each is a potential source of infection. While HIV/AIDS is on everyone's mind, the risk of catching hepatitis virus is far higher. Tuberculosis (TB) has re-emerged with increased virulence and resistance to drug therapy.

Viral hepatitis

Viral hepatitis causes inflammatory liver disease. If the inflammation is long standing hepatic fibrosis will result in chronic cirrhosis.

HEPATITIS A (HAV)

Previously called infectious hepatitis. It is common, transmitted by faecal-oral route, with a 20 - 40 day incubation. It does not progress to chronic liver disease, and can be prevented by pooled gamma globulin injection. It has a mortality less than 0.2 per cent and is not a major problem in recovery room. Vaccination against HAV is now available.

HEPATITIS B (HBV)

Previously called serum hepatitis. It is usually transmitted by contaminated blood such as needle stick injury (or sexual intercourse), with a 60 - 120 day incubation period. It progresses to chronic liver disease in 2 - 10 per cent of patients, and can be prevented by prophylactic immunization.

Transmission to non-immune staff after accidental needle stick injury with a hepatitis B (HBV) contaminated needle carries a 3 - 35 per cent risk infection. HBV can be transmitted through all body fluids, including breast milk, and it can enter the host via almost all surfaces, including mucous membranes. Risk of infection can be minimized by the use of gloves, aprons and masks, disinfectant, sterilization and vaccination. Wear goggles, or better still a full face screen to protect your eyes and mouth.

All staff should be immunized against Hepatitis B with the safe and effective genetically engineered vaccine. Five to ten per cent of recipients of the vaccine do not develop protective antibodies after the completion of the course, and remain at risk. Test for Hepatitis B antibody two months after completion of the initial three dose course. A protective level of antibody is greater than 10 milli IU/ml. Repeat the course if needed.

HEPATITIS C (HCV)
Previously called non-A, non-B hepatitis. This ribonucleic acid (RNA) virus is usually transmitted by contaminated blood, such as needle stick injury (risk is 2.5 - 10 per cent),[1] but has been reported to occur from conjunctival splash[2]. The incubation period is 30 - 70 days.

This is a disease to avoid! Over 2 to 5 decades, it causes slowly progressive fibrosing liver disease. Within 20 years for every 100 patients with chronic HCV, 15 will progress to cirrhosis, of which 10 will die from liver failure, and 10 will develop hepatocellular carcinoma. It affects one per cent of the population and is usually acquired through drug users sharing needles or, prior to 1990, from contaminated blood transfusions. More than one percent of people from Asia, Africa, Southern America and the peripheries of Europe carry the disease, having acquired it from inadequately sterilized needles used for immunization, or surgical or dental instruments. There is a more than a 50 percent incidence in male haemophiliacs who received blood transfusions before 1990,[3] and prisoners with a history injecting drug use[4]. The diagnosis can be difficult, but is greatly aided by HCV polymerase chain reaction (PCR). No vaccine is available.

Other hepatitis viruses include Hepatitis G (HGV).

HIV/AIDS
Human immunodeficiency virus (HIV) infection is acquired through sexual intercourse or drug users sharing needles. Until 1995 when routine blood testing was commenced, it was also acquired through blood transfusions. In Australia HIV is carried by about 1:330 of the population, although the incidence rises to 40:100 in some countries. On first exposure

to HIV there is typically a 2 - 4 week period of intense viral replication before the onset of an immune and clinical illness. The diagnosis can be confused with infectious mononucleosis, but in contrast to IM, HIV is usually associated with a skin rash and mouth ulcers, while pharyngitis is relatively rare. The patient then recovers and remains asymptomatic for about 5 - 7 years later progressing to the acquired immunodeficiency disease syndrome (AIDS) with progressive multisystem infections from many bizarre diseases including herpes zoster, herpes simplex, cryptosporidiosis, toxoplasmosis, cytomegalovirus, or one of the lymphomas or other cancers that eventually accumulate to cause death. Patients with AIDS syndrome are highly susceptible to hospital acquired (nosocomial) infections.

The main danger to staff is a *needlestick injury*. Seroconversion is uncommon, and estimated to occur in about 1:300 - 400 needlestick injuries[5]. Recapping needles is the commonest cause of needlestick injuries. Do not attempt to remove the needle from the syringe, simply put the whole unit into the sharps disposal container. Do not let your sharps containers become over filled so that staff have to force objects in to make room.

Never, never recap needles.

No vaccination against HIV is available but the early administration of zidovudine reduced the risk of infection in nearly 80 per cent. This must be administered within 3 hours of exposure and continued for 4 weeks.[6]

Tuberculosis
Tuberculosis (Mycobaterium tuberculi) is an airborn bacterial infection, which is common in many developing countries, and its incidence is rising sharply in developed countries. Worryingly, there are a number of strains which are resistant to all antibiotics. The bacteria is usually transmitted as an aerosol from coughing or sneezing. Occasionally a bronchoscopy is performed on a tuberculous patient. These patients should be recovered in the operating theatre and not in the recovery room. Wear gown, gloves, goggles and cover your head, as far as possible leave no area of your skin uncovered. Do not accompany the patient to the isolation unit. You should leave all your potentially contaminated clothing in the operating theatre and shower yourself thoroughly including washing your hair.

BCG vaccination is effective against TB. Regular Mantoux skin tests every 2 years are recommended where this disease is endemic. Other diseases for which vaccination is available include measles, mumps, rubella, tetanus, polio, diptheria, influenza and varicella. Recovery staff are advised to know their immunization status with regard to these diseases and if necessary protect themselves.

SOURCES OF INFECTION

POTENTIALLY INFECTIOUS BODY FLUIDS

MAJOR:
- blood;
- serous ooze;
- pus;
- faeces;
- sputum;
- saliva.

MINOR:
- urine;
- nasal secretions;
- gastric secretions;
- peritoneal dialysis fluid;
- ascitic fluid;
- pleural and pericardial fluid.

POTENTIALLY INFECTIOUS BODY SITES

MAJOR:
- wounds;
- skin lesions;
- drainage sites;

MINOR:
- nasal passages;
- mouth;
- intravascular access sites;
- perianal area.

CROSS INFECTION

The airborne viruses such as influenza A and B, and adenovirus are easily transmitted from patients to staff in recovery room. They can also be transmitted from staff to patients, and this is a very good reason that sick staff with a cold, 'the flu' or any other infection should stay at home until well. The fact that you are sick testifies to the virulence of the organism. Patients recovering from anaesthesia are particularly likely to catch airborne viruses that can cause major complications such as pneumonia. You may also infect other staff. One person with a upper respiratory tract infection who spreads it around can cause havoc with the rosters.

If you are sick stay at home.

Working in the recovery room demands concentration, and vigilance. Ill people cannot perform their jobs properly, and are more likely to make mistakes.

Principles for preventing cross infection

1. Set up an Infection Control Subcommittee as part of the organisation of your operating theatres. Its duty is to set standards, and write protocols for the prevention of cross infection.

2. Every person in recovery room needs proper protective clothing. Staff should not wear street dress, or their normal uniforms while attending patients.

3. When working in the recovery room do not wear wedding rings, and hand jewellery.

4. Design the recovery room to prevent dust from accumulating. Keep your recovery room as tidy as possible. Do not use it as a general storage area for bulky equipment. Put these things away somewhere else.

5. Keep to a regular cleaning schedule.

Germs don't fly - they hitch hike.
Wash your hands properly before,
and after touching a patient.

6. Place contaminated material in leak proof sealed containers which must be removed at scheduled intervals, and not just when they are full.

7. The most important point for the prevention of cross infection is proper hand washing. Use liquid soap from squirt containers. Do not use bar soap. Wet bar soap is a good growing medium for some bacteria. Use disposable, preferably paper, towels. Hot air hand driers are noisy and slow. They are not suitable for recovery room because they blow skin squames, germs and dust into the air.

8. Clean well fitting non-latex rubber disposable gloves should be freely available throughout the recovery room.

9. Use single-use sterile needles and syringes. Use these only once and then discard them. If you use pins for neurological testing then use once only.

10. Do not use multi-dose injectable drug containers.

11. Nebulizers can be a source of infection, because they spray fine aerosol into the air. This aerosol can carry infective particles.

STAFF EXPOSED TO CONTAMINATION WITH POTENTIAL PATHOGENS

Report all injuries or accidents involving blood or blood stained body fluids. Prepare a policy of how to manage and counsel staff who have had a needlestick injury, or accidental exposure to potentially contaminated substances.

If a member of the staff has been exposed to blood-borne pathogens then:
• wash the affected area well with soap and water;
• if the eyes are contaminated rinse gently with normal saline while the eyes are open;
• if blood gets in your mouth, spit it out and then rinse your mouth with water several times;
• apply an antiseptic solution such as 0.5% chlorhexidine in 70% alcohol, or a povidone iodine solution such as Betadine® to skin wounds. Do not use these solutions on mucosal surfaces or the eyes;
• seek immediate medical attention. Decisions about treatment options need to be made within two hours of exposure.

UNIVERSAL PRECAUTIONS

The underlying principle of universal precautions is that every single patient must be managed as definitely carrying an infectious disease. This makes sense, because it is superficially impossible to determine clinically which patient is carrying a disease such as hepatitis or HIV, and who is not.

All patients are potentially infectious.

The aim is to minimize hospital cross infection, and the risk of patients or staff acquiring disease. Written protocols for infection control are available in every hospital. Study these carefully and ensure full compliance from all staff. This will protect everyone in the recovery room from infection as a result of occupational exposure. Hand washing, appropriate vaccination and isolation of known infected cases will markedly reduce risks, not only safeguarding the livelihoods and incomes of the staff but their lives as well.

Handwashing
Wash your hands after any patient contact to remove transient surface organisms. Do not move from one patient to another without first washing your hands. This habit must become deeply ingrained.

Gloves
Use gloves if you anticipate contact with blood or body secretions. Dispose of them after a single use.

Gowns
Use plastic aprons and goggles, if there is any chance that blood or other body secretions could splash on to your face or clothing.

Linen
Place soiled linen, including blankets and pillows, in leak proof double bags for transport and disposal. The outside of the bag must never become moist with blood or faeces. Place these bags inside a big yellow plastic bag for transport. Clearly label this linen as infectious. Pillows and blankets which have been soiled with body fluids must not go back to the ward. Have an appropriate laundry facility for these items.

Waste
Treat all waste contaminated with blood or body secretions as potentially infectious.

Specimens
Send specimens for laboratory investigations in tightly sealed stout containers to prevent leakage during transport. Conventially these containers are coloured bright yellow with a biohazard emblem on them.

Sharing
Do not share items for individual use among patients. This includes shaving razors, inhalers, creams and ointments.

Cleaning
Routine cleaning with neutral detergent is sufficient to make surfaces microbiologically safe. Give your area a thorough clean every day. Check for damaged surfaces and report these. Insist on repairs to cut linoleum or broken woodwork are carried out immediately.

Spillage
- Throw a paper absorbent towel over the spill as soon as it occurs;
- apply 0.5% hypochlorite solution to this towel;
- wear gloves and carefully pick up this towel and discard;
- apply 0.5% hypochlorite solution to this area and leave to dry;
- rinse with clean water and leave to dry.

Sharps

Avoid injury from contaminated *sharps*:

- do not recap needles;
- do not remove needles from syringes, discard them in one piece;
- discard all sharps into *sharps containers*;
- do not over fill the sharps container;
- do not leave sharps in the drapes;
- never pass an unguarded needle to another person;
- ensure that others cannot be jabbed at any stage while assisting you, cleaning up afterwards or transporting the sharps.

PRINCIPLES FOR CLEANING AND STERILIZATION OF EQUIPMENT

Cleaning is a process which removes micro-organisms and biohazardous materials from the surface of an object. *Disinfection* is a process eliminating all micro-organisms except bacterial spores.

Normal hospital procedures, presently available, can not completely inactivate the prion protein responsible for variant Creutzfeldt-Jacob disease, the most common human form of bovine spongiform encephalopathy (BSE) also known as Mad Cow Disease.

Cleaning of instruments is extremely difficult if blood or any other proteinaceous tissue is allowed to dry and the prion protein is especially tenacious. A validated, automated, cleaning system should be used before disinfection and sterilization. This washes initially with a low temperature using ultrasonics which removes prion protein without coagulating it.[7]

Sterilization

Sterilization is a process intended to eliminate or destroy all forms of microbial life including viruses and bacterial spores.

Practical points:

1. If possible have a qualified person to supervise cleaning and sterilization of equipment.
2. Physically clean the equipment thoroughly before sterilization to remove blood and other debris. First rinse the instruments under cold running water. Do not use hot water because it coagulates proteins which stick to the equipment offering shelter to microrganisms.
3. Initial cleaning reduces the risk of infecting the staff handling the dirty instruments. Wear heavy duty gloves, and goggles or preferably visors,

to protect face, eyes and mouth from contaminated aerosols. Do not clean or wash instruments in hand basins.

4. Steam under pressure (autoclave) is the best method of sterilization. Heat destroys bacteria by coagulating protein in the cells. Boiling will disinfect but not sterilize instruments. Metal instruments (non-porous) require surface sterilization. Rubber, towels, hollow items and plastic (porous) require penetrating sterilization. To be effective autoclaves must meet the following criteria:[8]

   GRAVITY DISPLACEMENT STERILIZERS:
   - non-porous items 3 minutes at (or above) 132°C;
   - porous items 10 minutes at (or above) 132°C;

   PREVACUUM OR HIGH VACUUM STERILIZERS:
   - non-porous items 3 minutes at (or above) 132°C;
   - porous items 4 minutes at (or above) 132°C;

5. Chemical sterilization is necessary for items which are not suitable to be autoclaved.
   - Ethylene oxide is useful to sterilize heat sensitive materials such as plastic, electrical apparatus, endoscopes and sphygmomanometers;
   - Some equipment will need to be sterilized by soaking in gluteraldehyde;
   - The STERIS™ system which uses paracetic acid is excellent for fibreoptic equipment;
   - The STERRAD™ system uses hydrogen peroxide and radiofrequency and is suitable for sterilizing many unusual materials like polystyrene.

6. Review sterilization procedures regularly. Check the steam penetration of each load with a Bowie-Dick type test paper (Incheque™) which turns black after being exposed to steam. Autoclave tapes only show that items have been exposed to steam, but not if satisfactory sterilization conditions were met. For this reason use a spore strip of Bacillus stearothermophilus to monitor the autoclaves at least once a week.

7. Keep sterilizers in top working condition. Ensure regular maintenance by the hospital engineers. Ask the manufacturers to inspect, and submit, a report on the condition of the equipment each year.

8. Stamp the shelf life showing a use by date on the outside of packs.

9. Store sterile stock in dust free drawers or cupboards with doors.

10. Have the recovery room painted and thoroughly 'turned out' once a year.

1 Mitsui T, Iwano K et al. (1992) Hepatology 16:1109-14.

2. Rosen H. (1997). American Journal of Infection Control 25:242-7.

3. Williamson G, Wilson J et al. (1990) Australian Medical Journal 152:504.

4. Crofts N, Stewart, T et al. (1995) British Medical Journal 310: 285-8.

5. Rogers PL, Lane HC, et al. (1989). Critical Care Medicine, 17: 113-17.

6. Gerbeding JL. Prophylaxix for occupational exposure to HIV. Annals of Internal Medicine. 1996; 25 497-501.

7. Hill AF et al (1997). Nature 387: 448-50.

8. Fogg DM. (1989). AORN Journal, 50: 888-92.

7. PHARMACOLOGY

A wide range of drugs are needed in the recovery room, sometimes urgently. It is wise to have them near by. If you only have limited stocks of drugs in your hospital, then keep them in the recovery room rather than in the pharmacy. Having to send to the pharmacy when an emergency occurs, causes dangerous delays.

> *Ignorance can be lethal.*
> *If you are in any doubt…ask somebody!*

Many drugs are chemically incompatible with each other, and strange things can happen if you mix drugs, or dilute them with the wrong fluid. Most, but not all, drugs are stable in normal 0.9% saline or 5% dextrose. Never add drugs to blood, blood products, fat emulsions, parenteral nutrition fluids or sodium bicarbonate. Read the manufacturer's recommendations or check with your hospital pharmacist if you are in doubt. It is useful to save the drug manufacturer's package inserts and stick them in a book as a study guide and for reference. These inserts are updated regularly with new information. The correct dose of the drug is enough, it is unwise to exceed the dose recommended by the manufacturer.

COMMON PROBLEMS WITH DRUGS

- wrong dose;
- wrong drug;
- drug interactions;
- intramuscular injections causing nerve damage;
- adverse reactions;
- allergies;
- inappropriate drug;

FORMULARY
Get a good reference book about drugs, and keep it available. Tie it down if necessary. Two good references are: *British National Formulary*. Obtainable from the British Medical Association, Tavistock Square, London WC1H 9JP, England. *Australian Medical Handbook*. Copies can be obtained from AMH, PO Box 240, Rundle Mall, Adelaide, SA 5000, Australia. Other countries have their own formularies. Check your local medical authority. You will also need a drug interaction and compatibility guide.

THE BASICS OF PHARMACOLOGY

Pharmacokinetics is the study of drug absorption, distribution, metabolism, and excretion. *Pharmacodynamics* is the study of the effects of drugs, whether these be wanted *(therapeutic)* or unwanted and harmful *(side effects)*.

Pharmacokinetics is how the body handles the drug.
Pharmocodynamics is what the drug does to the body.

ABSORPTION

In the recovery room most drugs are injected either intramuscularly, where they are absorbed and released slowly into the blood stream, or intravenously where they are quickly carried to every tissue in the body.

DISTRIBUTION

Only a few drugs stay in the blood stream. Most pass quickly into the extracellular fluid and the tissues, especially fat muscle. When the concentration of a drug in the blood is measured it appears as though the drug has been diluted in a large volume and this calculated volume is called the *volume of distribution*.

Once the body has been given a proper loading dose, repeated smaller amounts will maintain the drug at a therapeutic level. The dose of drug needed to keep a constant *therapeutic level* is called the *maintenance dose*. A constant plasma drug level and its clinical effect, can only be sustained if the maintenance dose is given at the same rate as the body removes the drug.

PHARMACODYNAMICS

When the drug reaches its site of action it causes an effect. It may act on special structures called *receptors*, either on the cell membrane or within the cell. The effect depends on how much of the drug is given. All drugs are *toxic* if given in too great a dose, and ineffective if given in too small a dose. The right dose is called the *therapeutic dose*. With many drugs it is necessary to build up the concentration of the drug in the body to achieve its desired effect. The dose of drug needed to do this is called the *loading dose*. The dose range between the ineffective dose and the toxic dose is called the therapeutic margin. Safe drugs have a wide therapeutic margin.

The *potency* of a drug is the amount of drug needed to achieve a given effect. For instance one-thousandth of the amount of fentanyl is required to achieve the same level of analgesia as pethidine. Fentanyl is 1000 times more potent than pethidine.

Sometimes, despite a therapeutic level of a drug in the blood, the clinical effect begins to wear off. This phenomenon is called *tachyphylaxis* if it occurs over minutes or hours; or *tolerance* if it occurs over days or weeks.

ELIMINATION AND EXCRETION

The body immediately starts eliminating the drug by:
- metabolizing it in the liver or;
- excreting it through the kidneys, or;
- using enzymes to break it down, or;
- storing it.

The time taken to eliminate drugs varies from a second or two, to months. The time taken to eliminate half the dose given is called the *elimination half life*. In contrast, the clinical half life is half the time it takes for the effect of a drug to wear off.

The elimination half life of pethidine is close to its clinical half life. Compare this with action of drugs such as thiopentone that are terminated because they are diluted in the body fluids. These have a short clinical half life, but it takes much longer time for the liver to eliminate them from the body.

Clearance is that volume of plasma from which the drug is completely removed in a given time.

Clinical factors altering the pharmacokinetics and pharmacodynamics of a drug given in the recovery room are:
- cardiac failure will delay their distribution;
- bleeding, or shocked patients will alter their distribution;
- interaction with residual anaesthetic drugs;
- hypothermia will delay their metabolism and elimination.

Patient factors

1. Do not use a drug unless there is a clear reason to do so.
2. If a patient is pregnant do not use any drug unless it is absolutely necessary.
3. Check the patient's notes, and his *alert bracelet* for allergies and sensitivities.
4. If the patient is hypersensitive to a drug never give it, or another member of the same group of drugs.
5. Check if the patient has been taking any prescription drugs, or medicine that he has bought for himself especially aspirin, over the counter medication, or herbal remedies.
6. Use smaller doses in the elderly, or if the patient has liver or renal disease.

For elderly patients give half
the dose twice as slowly.

7. Prescribe as few drugs as possible.
8. Where possible use a drug that you are familiar with.

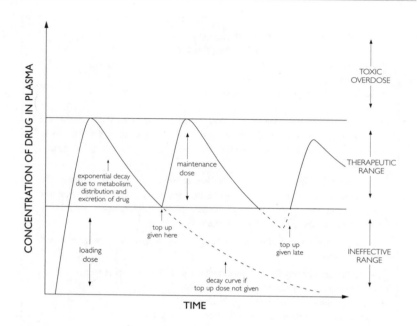

fig 7.1 Effect of drug dosing and its exponential decay

Staff factors

1. Most accidents happen because people make mistakes.
2. Never accept an illegible, altered or doubtful order for drugs.
3. Always check the dose and calculations with a second qualified person.
4. Discourage telephone orders for drugs. If this is unavoidable a second person should independently check the order.
5. Write the word *units* in full on a separate line for drugs such as insulin or heparin. Many disasters have occurred because a simple 'U' has been mistaken for '0', leading to ten times the dose being administered.
6. If a drug dose is a whole number do not use a decimal point when writing an order; for instance morphine 4 mg IV, not morphine 4.0 mg IV. Always precede a decimal point with a zero; for instance 0.4 mg, and not .4 mg.
7. Doses in micrograms should be written as *micrograms* because the abbreviation (µg) can be mistaken for milligrams (mg), which would amount to a 1000 fold overdose.
8. Some doctors' writing is barely legible. Drug orders must be printed in block capital letters, but even then it is sometimes difficult to tell whether IM or IV has been written. Intravenous orders should be written IV and intramuscular orders I/M.

9. Giving the wrong drug to the wrong patient is a very common error. Check the patient's identity bands, and drug sensitivity labels correspond with the name on the drug order sheet. Make sure that the drug is the correct drug, the strength is correct, the drug has not expired, and confirm the route of administration.

ADVERSE EFFECTS

Adverse, toxic or undesirable effects associated with the use of normal doses of a drug. This may be due to the pharmacological effects of the drug; or it might be an idiosyncratic response by the patient. Almost all drugs will have adverse effects in some patients. Sometimes we have to accept the adverse effect of a drug because the drug is needed to control a more serious problem. For instance patients are prepared to tolerate drowsiness rather than to put up with nausea and vomiting.

Factors predisposing to adverse effects include:
- elderly patients and neonates;
- the sick, the frail or a patient suffering from malnutrition;
- females are more susceptible than males, probably because of their smaller size;
- higher doses are more likely to cause problems than lower doses;
- the incidence of adverse effects increases if the patient is also receiving other drugs;
- genetic effects such as enzyme deficiencies can predispose o advers effects;
- previously encountered adverse effects with drugs increases the risk of subsequent problems.

Adverse effects can be life threatening (anaphylaxis), debilitating (prolonged nausea and vomiting), or annoying (itch).

Drug interactions

Drug interactions occur when two or more drugs are given concurrently that can result in increasing the effects (*synergism*), decreasing the effects (*antagonism*), or produce adverse effects.

Drug interactions can be expected, predictable, or obscure.

EXPECTED INTERACTIONS occur if two or more drugs are given that have the same effect, or act on the same receptors for instance: diazepam and midazolam will produce additive sedation; and metoclopramide will antagonize dopamine.

PREDICTABLE INTERACTIONS occur if two drugs are eliminated by the same pathway, produce similar clinical effects, or block a compensatory response. Volatile agents will delay the metabolism of ketamine because volatile agents slow liver blood flow; aspirin and warfarin will cause bleeding. ß-blockers will counteract the symptoms of insulin induced hypoglycaemia because these drugs block the sympathetic response to low blood glucose. Erythromycin and ketoconazole prolong the action of midazolam by many hours.[1]

OBSCURE INTERACTIONS occur where the mechanism is not well known. Lithium for instance can produce a fatal encephalopthy if combined with butyrephenones such as droperidol. Selective seritonin reuptake inhibitors (SSRIs) and tricyclic antidepressants fight in obscure ways with many drugs.

SIGNIFICANT DRUG INTERACTIONS IN THE RECOVERY ROOM INCLUDE:

PATIENT TAKING	DRUGS IN RECOVERY ROOM	INTERACTIONS/COMMENTS
Antihypertensives	pethidine, metocloparamide	hypotension
Antiparkinson drugs - L-dopa - pergolide - selegiline	metoclopramide, prochlorperazine.	rigidity tremor hypertension cardiac arrhythmias
SSRIs: - citralopram - fluoxetine - fluvoxamine - paroxetine - sertraline	pethidine fentanyl possibly morphine	Seritonin syndrome: agitation, sweating, hypertension, tachycardia, cyanosis, fever.
MAOIs - phenelzine - tranylcypromine - moclobemide	pethidine metaraminol ephedrine	fulminating hypertension
Other antipsychotics	Multiple interactions	Check carefully in your drug literature before giving any drugs.
digoxin	ß-blockers	arryhthmias
esmolol	morphine	heart block
methadone	opioids	respiratory depression
phenytoin	dopamine	hypotension

ALTERNATIVE REMEDIES

If confronted with a therapeutic puzzle ask your patient about over the counter, unprescribed or alternative remedies. Some surveys reveal than 30 per cent of the hospital outpatient population are taking unprescribed herbal remedies, or "over the counter" medication in one form or another. Herbal remedies such as gingko balboa, ginger concentrate, St John's Wort, can exacerbate bleeding tendencies. Ginseng enhances cardiac arrhythmias, and echinaccheae can precipitate asthma. Herbal remedies are untried, undocumented and untested drugs, some of which have unexpected effects. Just because it is a natural substance does not mean it is not harmful. Arsenic is a natural substance!

DRUG DOSES IN CHILDREN (SEE PAGE 385).

DRUG DOSES IN THE ELDERLY

Much of the body's mass in young people is muscle with a high water content. As the body ages muscle is progressively replaced by fat, with a low water content. Therefore the elderly have proportionately less body water than young people. A drug injected into an older person will have less water to dissolve in and is therefore more concentrated. This is the main reason the elderly require smaller doses of drugs to achieve the same effect.

Many drugs are transported partly bound to plasma proteins and partly free in the plasma. For example, fentanyl is 70% bound to protein and 30% is carried free in the plasma. Only the free portion is available to act on the receptors. If nutrition is poor there is less plasma protein available to bind the drug. This means there is more active drug free in the plasma which increases the potency of a given dose.

Liver and renal function decline, delaying the rate of metabolism and excretion of drugs and prolonging their action.

The elderly are often on multiple medications increasing the risk of adverse interactions and unwanted effects.

If the operation has lasted more than an hour, many elderly patients will be hypothermic. This delays the enzymatic degradation of drugs.

Fentanyl is thought to be bound to skeletal muscle protein. In the recovery room the elderly tend not to move about much; however, once back in the ward, when they start to move their limbs, the increased muscle blood flow washes the fentanyl back into the circulation. This sudden rush of fentanyl is thought to be the cause of the delayed respiratory depression sometimes seen many hours after the last dose.

DRUG DOSES IN OBESE PATIENTS (SEE PAGE 417)

1. Miller A., Olkkola K.T., *et al.* (1990) *British Journal of Anaesthesia,* 65:826-8.

8. INTRAVENOUS FLUIDS AND RENAL PHYSIOLOGY

Patients coming to recovery room from theatre have altered fluid status for many reasons. They have been fasted, received intravenous fluids, and lost fluids during their operation. Check that the blood volume of your patient is adequate.

• Check the blood pressure and pulse rate;
• assess perfusion status (see page 255).

In unstable patients:
• Measure the central venous pressure (CVP);
• measure the serum sodium.

These parameters will help you understand the adequacy of the patient's salt and water status and his blood volume.

On arriving in recovery room nearly every patient will have an intravenous infusion running, and even after minor surgery may be starting their second litre of saline or Hartmann's solution. Patients having major surgery may be receiving blood, or have received many litres of fluid.

Before the patient returns to the ward make sure there are formal written orders for his on-going fluid therapy. Do not remove any intravenous line until you have discussed it with the anaesthetist, and you are sure that the risk of vomiting is past.

Patients are occasionally ordered glucose immediately after surgery, and this is unnecessary. Contrary to popular belief, patients do not become hypoglycaemic when they are fasted.[1] The exceptions are very small babies, or newly delivered neonates with diabetic mothers.

PHYSIOLOGY OF BODY FLUIDS

Fluid distribution
The body is separated into two fluid compartments, the intracellular compartment (ICF) and the extracellular fluid compartment (ECF). The two compartments are separated by the cell membrane. Only water can freely pass between the two compartments. In contrast, isotonic fluid such

as Hartmann's solution or Ringer's solution is confined to the ECF and cannot pass into the cells.

The body has two sensor receptor systems that recognise the two types of fluids. These are *osmoreceptors* and *volume receptors*. Osmoreceptors recognize pure water containing no dissolved ions. Volume receptors recognize *isotonic fluids*.

MAINTENANCE FLUID REQUIREMENTS

The first 24 hours of postoperative fluid therapy is usually planned by agreement between the anaesthetist, surgeon and the recovery room nursing staff. If you understand the physiology involved in fluid and electrolyte balance it makes it easier to make sensible decisions.

Below is a "cook book" approach to maintenance fluid therapy. This will allow you to judge whether your tailor-made orders are approximately correct.

ADULT MAINTENANCE
Fluids = 40 mls + 1 ml/kg each hour.

A 70 kg man will require 40 + (70 x 1) = 110 ml/hr. This is 2640 mls. per day. Add 13.4 mmols of potassium per litre. For a routine adult patient who is expected to drink within a few hours maintenance fluids would be 1 litre of saline and 2 litres of 5% dextrose daily. Give each litre over 8 hours.

CHILD MAINTENANCE
A solution of 1/5 normal saline and dextrose is a commonly used fluid for small children.

For the first 10 kg give 4 ml/kg/hr
Add a further 2 ml/kg/hr for children weighing 10 - 20 kg
Add a further 1 ml/kg/hr for children over 20 kg

Examples:

- 5 kg infant would require
  5 x 4 = 20 ml/hour or 480 ml/day

- 15 kg child would require:
  for the first 10 kg give 4 ml/kg/hr = 10 x 4 = 40 mls
  add 2 ml/kg /hr for the next 5 kg = 5 x 2 = 10 mls
  total requirements = 50 ml/hr or 1200 ml/day

- 28 kg child would require:
  for the first 10 kg give 4 ml/kg/hr = 10 x 4 = 40 mls
  add 2 ml/kg/hr for next 10 kg = 10 x 2 = 20 mls
  then add 1 ml/kg/hr for next 8 kg = 8 x 1 = 8 mls
  total requirements = 68 ml/hr or 1632 ml/day

Consider putting these formulas on a wall chart in the recovery room.

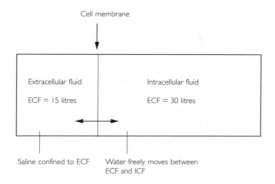

fig 8.1 Body fluid compartments

Water load

Infusing 5% dextrose is a way of giving water, because the dextrose is quickly metabolized. This water spreads itself through the 45 litres of body fluids, moving freely through the *extracellular fluid* (ECF) and into the *intracellular fluid* (ICF). In doing so the water (as 5% dextrose) dilutes the extracellular sodium ion.

A water overload shows up as a falling serum
sodium and water deficit as a rising serum sodium.

FLUID SPACES		
	EXTRACELLULAR FLUID	**INTRACELLULAR FLUID**
Volume	15 litres	30 litres
Sodium	140 mmol/litre	2 mmol/litre
Potassium	4 mmol/litre	140 mmol/litre
Other cations	3 mmol/litre	5 mmol/litre
Osmols*	294 mosmol	294 mosmol
Sensing mechanism	volume receptors	osmoreceptors
* An Osmol is a unit of osmotic pressure. It is the osmotic pressure generated by one mol of a substance. 1 Osmol =1000 milli Osmol (mOsmol).		

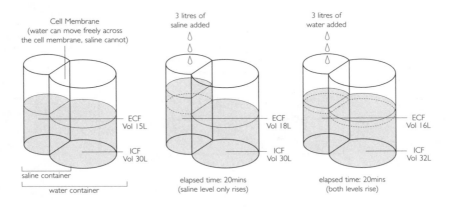

fig 8.2 Distribution of body fluids

A simple proportion calculation will reveal that in an adult a rise of 3 mmol of sodium (say from 140 mmol/l to 143 mmol/l) indicates a deficit of one litre of water. The *hypothalamic osmoreceptors* detect this change, and *antidiuretic hormone* (ADH) adjusts the kidney tubules to reabsorb water.

Water deficit

In contrast a fall in plasma sodium concentration of 3 mmol (say from 140 mmol/l to 137 mmol/l) indicates an excess of one litre of water. The hypothalamic osmoreceptors detect this change and turn off the release of antidiuretic hormone to allow the kidney to excrete the water load.

ISOTONIC SOLUTIONS					
Solution	Na+	K+	Lactate	Cl-	Ca++
Saline 0.9%	150			150	
Hartmann's solution*	131	5	29	111	2
Ringer's lactate	131	5	29	111	2
Ringer's solution	147	4		156	2.2

* Hartmann's solution is used in Australia, New Zealand and Oceania as a substitute for Ringer's solution. Hartmann's solution (Ringer's lactate), Ringer's solution and normal 0.9% saline are isotonic solutions.

Saline load

Saline-like isotonic solutions expand the extracellular fluid space. Unlike water, these solutions do not move into cells. They are confined to the

15 litres of extracellular fluid. Once a bolus of isotonic solution enters the circulation it equilibrates, within about 10 - 15 minutes, throughout the extracellular fluid volume. If infused quickly, the blood volume rises initially and then falls again as the saline re-distributes throughout the extracellular fluid space. It does not dilute the extracellular sodium, so the measured plasma sodium concentration remains unaltered. Low pressure receptors in the right atrium and great veins detect a change in pressure in these vessels. These receptors respond in a variety of ways involving atrial naturetic peptide, blood pressure, and other mechanisms, to prompt the kidneys to excrete the equivalent amount of near isotonic urine. Given a mean blood pressure above 75 mmHg, a normal well oxygenated kidney will competently adjust the extracellular volume.

Natural diuretics and antidiuretics

ATRIAL NATURETIC PEPTIDE (ANP) is one of the body's natural diuretics and provides an important mechanism for getting rid of excess isotonic fluid. ANP is released by the right atrium and ventricular myocytes as they are stretched by the increase in blood volume. ANP increases urine output, and by excreting isotonic fluid reduces ECF volume.

ANTIDIURETIC HORMONE (ADH) prevents the kidney losing water. Specialised neurones called osmoreceptors in the hypothalamus detect excessive water in the extracellular fluid. They send a message to the posterior pituitary gland, to trigger the release of ADH. The ADH allows water to diffuse back from the nephron to the bloodstream.

Fluids other than normal 0.9% saline, Ringer lactate and dextrose are sometimes given to patients.

Colloids

Blood and the colloids are initially confined to the 5 litres of vascular space, and do not spread right through the extracellular fluid. Protein solutions such as plasma take about 18 hours to clear from the circulation, and polygeline (Haemaccel®) about 8 hours.

Mixtures

The body recognizes mixtures of water and isotonic fluids as being a certain proportion of isotonic fluid, and a certain proportion of water. For instance the sensor systems recognise a litre of 4% dextrose and 1/5th normal saline as equivalent to 200 mls of saline and 800 mls of water.

DIURETICS USED IN RECOVERY ROOM

LOOP DIURETICS

Frusemide and ethacrynic acid, work by inhibiting the uptake of chlorine in the ascending loop of Henle in the kidney. They cause loss of sodium, potassium and magnesium ions. They are all nephrotoxic. If given in high doses or too fast intravenously, they will cause ringing, or humming, in the ears (tinnitus); giddiness (vertigo), and occassional hearing loss. This is more likely if the patient is also receiving an aminoglycoside such as gentamicin. The cephalosphorins are another group of drugs that increase their toxicity.

FRUSEMIDE (Lasix®) (furosemide in USA) is the most commonly used of the loop diuretics. It is especially useful in pulmonary oedema as it dilates the venous side of the circulation, causing a decrease in the right heart filling pressure (preload). This vasodilation is a bonus, it lowers the pressures in the pulmonary capillaries and the patient gets quick relief from his dysnoea. If a large dose is given rapidly, intravenously, hypotension can occur. Frusemide reaches its peak effect in 30 minutes and a single dose wears off in 3 hours. A healthy young person with normal kidneys can achieve a diuresis of more than 1000 ml in the first hour after 5 mg of frusemide. After a dose of frusemide, the urine will contain 120 mmol/l of sodium ion (or even more). The initial dose in pulmonary oedema or renal failure 40 mg intravenously given at 5 mg per minute. If there is no effect after 20 minutes check that the catheter is not blocked, then double the dose to 80 mg. If, after another 20 minutes there is little or no diuresis then slowly give 120 mg. After this large dose it is unlikely that frusemide can achieve an effect and there is a risk of toxicity. Frusemide can be diluted in normal 0.9% saline, but is incompatible with solutions containing glucose (dextrose).

ETHACRYNIC ACID is sometimes used because it rapidly reaches its peak effect, in about 5 minutes, and wears off in about 2 hours. It is considered more toxic than frusemide.

OSMOTIC DIURETICS

MANNITOL is an inert sugar useful as an osmotic diuretic. It is available in a 10% and 20% solution. Mannitol increases plasma osmolarity and draws water from the intracellular to the extracellular spaces. This is useful to relieve increased intracranial pressure and cerebral oedema after neurosurgery It is also used in patients at risk to prevent hepatorenal syndrome (see page 138). An infusion of 0.5 to 1 gm/kg is used as a diuretic to remove undesirable molecules from the blood.

ACETOZOLAMIDE (Diamox®) is a carbonic anhydrase inhibitor. It is useful to relieve increased intraocular pressure after eye surgery especially after the removal of cataracts and implants of intraocular lens. The usual dose of acetazolamide is 500mg IV.

Hypertonic fluids

Hypertonic fluids that contain concentrations of sodium ion higher than the extracellular fluid will suck water from the cells to dilute the ions. In this way they steal from the intracellular volume to expand the extracellular volume. They are sometimes used by neurosurgeons to reduce the volume of the brain. Their use requires guidance from a specialist physician or an intensivist.

DISORDERED FLUID BALANCE

The priorities in correcting disordered fluid balance are:
• Correct the blood volume to preserve the brain, heart and kidneys;
• adjust the isotonic fluid balance;
• adjust water balance;
• correct other electrolyte disturbances.

Correct the blood volume

DEPLETED BLOOD VOLUME

After major surgery, especially major vascular surgery, patients are often haemodynamically unstable with a depleted blood volume. Moving the patient from theatre to the recovery room exaggerates this. At the end of the operation the patient may have a good blood pressure, good perfusion, and stable pulse rate. Transfer to the recovery room can cause this to change rapidly and dramatically, presenting as hypovolaemic shock.

The signs of a depleted blood volume are:
• Tachycardia;
• urine output of less than 0.5 ml/kg/hr;
• pallor;
• cold hands and feet;
• hypotension may or may not be present. The *pulse pressure* (gap between systolic and diastolic pressure) may narrow.

Your immediate aim is to restore the circulating blood volume, and ensure good perfusion and oxygenation of the kidneys. Give blood (see page 259), or colloid if the patient has lost blood. This will stay in the intravascular space. Replace what the patient has lost.

BLOOD VOLUME OVERLOAD

If the patient has received too much blood or colloid during the operation, he will present with signs of left ventricular failure (see page 281). Sit him up, give him high flow oxygen, frusemide and sometimes a small dose of morphine 2mg IV if he is distressed by extreme dysnoea.

Correct the isotonic fluid balance

SALINE DEPLETION

In an adult patient the signs indicating that 0.9% saline is needed are:

- Urine output less than 60 mls per hour;
- postural drop in systolic blood pressure of more than 20 mmHg when the patient is sat up;
- tachycardia with a pulse rate greater than 100 per minute;
- low jugular (central) venous pressure;
- evidence of extracellular fluid loss such as: nasogastric loss, vomiting, burns, fistulae, bowel obstruction, and diarrhoea.

SALINE OVERLOAD

This may be chronic, if the patient has come to theatre with ankle or sacral oedema, shortness of breath on exertion, and a slightly enlarged heart on chest X-ray; or acute if too much isotonic fluid has been given during the operation.

Raised jugular pressure, added heart sounds, creps in the lungs, peripheral pitting oedema and pulmonary oedema are all serious signs of saline or blood volume overload. Treat them urgently (see above).

Correct the water balance

WATER DEPLETION

Signs indicating 5% dextrose is needed are:

- A serum sodium greater than 142 mmol/l;
- concentrated urine with a urine specific gravity of 1030. This is equivalent to a urine osmolarity greater than 1000 milli-osmol.

For instance a serum sodium of 143 mmol/l indicates a water deficit of about 1000 mls. This can be replaced with a litre of 5% dextrose over the next 8 hours.

WATER OVERLOAD

A serum sodium of less than 135 mmol/l is a sign that too much water or 5% dextrose has been administered.

WATER INTOXICATION

Water intoxication (see also TURP syndrome, page 79) occurs when the serum sodium falls to less than 130 mmol/l. It is more serious if the onset is sudden, for instance, after urological surgery, than if it occurs slowly over a number of days. Suspect water intoxication in the recovery room with an obtunded urolology patient who is slow to rouse, or who has muscle twitches. Fitting and coma may occur if the serum sodium falls from 140 mmol/l to less than 125 mmol/l.

The causes are:
- Irrigation of the bladder during transurethral resection of the prostate (TURP) allowing water to enter the open prostatic veins. Even if glycine 1.5% is used instead of water this may still occur.
- Hysteroscopy, where large amounts of fluid are used;
- endoscopic endometrial cautery, where water is used as the irrigating solution;
- excessive use of 5% dextrose solutions;
- rarely, inappropriate antidiuretic hormone secretion.

In the recovery room the patient complains of:
- dizziness;
- headache;
- nausea;
- a tight feeling in the chest;
- shortness of breath;
- sometimes abdominal pain.

He may become
- restless;
- confused, and disoriented;
- start retching;
- develop muscle twitching;
- start wheezing from acute left ventricular failure.

Then
- the blood pressure rises;
- the urine may turn brown due to haemolysis;
- if fitting occurs it can lead to a respiratory arrest;
- pulse slows to a bradycardia;
- ECG shows a widening QRS complex, and T-wave inversion.

If not treated, the patient will become cyanotic, hypotensive, and have a cardiac arrest. Acute water overload is particularly dangerous in children, especially if the serum sodium drops below 125 mmol/l. The mortality is high, and survivors are often brain damaged. Pathology tests will reveal haemolysis, haemoglobinuria, and hyponatraemia.

MANAGEMENT
1. Initially give high flows of 100% oxygen by mask.
2. Monitor blood pressure, pulse, respiratory rate, oxygen saturation and ECG.

3. Stop any infusions containing dextrose.

4. Measure the serum sodium if you suspect acute water overload. A serum sodium of less than 130 mmol/l is diagnostic. In a 70kg adult each decrement of 3 mmol/l of sodium ion indicates approximately a one litre water overload.

5. If the patient is stable, and the serum sodium is greater than 120 mmol it can be managed conservatively by simply witholding water and 5% dextrose, for the next few days. Do not simply *fluid restrict* the patient as he still may still need saline. To deprive a water overloaded patient of saline will cause acute renal failure.

6. Give frusemide 40 - 120 mg

7. A dopamine infusion may be needed if cardiac failure develops.

8. Transfer to a high dependency unit where the patient can be monitored.

9. If the patient is confused, or the serum sodium is less than 125 mmol per litre, then consider using hypertonic *3 normal saline* (3N saline) to correct the water overload. Proceed cautiously. Each litre of 3N saline will convert 2 litres of water overload to 2 litres of saline overload and add a further litre of saline. Readjust the fluids slowly because it is easy to precipitate cardiac failure with this regime. Frusemide will remove the excess saline. Patients with this degree of water overload should be transferred to a high dependency unit as soon as possible.

SYNDROME OF INAPPROPRIATE ADH SECRETION (SIADH) is a rare cause of water overload normally only seen in patients who were very sick preoperatively. Consider the diagnosis if the urinary sodium concentration is higher than the serum sodium concentration.

Correct other electrolyte disturbances
HYPOKALAEMIA

Hypokalaemia may aggravate residual paralysis following the use of muscle relaxant drugs. The patient will have a weak hand grip and be unable to sustain a 5 second head lift from the pillow. Suspect hypokalaemia if the ECG shows flattened or inverted T-waves, increasing prominence of the U-wave, and sagging of the ST segment.

Hypokalaemia is more likely to cause problems if the oxygen saturation is low, the PCO_2 high, or there is an increase in circulating catacholamines or anticholinergic drugs. Treat hypokalaemia by adding 2 grams (26.8 mmol) of potassium chloride to 1000 mls of dextrose or saline, and give it at a rate of not more than 1 gm/hr, and then only with ECG control. If extrasystoles occur, slow the infusion rate.

Acute hypokalaemia causes muscle
weakness and cardiac arrhythmias.

HYPERKALAEMIA

Patients with renal failure may come to the operating theatre with a high serum potassium. Others at risk are patients with: burns, severe crush injuries, established paralysis, saline depletion, incompatible blood transfusions or where haemolysis has occurred.

In the recovery room the ECG shows high peaked T-waves, especially in the precordial leads, but there should be no prolongation of the QT-interval as occurs with other causes of peaked T-waves. Later there will be prolongation of the PR interval, progressing to heart block, with widening of the QRS interval and finally asystole.

Should arrhythmias occur give calcium gluconate 1 gram intravenously over two minutes, which may be repeated once if needed.

Give calcium slowly into a fast running large bore infusion.
Failure to do this can cause horrific tissue damage.

If the serum potassium remains high, above 6.5 mmol/l treat it with:
- insulin and a glucose infusion which moves the potassium into the cells; One unit of insulin can be given for every 2 - 5 grams of glucose. Set up an infusion of insulin running at 2 units per hour. Measure the glucose and potassium levels every half an hour. Watch for signs of hypoglycaemia which are sweating, confusion and tachycardia;
- Slower control can be gained by using a calcium resonium enema;
- peritoneal or haemodialysis. To treat these patients you will need guidance from intensive care staff.

Hypokalaemia is easy to correct but hyperkalaemia
is dangerous and requires intensive care.

DRIP SETS

STERILITY

Be careful to maintain sterility if you are connecting a new drip set to a cannula that is already in the patient. Wear sterile gloves, swab the drip cannula and site with poviodine Betadine® and give it 90 seconds to work.

Wear gloves when handling blood.

Read about administering a blood transfusion on page 352.

BURETTES

Always use a burette when putting additives into a flask or bag or giving fluids to children. Check the order is written in full, because using abbreviations or symbols may cause errors. The order should state:

*   flask or bag number;
*   substance to be added;
*   dose, write this carefully if it is 5mg do not write 5.0mg. The decimal point can get lost so there is a danger that 5.0 could be read as 50. Always use the zero if it is 0.5mg. This attention to detail makes your work safe.
*   time to start;
*   duration of infusion;
*   route; that is whether the additive is added to the flask or to the burette;
*   dilution.

Always use an additive label. These are usually coloured red to signal that something has been added to the flask. Mix the added drug well, or it will pool at the bottom of the bag.

Patient's name.......................	Unit record number ....
Ward .... Date..........	Time prepared ....
Prepared by........................	Checked by ....
DRUG AND DOSE ADDED	
Concentration.......................	Duration of infusion ....
Time started	Time to finish ....

Do not write straight onto the bag.
The solvent may penetrate the solution.

Two trained staff should check and sign the additive label. Commercial additive labels are available. Before adding any substance to an intravenous infusion check that the drug and the solution are compatible. The necessary information should be on the drug information leaflet packed with the drug. If you have doubts about the compatibility of the solution with the drugs, contact your pharmacy.

THROMBOPHLEBITIS[3]

In some cases patients will come to theatre with intravenous lines which have been in place for several days. Check them on admission to recovery room. Thrombophlebitis is potentially lethal. It can lead to septicaemia. If there is any sign of thrombophlebitis, re-site the cannula, and put up a new infusion and giving set. Write the date on the plaster dressing if the cannula is expected to stay in more than 24 hours.

Send the tip of the old cannula to the laboratory for culture.

There are many causes of thrombophlebitis.

- If the antiseptic skin prep is not properly dry, it can be dragged into the vein as the cannula is inserted and irritate the endothelium;
- Improper aseptic technique is another potent cause. Always use a sterile technique and wear sterile gloves when inserting a drip;
- Movement of the cannula in the vein;
- Hypertonic fluids such as 50% dextrose (even 5% dextrose is irritating to the vein) or intravenous parenteral feeding formulas;
- Many drugs are irritant and some like vancomycin dangerously so.. Check the manufacturer's recommendations.

SETTING UP AN INFUSION (SEE APPENDIX I)

FLUIDS AFTER SURGERY

Bowel surgery

For some days after bowel surgery isotonic fluid transudates into the gut. An atonic bowel may contain 6 litres or more. As this fluid is lost from the extracellular space it is no longer available to interchange with the circulation and is sometimes called the *third space loss*. It takes up to 6 or more days for the bowel to recover its function. If the patient drinks fluids during this interval he runs the risk of acute gastric distension and vomiting. Replace four-fifths of the fluid requirements following bowel surgery with isotonic solutions, such as saline or Hartmann's solution. The patient will need additional potassium supplements. The basic potassium requirements is 1 mmol/kg/day. Make sure this has been prescribed but do not begin its administration in the recovery room.

INTRAVENOUS CANNULA AND THEIR INSERTION

1. The chosen cannula should be appropriate to the task.

- Blood transfusion size 14 to 16 G. Blood can be infused through smaller cannulas, but only slowly. Cannulas as large as 10 G are available. For a rapidly running drip use a short, wide bore cannula and a high drip stand. To increase the rate further use an in-line pump, or an inflator bag.

- Electrolyte solutions   size 18 - 20 G

- Drug administration   size 22 - 24 G

2. If you are inserting a cannula larger than size 22, then use a 30 G needle to raise a skin bleb with local anaesthetic. An alternative is to use an insulin syringe, with its a tiny needle that can barely be felt as it enters the skin.

3. Choose a vein on the forearm well away from the elbows.

4. Do not put cannulas in veins near flexures such as the elbow or wrist joint, because as the joint moves the cannula will abrade the inside of the vein causing inflammation. They are also likely to kink off. If you insert a drip near a joint, then use a splint.

5. Use a sterile technique for insertion. Use gloves and allow enough time (about 90 seconds) for the skin prep to dry. If skin preparation fluid enters the vein it can cause thrombophlebitis.

6. A transparent dressing is useful to protect the insertion site. If these are not available, use a small adhesive dressing over the puncture wound and fix the cannula with tape on top of this.

7. A valuable approach in an emergency is to insert a large bore cannula into the femoral vein using a Seldinger wire technique and 8.5 F sheath.

8. In the complete absence of veins in children an intramedullary or intraosseous infusion can be used[2] (see fig 20.1, page 397). Insert a large bore, short bevelled needle into marrow of the tibia taking care to avoid the epiphysial plates. Use an infusion pressure of up to 300 mmHg.

9. Sometimes lines are flushed with heparinised saline. This can cause bruising and haemorrhage if it extravasates into the tissues. Apart from arterial cannulae it is not necessary to use heparinised saline; instead, flush the lines with normal saline. This will reduce the incidence of heparin induced thrombocytopaenia (HITS).

Urological surgery

Clots may form in the bladder after urinary tract surgery. A bladder washout will flush these away. If this is not in place keep the urine output high by increasing the intravenous fluids to 3000 ml/day. Water intoxication is a serious complication of prostate surgery (see page 79).

Neurosurgery

Many neurosurgeons prefer to keep their patients water depleted, with their serum sodium ion concentration higher than normal. There is little evidence that this reduces the incidence of cerebral oedema. Indiscriminate fluid restriction may cause saline depletion, and jeopardize the patient's kidney perfusion resulting in renal failure. Remember these patients still require saline to preserve renal function, even if they need less water.

Chronic renal failure

Patients with renal failure who have been recently dialysed, should be able to cope with a litre of saline during their procedure and the immediate postoperative period in recovery room. However their problems are often complex. If in doubt, give 700 mls of 5% dextrose per day in addition to their urine output and consult the renal physicians. After a long procedure, monitor their electrolytes. Check that they have not become saline overloaded.

Cardiac failure

Patients with potential cardiac failure need frequent attention to the balance of the fluid given and the urine produced. Listen to their chests for the fine moist sounds, and added heart sounds indicating fluid overload. Recovery room staff should be alert for a rising respiratory rate, wheezing, breathlessness and a reluctance to lie flat which are sign of fluid overload or confusion and restlessness that warn of hypoxia.

Febrile patients

Patients with temperature greater than 39°C need an additional 500 mls of saline daily to make up for their sweat loss. Sweat is about half saline and half water.

THE KIDNEY

Physiology

The kidney filters the blood, and reabsorbs most of its useful components back into the blood stream, excreting the unwanted wastes in the urine. Most of the waste products are protein break-down from food and cellular metabolism, but the kidney also has an important role in metabolising and excreting drugs. The kidney controls the volume and composition of the extracellular fluid by regulating the balance of water, sodium, potassium, hydrogen ion and other water soluble substances in the body. It also produces hormones, erythropoietin, activated vitamin D, renin and prostaglandins.

The kidney receives 20 - 30 per cent of the cardiac output (about 1250 - 1500 mls passes through the kidney each minute), which is far more than the amount needed to preserve its viability, but is important for its role as an excretory organ. If the extracellular fluid volume falls, the kidney will help correct this by retaining sodium and water and diverting up to a litre per minute of its blood supply to boost the central circulation.

The kidney can survive for 30 minutes to an hour on a circulation of as little as one tenth of its normal blood flow, but its ability to function becomes progressively impaired. The kidney can maintain a urine output while its blood supply is reduced, until it reaches a point where it becomes so starved of oxygen that its tubules fail to function and *acute tubular necrosis* (ATN) occurs. In the recovery room this is an important clinical point, because we must aim to prevent renal hypoxia.

If the patient has cold hands,
then their kidney's blood supply
may be critically low.

A hypoxic kidney can still produce urine for a short while before developing ATN. In the recovery room just because the patient is producing urine, does not mean that the kidney is safe. There is a small window of opportunity which presents in the first 20 minutes of so in the recovery room where restoration of renal blood flow will save the kidney. It is vital to make sure that the patient has a good perfusion status (see page 255). If not then give fluids, oxygen, restore blood pressure, reduce adrenergic drive with good pain relief, increase cardiac output and renal blood flow with dopamine; and avoid frusemide and mannitol.

If the patient is producing urine and has warm hands and feet, mean blood pressure over 100 mmHg or more, and does not have a tachycardia then their kidney has an adequate blood supply. If not, find a the reason for the poor perfusion and treat it.

To further check the health of the kidney we need to look at the composition of the urine, especially its concentration and sodium content. A healthy kidney will respond to hypovolaemia by concentrating the urine, removing almost all the sodium and most of the water. The urine will be concentrated (high osmolarity), but with a low sodium concentration. If the kidney is hypoxic the tubules stop retaining sodium, and produce a dilute urine with a high sodium concentration.

HYPOVOLAEMIA AND RENAL FAILURE

There is an ordered progression from hypovolaemia to renal failure. It starts with afferent arteriolar vasoconstriction, and cortical hypoxia; and progresses with impairment of autoregulation failure of efferent arteriolar constriction, with reduction in glomerular pressure; and finally neural and humoral effects on blood flowing to the kidney tubules. This progression is accelerated by renal vascular disease, diuretics and nephrotoxins such as gentamicin[1].

The fractional excretion of sodium (FeNa+) is a useful indicator of established acute renal failure.

$$FeNa+ \ = \ \frac{\dfrac{Urine\ [Na^+]}{Plasma\ [Na^+]}}{\dfrac{Urine\ [Cr]}{Plasma\ [Cr]}}$$

[Cr] = creatinine concentration   [Na+] = sodium ion concentration

Hypoxic injury   FeNa+ < 0.01

Acute renal failure   FeNa+ > 0.01

Drugs and renal disease

As a general rule if more than 50 per cent of a drug is excreted unchanged by the kidney reduce the dose. If there is an active or toxic metabolite then alter the frequency of administering the dose to allow for the clearance of that metabolite. In the recovery room pethidine is the drug most likely to cause problems.

As a useful generalization:
- renal impairment is a creatinine 12 - 20 mmol/l;
- renal failure is a creatinine greater than 20 mmol/l;

or
- renal failure is a creatinine clearance less than 10 ml/min;
- moderate impairment is a creatinine clearance 10 - 25 ml/min;
- mild impairment is a creatinine clearance 25 - 50 ml/min.

The Cockcroft and Gault Formula (1976) can be used to estimate creatinine clearance from the plasma creatinine level.

$$Creatinine\ clearance = \frac{(140 - age) \times lean\ body\ weight\ in\ kg}{815 \times serum\ creatinine\ (mmol/l)}$$

for females the value is 85% of that estimated by the equation.

Check renal function before prescribing any drug that is excreted by the kidney. Even mild renal impairment in the elderly indicates a degree of significant renal disease. After you have given a drug to a patient with renal impairment observe him carefully for untoward effects.

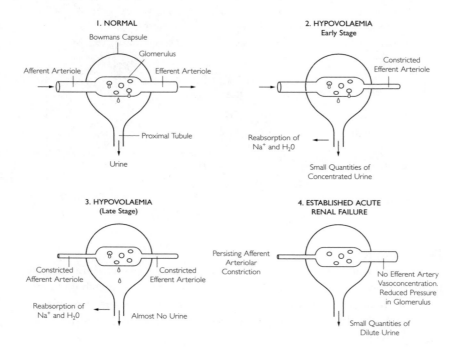

fig 8.3 Renal changes in hypovolaemia

CAUSES OF RENAL FAILURE

Oliguric renal failure

Without doubt the major cause of renal dysfunction in the recovery room is renal hypoperfusion with associated hypoxia, and the causes of this are in order: hypovolaemia, hypoxia, and hypotension. Hypovolaemia is the most likely cause of postoperative acute renal failure. These problems compound, for example, a fit young patient can tolerate hypotension mean BP down to 60 mmHg, providing the patient is not also hypovolaemic.

NORMOVOLAEMIC RESPONSE: Hypotension induced by epidural anaesthesia, or deliberate vasodilation, may result in little urine being formed. This is because the kidney's autoregulation of blood flow ensures that perfusion and oxygenation are maintained, even though the blood pressure in the glomerulus may not be enough to force fluid through the sieve to produce urine.

Renal hypoperfusion causing hypoxia
is the most important cause of acute renal failure.

HYPOVOLAEMIC RESPONSE: If the patient is hypovolaemic or is in cardiac failure the kidney is at risk. The patient's autonomic nervous system controls renal blood flow and the kidney is exquisitely sensitive to adrenaline and noradrenaline. It responds to hypovolaemia by progressively shutting down its blood flow. For a short time the kidney may be hypoxic and failing and still produce urine. You cannot simply rely on a urine flow of 0.5 ml/kg/hr as a sign of a properly oxygenated kidney.

Clinically we are warned of this renal hypoperfusion when the patient has cold hands, a poor perfusion status, a tachycardia and a low blood pressure.

Cold bloodless hands = cold bloodless kidneys.

High output renal failure

A second major cause of impaired renal function in the recovery room is drug toxicity. In this situation acute renal failure can occur when there is a good urine output. This is called *high output failure*.

The hypoxic kidney is sensitive to toxins and many antibiotics, especially aminoglycosides such as gentamicin, some of the cephalosporins, and radiocontrast solutions used during angiography. Other toxins are frusemide, non-steroidal anti-inflammatory drugs (NSAIDs), especially ketorolac, and endotoxins from sepsis. Patients who, preoperatively, were taking *angiotensin-converting enzyme* (ACE) inhibitors (drugs with the suffix - pril eg. captopril) are also at risk.

The combination of gentamicin,
frusemide and hypovolaemia is harmful
to the underperfused kidney.

Other risk factors:
- patients having aortic or cardiac surgery, especially if the surgeon has had the aortic clamps on for more than 30 minutes will cause renal hypoxia;
- adrenaline and noradrenaline infusions, which in high doses decrease tubular blood flow and cause renal hypoxia;
- patients taking antihypertensive drugs;
- diabetic patients who have diseased blood vessels serving their kidneys.

If a patient has received frusemide in theatre,
make sure he does not become hypotensive
while in the recovery room.

Hepatorenal syndrome

The hepatorenal syndrome is the association of severe liver disease with renal impairment. Usually the patient is jaundiced with cirrhosis and ascites. It may be precipitated by surgery and anaesthesia, particularily if there has been hypotension or hypoxia; or if there has been a shower of bacteria released from an abscess or source of infection uncovered during surgery. It is characterised by low urinary sodium concentrations. It is probably, in part, due to intense renovascular constriction causing tubular hypoxia. It is better to attempt to prevent the problem by :

- giving prophylactic mannitol in theatre (see page 140);
- maintaining good oxygenation;
- limiting the use of nephrotoxic drugs;
- lumbar sympathetic blockade can partially reverse renal dsfunction;
- using epidural analgesia.

Prevention of oliguria

- identify the patients at risk;
- as far as possible avoid the risk factors.

Management of oliguria secondary to hypovolaemia

What to do when your patient has a urine output of less than 0.5 ml/kg/hr

1. Give oxygen, and aim at a PaO_2 of at least 97 mmHg (13.2 kPa).

2. Monitor blood pressure, oxygenation and perfusion status.

3. Restore blood volume as quickly as possible. Aim for a mean blood pressure of at least 90 - 95 mm Hg to compensate for the impaired autoregulation of renal blood flow and to reduce sympathetic discharge.

NEPHROTOXINS

GENTAMICIN[5]

Gentamicin is frequently used during urological surgery. It is an aminoglycoside which is excreted exclusively by the kidney and is toxic to the renal tubules. Other factors that aggravate renal toxicity (and ototoxicity) are hypoxia, hypovolaemia, diuretics, hypokalaemia, and hypomagnesaemia. This combination of factors is more likely to be encountered in the elderly. The loading dose for both normal patient, and patients with renal impairment is gentamicin 1 - 2 mg/kg. Gentamycin should not be given more than once every 12 hours.

Do not give gentamycin in recovery room without first checking when the previous dose was given.

The major site of damage is in the tubules, so the earliest signs of toxicity are impaired acid excretion, and depressed urine concentrating ability. A rising serum creatinine is a late sign. Gentamicin is also ototoxic and vestibulotoxic and this is exacerbated by diuretics.

ASPIRIN

Aspirin should be stopped about 7 - 10 days before surgery. Aspirin inhibits cyclo-oxygenase, that is needed to maintain autoregulation of the kidney's perfusion and stops the renal blood vessels dilating in response to early hypovolaemia or hypotension. Elderly patients often have heart failure, or atherosclerosis that decreases renal perfusion. They are also often taking aspirin for its prostaglandin mediated antiplatelet activity to prevent stroke and coronary ischaemia. These patients are at high risk of acute renal failure if they become hypovolaemic, hypoxic, or hypotensive while they are taking aspirin. Antiplatelet activity in patients with angina can be achieved with transdermal nitroglycerine[6].

NSAIDS

These drugs cause similar damage to aspirin, and no NSAID is exempt from this problem. Ideally NSAIDs should be withdrawn about 5 days before surgery. Paracetamol can be used as a substitute for pain relief.

RADIOCONTRAST MEDIA

Acute tubular damage by radiocontrast media used during vascular surgery in the elderly may be as high as 80 - 90%[7]. Hypovolaemia is the major avoidable risk factor. The problem is also exacerbated by co-existent diabetes, vascular disease, and age-related reduced renal function, and drug therapy with gentamicn or vancomycin. The effects can be minimized in the recovery room by ensuring adequate hydration.

HIGH DOSE FRUSEMIDE OR ETHACRYNIC ACID

These drugs are sometimes given to encourage urine output. They have not been shown to protect the kidney from hypoxic or toxic damage.

4. Use low dose dopamine (3 - 5 microgram/kg/minute) to maintain blood pressure.

> ### DOPAMINE
>
> It is controversial whether dopamine is an effective renal vasodilator, and what role it plays in improving renal perfusion in impending renal failure. At low doses of 3 - 5µg/kg/min it usually dilates the renal vascular bed, improving renal blood flow. As the dose increases the effects progressively are due to, increasing cardiac output, and rising renal perfusion pressure. It also has a direct diuretic effect on renal tubular function[8]. Clinically, although not proven, it is a useful drug for the preservation of renal blood flow, and the prevention of renal hypoxia.
>
> The only therapy proven by clinical trials to improve renal function in critically ill patients is the augmentation of renal blood flow. Achieve this by supporting the mean arterial pressure with inotropes and colloid fluid loading.

5. Frusemide (Lasix®) is a potent diuretic used in both renal and cardiac failure. Use frusemide cautiously. Start with 0.5 mg/kg intravenously and repeat every 20 minutes until a dose of 4 mg/kg has been reached. Doses beyond this are unlikely to be successful and may be nephrotoxic or ototoxic.

6. Consider mannitol, an osmotic diuretic, used mainly in neurosurgery, but also for the prompt removal of renal toxins. Mannitol is useful to flush pigments through, such as in patients with myoglobinuria or haemoglobinuria. Another use is during or after hepatic surgery. Dose limits are less than 1 gm/kg in healthy patients, and less than 0.5 gm/kg in those with renal dysfunction. High doses of mannitol can damage kidneys.

> *If a patient has received gentamicin in theatre,*
> *make sure he does not become hypovolaemic*
> *in the recovery room.*

7. Prevent non-oliguric renal failure from converting into oliguric renal failure. Non-oliguric renal failure is a milder disease, with a shorter duration, and a lower mortality. The commonest cause of non-oliguric renal failure is an aminoglycoside antibiotic.

RENAL DISEASE

These are patients with impaired renal function who produce very little urine. and those you have lost the function of their kidneys totally and have no way of naturally removing fluid from their bodies.

These patients also have problems with:
- fluid overload;
- delayed excretion of drugs;
- hypertension;
- impaired tissue oxygenation;
- anaemia and coagulopathies;
- chronic steroid dependance;
- susceptability to infection.

There is another group of patients with high output failure. These patients cannot concentrate their urine and suffer the same problems with the additional one of losing too much ECF volume.

FLUIDS: Take care not to overload these patients with fluids. Up to one litre of intravenous saline is usually safe. If the patient comes to the recovery room with a second litre running, slow it to a 12 hourly rate unless you receive authoritative instructions and reasons for an alternative regime. Renal patients have no way of excreting fluid. All drips should be attached to burettes or infusion pumps to limit the rate of administration.

If there is any doubt about the management
of renal patients. Consult the renal physician.

DRUGS: Drug excretion is increasingly delayed as the glomerular filtration rate falls below 30 mls per minute. With the exception of atracurium and cis-atracurium, the action of all the long acting muscle relaxants is prolonged in renal failure. If partial curarization returns (neostigmine has a shorter half life than some of the relaxant drugs), it is better to sedate and re-intubate the patient; and ventilate him until the effects wear off, than to try other pharmacological measure to reverse the muscle relaxants.

Intra-operative fentanyl is well tolerated, and rarely lingers to cause a problem in recovery room. Morphine is partly metabolized in the kidneys. It is well tolerated in small doses, administered at longer intervals between each dose. Pethidine is poorly tolerated by patients with renal failure as one of the metabolites, norpethidine, is toxic and is excreted only by the kidneys. Norpethidine rapidly accumulates causing irritability, confusion, and eventually convulsions and coma.

Small doses of morphine given at
frequent intervals is the analgesic of choice
for patients with renal disease.

HYPERTENSION: Be wary of reducing the cardiac output in an anaemic renal patient, because he needs his high output to deliver oxygen to his tissues. Use vasodilators rather than ß-blockers (see page 264). Excessive hypertension is often due to saline overload. CVP is useful to guide fluid management in renal patients

OXYGEN DELIVERY is compromised by anaemia and any form of heart failure. Confusion, restlessness or agitation should be regarded as hypoxic in origin and treated with oxygen.

ANAEMIA: The haemoglobin may be only 50 - 70 gm/l. If anything depresses patients cardiac output they will be severely compromised.

BLEEDING: If the creatinine is above 600 mmol/l the patient is likely to bleed. Avoid major regional nerve blockades because of the risk of haemorrhage into a neurovascular bundle.

Veins are precious. Avoid lower arm veins because they may be needed for future haemodialysis. Do not use subclavian veins for central lines as there is a risk of thrombosis, internal jugular veins are preferable. Use small cannulae. Insert drips using strictly sterile techniques. Check to ensure intravenous access is no longer needed before removing it.

Thrombophlebitis must never occur. Remove the drip at the first sign of tenderness along a vein and reinsert it at another site. These patients are immunocompromised and very susceptible to infection. All dressings should be done as a strictly sterile procedure.

Avoid using radial artery punctures for blood gases, because this site may be needed for future access for haemodialysis and any stenosis or damage to the artery will preclude it use.

LIVING DONOR TRANSPLANTS

These may be related, or non related but involved, spouse or partner, as well as true family.

The donor

This patient is a healthy person who has undergone an operation to donate a kidney. There is a huge emotional involvement. Be very considerate and tell him all you can about the recipient while he is with you in recovery room. The recipient will probably still be in theatre while you are recovering the donor but there will be some news you can offer. The donor is often in severe pain because many muscles and nerves have been severed. This can be well controlled if a continuous epidural is in place, There is likely to still be some pain, above the level of the block. Give small increments of morphine, 2 mg at minute intervals or set up a PCA (see page 200).

The recipient

This patient has been in chronic renal failure, perhaps for years, before this operation. He will still be suffering from all the complications of this disease. Your job is to make sure he returns to the ward with a functioning kidney. A central venous catheter (CVC) is mandatory. Monitor this constantly and keep the central venous pressure (CVP) above 8 - 10 cm of water from the isophlebotic line. Measure, and accurately record, the urine output every 30 minutes once it begins. Check the haemoglobin, because many of these patients are chronically anaemic. Check with the renal physicians before transfusing him with blood.

1. Burnett YL, Lubicky JP, Podraza A, *et al.* (1993) *Anaesthetic Analgesia*, 76: S31.
2. Fisher DH. (1990). *New England Journal of Medicine*, 322: 1579-81.
3. Elliot TS, Faroqui MH. (1992). *British Journal of Hospital Medicine*, 48: 496-503.
4. Badr KF, Ichikawa I. (1988). *New England Journal of Medicine*, 319:623-9.
5. Walker R. (1994). *The New Zealand Medical Journal*, 107: 54-5.
6. Lacost L. (1994). *American Journal of Cardiology*, 73: 1058-62.
7. Thomson N. (1995). *The Medical Journal of Australia*, 62: 543-7.
8. Duke GJ, Bersten AD. (1992). *Anaesthesia and Intensive Care*, 20: 277-302.

9. METABOLISM

TEMPERATURE

A patient is *normothermic* when his core temperature is between 36.5 - 37.2°. Hypothermia becomes a clinical problem when the core temperature falls below 36°C.

Monitoring (see page 32)

HYPOTHERMIA

Thermoregulation is disabled during both general and regional anaesthesia and the body cools down. Apart from the severe metabolic stress imposed by hypothermia, just waking up and feeling cold after an anaesthetic is most unpleasant, particularly for those who live in warmer climates.

PHYSICS OF HYPOTHERMIA

Hypothermia is defined as a core temperature of 35°C or less. At a basal metabolic rate of 40 Kcal/m²/hr, normal metabolic activity uses about 72 Kcal/hr for an average adult. A *neutral thermal environment* occurs where the naked exposed body in still air neither loses, nor gains heat from the environment. This is in a fairly narrow range of temperature and humidity and changes with age. In a young adult it is about 29°C with a relative humidity of about 60%, but in a baby it can be 32 - 35°C. The usual operating theatre temperature is well below the neutral thermal environment, and is about 19 - 21°C with a relative humidity of 50 - 60 per cent. This suits surgeons wearing gowns and gloves, but during a general anaesthetic the patient loses the ability to maintain his body temperature and will slowly cool down as the operation progresses. He loses heat by *radiation, conduction, convection* and *evaporation*. The temperature stays stable for the first twenty minutes or so, then drops rapidly for two hours then more slowly again.

The side effects of perioperative hypothermia extend beyond the immediate postoperative period; impairing wound healing and increasing the risk of infection,[1] increasing the risk of deep vein thrombosis, and contributing to myocardial ischaemia.[2] Heat can be lost from the body by radiation, convection, conduction, and evaporation. All these mechanisms occur in the operating theatre.

Elderly people and babies are particularly susceptible to hypothermia. Other patients who easily become hypothermic are burn victims, and those who have had major vascular, abdominal, thoracic, or trauma surgery. Also those unable to shiver (paraplegics, quadraplegics, and those temporarily rendered so by spinal or epidural anaesthetics). Surgery lasting more than 3 hours, blood loss and transfusion, and the use of cold fluids (urology) also contribute to hypothermia.

The cough reflex is reduced in hypothermia increasing the risk of aspiration. Anaesthetic agents are more soluable and therefore leave the patient more slowly. Liver function is depressed in cold patients affecting most enzymatic and detoxifying processes. Avoid giving lactated Ringer's solution as the liver will not metabolise the lactate. Metabolism of drugs given during anaesthesia is slowed. Central nervous system processes are also slowed keeping the patient asleep longer. Take care to use small increments of drugs in cold patients. Drugs can accumulate and cause problems later.

Sympathetic stimulation with mild hypothermia will cause a tachycardia and an increase in cardiac output. If the temperature continues to fall there will be a reduction in tissue perfusion and atrial fibrillation can occur. Stimulation such as the insertion of a CVP line or intubation can also cause fibrillation in a cold patient.

The metabolic response and haemodynamic changes associated with even mild postoperative hypothermia include:
- physiological stress with rises in catecholamines and cortisol secretion;[3]
- delay in the metabolism and excretion of drugs;
- prolonged action of sedative drugs and opioids;
- failure of the kidneys to concentrate urine; urine output increases by about a litre an hour;
- coagulopathies, platelets are sequestrated in the liver;
- a reduction in the activity of clotting enzymes;
- a rise in blood viscosity impeding flow through the microcirculation;
- a slow return to consciousness and poor airway maintainance.

Patients may cool further before they begin to warm and this phenomenon is called *after fall*. It is caused by cold blood returning from the muscle beds and skin as circulation to these areas is restored.

Shivering

Shivering is a response to cold. A normal patient will shiver in response to mild hypothermia, shutting down the blood flow to his skin so that heat production will exceed heat loss. Shivering muscle produces large amounts of heat, by increasing the metabolic rate and oxygen consumption five- to seven-fold. To deliver oxygen to the highly active muscle tissue, the heart must increase its cardiac output proportionately.

Hypothermia causes peripheral vasoconstriction, so the heart has to work even harder to pump blood through constricted vessels. This can result in myocardial ischaemia, tissue hypoxia, and lactic acidosis.

MECHANISMS OF HEAT LOSS

EVAPORATION

It requires an astonishing amount of heat to turn water into a vapour - about 580 Calories per litre of water. Evaporation (sweating) is the only way heat can be lost from the body against a thermal gradient. This is useful in the desert, but catastrophic in the operating theatre or recovery room. The evaporation of one litre of fluid from an open abdomen uses about 25% of the body's total daily heat production.

CONDUCTION

Heat is transferred from molecules of higher kinetic energy to molecules of lower kinetic energy down a temperature gradient. It can occur during the infusion of cold fluids, or contact with a cold medium such as immersion in cold water. Two units of cold blood at 4°C can cool the core temperature by 0.5°C. Warming blankets can delay heat loss by conduction.

CONVECTION

Convective losses are really a special form of conduction. As heat is transferred from a place of higher temperature to one of lower temperature it is moved away from the point of transfer. Convective heat losses occur during exposure during positioning and draping a patient, pulmonary ventilation, dialysis or bypass. Air velocity, ambient temperature, and exposed surface areas determine convective losses.

RADIATION

Energy is lost from the body by transfer of electromagnetic infra-red waves. No direct contact is needed. Put your warm hand near a cold object and you will feel the transfer! Babies can develop cold injury (sclerema) if their cots are placed too close to a cold outside wall; they just radiate their heat to the wall. Radiant heat loss is proportional to the fourth power of the area exposed.

Cocoon the patient in a metallic (Mylar®) space blankets. These do not actively warm the patient, but prevent heat loss by radiation and convection. Separate the space blanket from the patient's skin by at least a cotton sheet. Place the reflective side towards the patient, and cover it with warm blankets.

Once the temperature falls below 33°C, the patient ceases to shiver, and his conscious state becomes increasingly obtunded.

Epidural opioids depress shivering and increase heat loss, particularly after Caesarian section.[4] The patient does not feel cold and does not ask for blankets. The endocrine and metabolic response to the fall in temperature is atttenuated[5] and the patient is vasodilated. Rewarming is therefore slow. Interestingly, cold patients with epidurals require larger top ups to achieve the same pain relief as warm patients.

Neonates (see page 384)

Hypothermia during blood transfusion (see page 353)

Initial management[6]
MONITOR: Core temperature, blood pressure, pulse rate, ECG, glucose level, and urine output.

Many patients remember being 'freezing cold' when they wake. They are comforted by a warm blanket. Unless myxoedaemic or hypoglycaemic, most postoperative, mildly, hypothermic patients will warm themselves up if they are protected from further heat loss. Infants and neonates are very slow to warm. Everything possible should be done in theatre to prevent them from cooling. Patients with temperatures less than 34°C should remain intubated and sedated until rewarmed. In the elderly, or sick patient; or after major surgery, the patient should remain intubated, paralysed and ventilated until his core temperature has risen to at least 35.8°C.

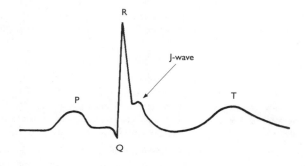

fig 9.1 J wave seen on ECG in hypothermia

It can take 12 hours, or more to rewarm a severely hypothermic patient. Proceed slowly, active rapid warming beyond the use of a forced air convection heater such as Bair Hugger™ (see page 493), or a heated humidifier, can cause complications. There is no place for domestic heating, hot water bottles etc. If you do not have a Bair Hugger™ use a metallic (Mylar®) space blanket (see page 488). Rewarm at a rate no faster than 0.8°C an hour. Give high concentrations of oxygen, because shivering increases oxygen consumption by 5 to 8 fold, and the patient may become hypoxic.

Watch for ECG changes. At temperatures of about 33°C the ECG will show prolongation of the PR and QT interval, and J-waves.

Be prepared to give additional fluids during the rewarming phase to prevent hypotension.

Warm the intravenous fluids by passing them through an 'in line' blood warmer. As the patient rewarms in the recovery room he will vasodilate, because shivering increases blood supply to the muscles. Use a heated humidifier if the patient is still intubated. Neonates and infants need incubators, if these are not available use overhead infrared heaters.

For interpretation of blood gases in hypothermic patients (see page 162).

Do not send a patient back to the ward until
his core temperature is above 36.5°C.

HYPERTHERMIA[7]

Fever (pyrexia) refers to a core temperature of 37.8 - 40°C. *Hyperthermia* usually refers to a core temperature greater than 40°C. At about 42°C brain enzymes are damaged. and muscle tissue breaks down (*rhabdomyolysis*) releasing myoglobin into the blood stream.

Fever occurs because the patient's heat
production is faster than his heat loss.

It is rare for a patient to become febrile in the recovery room but it is always serious when it does happen. Normally the body produces about as much heat as a 100 watt light globe to keep the body temperature at about 37°C. For every degree Celsius rise in temperature that the body temperature goes up, oxygen consumption increases by about 15 per cent. The heart needs to increase its stroke volume and heart rate to meet the increasing tissue demands; to compensate for vasodilation, and the increased work of breathing. Arryhythmias and cardiac failure occur if the heart is unable to increase its output.

A rise in body temperature can be generated by:
1. A rise in metabolic rate due to:
   • sepsis following urinary surgery, bowel surgery, drainage of an absess or from aspiration pneumonia;
   • thyroid storm;
   • reaction to blood or blood products;
   • phaeochromocytoma.

2. Increased muscle activity:
   • shivering and shaking (see page 451);
   • malignant hyperthermia.

3. Drug reactions:
   • LSD;
   • amphetamines;
   • cocaine (these drugs cause an adreneric storm);

4. Decreased heat loss:
   • atropine or other anticholinergic drugs preventing sweating;
   • obesity where the fat prevents dissipation of heat from a hot core.

MALIGNANT HYPERTHERMIA (MH)

Malignant hyperthermia (also called *malignant hyperpyrexia*) is a rare syndrome characterized by an enormously high metabolic rate It is triggered by many drugs including all the volatile anaesthetic agents and suxamethonium. The full syndrome is probably as rare as 1:260000 cases where volatile agents are used and about 1:60000 from the use of suxamethonium.[8] It tends to run in families as an autosomal dominant gene. Both a genetic disposition and one or more of the triggering agents are necessary to evoke this life threatening disorder. It develops during or after general anaesthesia. A rising end tidal CO_2 and muscle spasm suggests the diagnosis, but it may not be obvious until the patient comes to the recovery room.

Those patients who are at risk tend to have musculoskeletal disorders especially one of the many muscular dystrophies. They are often short and stocky, with bulky muscles and rounded bellies. They may have one or more of the following: kyphoscoliosis, squints, hypermobile joints, clubbed feet, atrophied muscle groups; or diseases such as myotonia congenita, arthrogryposis multiplex, or osteogenesis imperfecta.

MH presents with several or more of the following: muscle (especially masseter) spasm, hypercarbia, skin mottling, profuse sweating, core temperatures rising to exceed 40°C and perhaps rising to 43°C, tachycardia, cardiac arrhthmias. rapid respiratory rate, cyanosis. Laboratory tests reveal signs of disrupted muscle membranes: hyperkalemia, a raised creatine kinase and myoglobinuria.

A MH crisis is a hypermetabolic state where all the voluntarily muscles start producing large quantities of heat. Muscle rigidity occurs in 75 per cent of cases, while the remaining 25 per cent may not develop this helpful sign. The muscle rigidity occurs as calcium ions flood into the muscle cells activating actin and myosin filaments. A tightly clenched jaw is an early sign of a MH. The high metabolic rate causes a huge increases in muscle oxygen consumption and carbon dioxide production; and results in hypercarbia, hypoxia and a metabolic acidosis. If the patient's minute volume remains constant his end expired PCO_2 will rapidly rise. In recovery room we miss this sign as we do not normally monitor the end tidal CO_2.

> *Diagnostic signals include masseter spasm and a*
> *rapidly rising end tidal CO_2, hyperthermia comes later.*

Intravenous dantrolene is the drug to use in this crisis. It is an expensive drug with a limited life, so groups of hospitals find it cheaper to pool their resources instead of keeping a full stock at each hospital. Keep the instructions for using the drug, plus a MH protocol with the dantrolene. Do not lock the dantrolene away in the pharmacy. It must be immediately available at all times. Keep a starting dose of dantrolene in your refrigerator. Make sure you have enough solvent. Up to 20 vials will be required as a starting dose to treat one case. Dantrolene is an orange powder which requires a special solvent containing mannitol and sodium hydroxide.

Management

A guide to the preparation of a suitable trolley in anticipation of this emergency can be found in Appendix VII.

WHAT TO MONITOR: Pulse rate, ECG, blood pressure, (insert an arterial line), core temperature, urine output, end tidal CO_2, (if you can intubate or place a laryngeal mask, otherwise this is not possible), central venous pressure, and perhaps pulmonary artery wedge pressures.

LABORATORY: arterial blood gases, sodium, potassium, bicarbonate, creatinine, urea, glucose, lactate, ketones. Repeat blood gases and electrolytes every 15 minutes.

IMMEDIATELY

1. Give high flow oxygen and continue it in an attempt to keep up with the enormous rise in oxygen consumption.
2. Summon help.
3. Insert a new large bore intravenous line and attach a new drip with extensions which should lie in a bucket of ice. If you have a blood warmer which will function as a blood cooler, use that. Keep at least 12 litres of ice cold saline available in your fridge.

FURTHER MANAGEMENT

WHAT TO MONITOR: Continue as above, plus DIC screen, clotting profile, serum Ca^{++}, CXR, myoglobin and haptoglobin.

1. Arrange for transfer to an intensive care unit.

2. Reintubate and hyperventilate vigorously. Start with a minute volume of 12 - 14 litres per minute. Use the blood gases and end tidal CO_2 monitor as your guide. The arterial PCO_2 is roughly inversely proportional to the patient's minute volume.

3. Sedate the patient with morphine.

4. Commence the dantrolene infusion starting at 2 mg/kg and repeat this every 7 minutes until the muscle rigidity resolves. Give at least 6 mg/kg[9] but do not exceed 10 mg/kg.

5. Aggressively cool the patient with ice packs in the axillae and groin. Infuse cold but not iced solutions. Give 1 litre every 10 minutes for the first 30 minutes.

6. If the pH is less than 7.10 correct the acidosis with sodium bicarbonate 0.5-1.0 mmol/kg, and then recheck the blood gases and pH. It may be necessary to repeat the sodium bicarbonate at intervals.

7. Keep the arterial $PaCO_2$ between 35 - 45 mm Hg (4.6 - 5.9 kPa) by hyperventilating the patient.

8. Check electrolytes and treat hyperkalaemia with sodium bicarbonate, 50% glucose and insulin.

9. Treat arrhythmias with procainamide 100 mg intravenously over 5 minutes then 15 mg/kg until arrhythmia is controlled or up to 1000 mg or amiodorone 150 - 300 mg intravenously over 1 - 2 minutes followed by an infusion 5 mg/kg over 20 minutes. Do not use both procainamide and amiodorone as toxicity is enhanced. Avoid calcium channel blockers as these antagonise dantrolene.

10. To prevent myoglobin and haemoglobin from sludging up the kidneys, maintain the urine output over 1.5 ml/kg/hr

Late complications include: disseminated intravascular coagulopathy (DIC), acute renal failure, hyperkalaemia, hypocalcaemia, hypothermia, pulmonary oedema, cardiac failure, neurological sequelae, and continuing rahbdomyolysis.

THYROID STORM

Thyroid storm is a life threatening exacerbation of hyperthyroidism that typically occurs after an operation on the thyroid gland of a patient with inadequately treated thyrotoxicosis. It may occur in patients with unrecognized thyrotoxicosis. A large flush of thyroid hormone into the circulation causes a hypermetabolic state similar to malignant hyperthermia: hot flushed skin, sweating, tachycardia, atrial arrythmias, hypotension, pulmonary oedema, nausea, vomiting and perhaps diarrhoea. As the temperature rises, convulsions and coma will occur. The temperature will probably be in the region of 38 - 41°C. Females in their late 30s or 40s are the most susceptible. It usually occurs 8 - 16 hours after severe stress or an operation. It is more likely to be seen in recovery room if there has been preoperative stress which acutely raises thyroid hormone levels such as: anxiety, apprehension, iodine withdrawal, pain, trauma, or infection.

MANAGEMENT

What to monitor: blood pressure, pulse rate, ECG, core temperature, urine output, arterial blood gases, central venous pressure.

Laboratory: sodium, potassium, bicarbonate, creatinine, glucose, lactate, ketones, and blood gases.

TREATMENT

1. Support oxygen and fluid requirements and reduce the patient's temperature as outlined in the treatment of malignant hyperthermia.

2. Control arrhythmias with metoprolol 0.15 - 0.3 mg/kg intravenously every 10 minutes until tachycardia drops below a rate of 100 per minute.

3. Give propylthiouracil 12.5 mg/kg loading dose down a nasogastric tube; followed by 0.5 mg/kg every 8 hours.

4. Give sodium iodide 30 mg/kg intravenously. Theoretically this should not be given until the propylthiouracil has had time to reduce the iodine uptake by the thyroid gland. One hour after administration is sufficient.

5. Dexamethasone 4 mg or hydrocortisone 3 - 5 mg/kg intravenously will inhibit further thyroxine release. Adrenal insufficiency is a feature of thyroid and adrenergic storms.

HYPOGLYCAEMIA

Patients experience symptoms when the blood glucose concentration falls below 2.5 mmol/litre (30 - 45 mg/100ml) This may occur in:
- diabetes (see page 416);
- alcoholics (see page 410);
- neonates (see page 385);
- infants (see page 398).

Symptoms and signs are mostly those of excessive sympathetic discharge, these include:
- sweating;
- tachycardia;
- hypertension;
- confusion;
- restlessness;
- slurred voice;
- aggressive behaviour;
- obtunded mental state progressing to coma and convulsion;
- brain damage and death.

MANAGEMENT

What to monitor: blood pressure, pulse rate , ECG, urine output.
Laboratory: glucose, sodium, potassium, bicarbonate, creatinine, lactate, ketones.

1. Measure blood sugar with test strips or a glucose meter. To get accurate results, follow the maker's instructions exactly. Send blood for a formal laboratory measurement.
2. Treat hypoglycaemia if the blood glucose is less than 3 mmol/litre. Give 0.5 - 1ml/kg of glucose 50% intravenously into a large vein, and the patient will improve within minutes. This hypertonic glucose will damage veins unless titrated into a freely running infusion.

HYPERGLYCAEMIA (SEE DIABETES PAGE 416)

ACID BASE DISORDERS

Acid base physiology has a reputation for being difficult. To simplify it take the maths out. Here are the absolute basics, which are enough to solve most problems. Forget about pH and work in hydrogen ion concentrations just as you would for any other ion. Ask your laboratory to give blood gas results as hydrogen ion concentration as well as pH.

---

pH

pH is defined as the negative logarithm to base 10 of the hydrogen ion activity. It was introduced as a way of manipulating huge numbers of hydrogen ions; but the term and the concept usually confuse more than it enlightens. A hydrogen ion is just an ion, as are sodium and potassium. It has not been given special powers because it is described in terms of pH. Just as we think of sodium ions in millimols/litre, it is easy to think of hydrogen ions in nanomols/litre.

1 000 000 nanomols = 1 millimol.

Too much or too little hydrogen ion disrupts cellular metabolism.

Hydrogen ions are positively charged sub atomic particles. Many organic compounds, such as proteins, and lipids are polarized so that they have a more positive charge in one part of their molecule and a more negative charge on another part of the molecule. The balance between acids and bases in the body is important because hydrogen ions alter the 3-dimensional shape of all proteins, but especially *enzymes*. They do this by repelling positive charges and attracting negative charges on the enzyme molecule.

Enzymes are organic catalysts which facilitate biochemical reactions. Each enzyme has a very specific shape, and if it is bent by too much, or too little hydrogen ion then it will not function properly. This disrupts metabolic pathways.

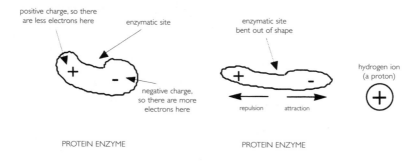

fig 9.2 How a hydrogen ion alters the shape and function of an enzyme

The body always compensates for an acidosis or alkalosis in an attempt to maintain a normal hydrogen ion level. To do this it either excretes or retains carbon dioxide through the lungs (*respiratory component*); or it uses the kidneys to excrete or retain bicarbonate and hydrogen ions (*metabolic component*).

Acids are substances that release hydrogen ions.
Bases are substances that accept or react with hydrogen ion.

The body hates alkalosis, but tolerates acidosis quite well. Mild to moderate acidosis, for a short time, improves tissue oxygenation. Severe alkalosis on the other hand can kill.

There are three chemicals which always adjust themselves to balance: carbon dioxide, hydrogen ion and bicarbonate ion. The balance is described by the Henderson equation.

Given good kidney and liver perfusion the normal body will sort itself out by manipulating bicarbonate, or carbon dioxide levels to restore the hydrogen ion concentration to normal. You may need to actively treat a hydrogen ion concentration at a 'cut off point' less than 25 nanomol/l (pH > 7.55) or greater than 80 nanomol/l (pH < 7.12). Initially just restore the levels to 'the cut off point' and allow the body to do the rest.

THE HENDERSON EQUATION

This equation simply says that if you know two of the values, you can calculate the third. The often quoted Henderson Hasselbach equation is derived by logarithmically converting the simple Henderson equation, but it is cumbersome and difficult to use in a clinical situation.

$$[H^+] = \frac{24\ PCO_2}{[HCO_3^-]}$$

where:

$[H^+]$ = hydrogen ion concentration in nanomols/litre.

PCO_2 = partial pressure of CO_2 in arterial blood measured in mmHg

$[HCO_3^-]$ = actual or measure bicarbonate ion concentration in millimol/litre

Do not use the standard bicarbonate for this value. You will need the actual bicarbonate ion concentration from a serum electrolyte analysis; you may need to ask the lab especially for this.

You can use this equation as a guide on how to use the ventilator to control PCO_2 and hence hydrogen ion concentration (pH). For example if a patient has an actual bicarbonate of 18 mmol/l, using the equation you can calculate that to achieve a normal hydrogen ion concentration (40 nm/l) you would need to adjust their ventilator to achieve a PCO_2 of 30 mmHg.

The equation is also useful to work out the effects of various components of an acid base disorder and the compensatory mechanisms.

Treat respiratory acidosis by improving ventilation. Treat metabolic acidosis by improving tissue perfusion and oxygenation.

ACIDAEMIA AND ACIDOSIS

The -aemias are what we measure in the blood, while the -oses are the effects in the tissues. The -aemias are can be affected by compensatory mechanisms. Thus a man with severe chronic bronchitis and a chronically raised $PaCO_2$, but a normal pH would have a chronic respiratory acidosis but no acidaemia.

Acidosis and alkalosis are further defined by what causes them. An excess or deficiency of carbon dioxide in the body results in a respiratory acidosis or a respiratory alkalosis; while an excess or deficiency of bicarbonate ion (HCO_3^-) results in a metabolic acidosis or alkalosis. The levels of carbon dioxide are controlled by the lungs, and the absolute levels of bicarbonate ion are controlled by the kidneys.

Respiratory causes of acid base disturbances.

Total body stores of carbon dioxide are about 120 litres. Normally the pressure exerted by this carbon dioxide in arterial blood is about 40 mmHg (5.3 kPa). If a patient hypoventilates and fails to excrete carbon the excess dioxide dissolves in the body water, releasing hydrogen ion (a strong acid) and bicarbonate ion (a weak base) causing a *respiratory acidosis*.

If the patient hyperventilates and carbon dioxide is blown off then there will be insufficient hydrogen ion and the patient will be said to have a *respiratory alkalosis*.

Common causes of respiratory acidosis in the recovery room are, those that cause the patient to hypoventilate, such as:

* excess opioids;
* inadequate reversal of muscle relaxants;
* uncommonly, drugs such as midazolam, or diazepam.

Respiratory alkalosis is uncommon in the recovery room, and is usually due to excessive hyperventilation during the anaesthetic. If a lot of carbon dioxide has been washed out of the body by excessive ventilation, it takes some time for the carbon dioxide to build up in the tissues again.

Another, but uncommon, cause of hypocarbia is *interstitial pulmonary oedema* which triggers the patient to hyperventilate. The causes of fluid collecting in the lung tissue as oedema include: fluid overload, cardiac failure, septicaemia, fat emboli, or early adult respiratory distress syndrome. These events result in reflex hyperventilation. The patient feels breathless, his respiratory rate rises and his $PaCO_2$ falls.

Metabolic causes of acid base disorders

If the liver fails to metabolize lactate, or the kidneys fail to excrete acids, a metabolic acidosis will occur. The causes are:

* hypoxia where lactic acid from anaerobic metabolism accumulates in the tissues faster than it can be metabolized by the liver;
* unstable diabetics where keto acids accumulate;
* serious sepsis where bacterial endotoxins have damaged the liver so it cannot metabolize organic acids;
* renal failure where the kidney cannot excrete acids.

Metabolic alkalosis is uncommon, and is usually due to severe preoperative potassium depletion, or the injudicious use of sodium bicarbonate. Occasionally it follows massive blood transfusion, as the liver is slow to metabolise sodium citrate, used as an anticoagulant in the stored blood, to bicarbonate.

Management of acid base disorders

What to monitor: blood pressure, pulse rate, ECG, urine output, temperature.

LABORATORY: pH, hydrogen ion concentration, PO_2, PCO_2, bicarbonate, sodium, potassium, chloride, creatinine, urea, actual bicarbonate, anion gap, lactate, glucose.

ACUTE OR CHRONIC DISORDER?

Disturbances can occur within minutes or hours, and these are known as acute disturbances. Others creep up slowly on the patient over days or weeks, and are known as chronic disturbances. Patients with acute disturbances either in the production or excretion of hydrogen ion tend to have an abnormal level of hydrogen ion (pH) in their plasma. Those with stable chronic disturbances have normal hydrogen ion concentrations, because the body always attempts to compensate to restore pH to normal levels in order to maintain the function of enzymes.

pH	HYDROGEN ION CONCENTRATION	EFFECT
6.80 - 7.00	160 - 100 nanomol/litre	life threatening acidosis
7.00 - 7.20	100 - 64 nanomol/litre	severe acidosis
7.20 - 7.30	64 - 50 nanomol/litre	moderate acidosis
7.30 - 7.35	50 - 45 nanomol/litre	mild acidosis
7.35 - 7.42	54 - 38 nanomol/litre	normal limits
7.42 - 7.50	38 - 32 nanomol/litre	mild alkalosis
7.50 - 7.55	32 - 38 nanomol/litre	moderate alkalosis
7.55 - 7.65	28 - 22 nanomol/litre	severe alkalosis
7.65 - 7.80	22 - 16 nanomol/litre	life threatening alkalosis

ACIDOSIS

Most acidaemia is caused by tissue hypoxia with excessive production of lactic acids.

This lactic acidosis is treated by improving tissue oxygenation. Depending on the cause, this includes: replacement of body fluids, support of cardiac output, correction of anaemia, and improvement of lung function, correction of electrolyte, and temperature disorders.

Ketoacidosis occurs in diabetics who have not had enough insulin. Insulin aids in the uptake of glucose into muscle, fat and heart. If insulin is absent these cells metabolize fat, instead of glucose, as their energy source. Large quantities of keto acids are produced which contribute to the metabolic acidosis. The excessive glucose is unable to get into cells. It remains in the blood stream to cause an *osmotic diuresis*, and as fluids are lost in the urine the patient becomes clinically shocked. This combination of events is life threatening.

Mild to moderate acidosis improves tissue blood flow and cardiac output, and improves tissue oxygen delivery. Enzyme systems do not begin to fail until the hydrogen ion concentration exceeds about 80 nanomols/l (pH < 7.12). Carefully consider the consequences before treating a metabolic acidosis until the hydrogen ion is greater than 80 nanomol/l (pH < 7.12) or there are signs of cardiac failure. The key to therapy is to improve tissue oxygenation and allow the body to correct the problem for itself. Occasionally, particularly in severe diabetic, ketoacidosis, or grave haemorrhagic shock you may need to give a small dose of bicarbonate slowly intravenously over 5 - 10 minutes. To prevent too rapid a change in hydrogen ion concentration, dilute 100 mls of 8.4% $NaHCO_3$ (100 mmol) in a 900 mls of 5% dextrose. Start with a dose of 150 mls of this mixture in an adult. Restore the hydrogen ion to about 75 nanomol/l (pH 7.15) and allow the body's homeostatic mechanisms to sort out the rest.

While metabolic acidosis may be corrected by sodium bicarbonate, a respiratory acidosis must be treated by removing carbon dioxide from the body. To do this you must improve the patient's ventilation.

ALKALOSIS

While acidosis is well tolerated, alkalosis is both dangerous and not well adjusted by body buffers. Postoperatively metabolic alkalosis is usually caused by excessive administration of sodium bicarbonate. Occasionally excessive vomiting with the loss of excessive hydrochloric acid, can cause a metabolic alkalosis.

Alkalosis causes major metabolic disorder:

- haemoglobin binds oxygen more firmly, so that it is not released readily to the tissues;
- body enzyme systems are disrupted;
- phosphate energy dependent pumps in the cells fail;
- cardiac arrhythmias occur;

- increased binding of calcium by proteins cause tetany and cardiac dysfunction;
- urinary potassium and chloride losses can rapidly cause potentially fatal hypokalaemia.

MANAGEMENT OF METABOLIC ALKALOSIS:

- If the pH is greater than 7.55, aim to increase the hydrogen ion concentration to 25 - 30 nanomol/l;
- Acetazolamide (Diamox®) can be used to prevent the kidney excreting hydrogen ion. Initial dose is 500 mg given slowly over 5 minutes;
- If the patient is haemolysing due to the alkalosis you may need to give 0.1M hydrochloric acid infused into a central vein.

SODIUM BICARBONATE

Sodium bicarbonate will correct an acidosis, but use it cautiously.

Disadvantages:

- It carries a large sodium load: 100 mls of 8.4% $NaHCO_3^-$ contains 100 mmol of Na^+. This osmotically drags water rapidly out of the intracellular volume. Once equilibrated it is equivalent to giving approximately 660 mls of normal saline. It is easy to saline overload your patient, and cause pulmonary oedema.
- It causes disequilibration of hydrogen ion across the blood brain barrier and may paradoxically increase the concentration of hydrogen ion in cerebrospinal fluid.
- It alters the shape of the haemoglobin molecules, so that it is reluctant to give up oxygen to the tissues. This may aggravate tissue hypoxia in a shocked patient.
- Renal excretion of the bicarbonate is very slow.

HOW TO INTERPRET ARTERIAL BLOOD GASES

There are five steps:

STEP 1: What is the hydrogen ion concentration (H^+) ?
If [H+] > 45 nanomol/l (pH< 7.35) the patient has an acidaemia
If [H+] < 35 nanomol/l (pH > 7.42) the patient has an alkalaemia

STEP 2: What is the arterial PaO2 ?
If PaO_2 < 60 mmHg (7.9 kPa) then the patient is hypoxaemic.
If PaO_2 < 35 mmHg (4.6 kPa) then the patient is dying.

STEP 3: What is the arterial $PaCO_2$?

If $PaCO_2$ < 35 mmHg (4.6 kPa) then the patient is hyperventilating.

If $PaCO_2$ > 45 mmHg (5.5 kPa) then the patient is hypoventilating.

STEP 4: What is the actual bicarbonate?

If it is nearly normal then there is a respiratory component.

If it is abnormal then there is a metabolic component.

STEP 5: Does the patient have a pulmonary shunt?

This can be roughly determined by assuming that if a patient is hypoxic while receiving supplemental oxygen then a shunt is present. See also page 299.

CASE STUDY

Edith, aged 35, has had a severe post partum haemorrhage, and is admitted to the recovery room shocked with a blood pressure of 100/60, and a pulse rate of 140. Her perfusion status is poor. Blood gases reveal pH 7.20, PaO_2 40 mmHg on 100% oxygen, $PaCO_2$ 20 mmHg, HCO_3- 7.5 mmol/l. Her core temperature is 36°C.

ANALYSIS: Edith is acidaemic (pH of 7.20) and hypoxaemic (PaO_2 of 40 mmHg) breathing 100% oxygen. She is hyperventilating ($PaCO_2$ of 20 mmHg). The actual bicarbonate of 7.5 mmol/l reveals a severe metabolic acidosis. The fact that she is hypoxaemic on 100% oxygen shows she has a large shunt in her lungs with a lot of blood not being oxygenated because it is bypassing oxygenated alveoli.

NORMAL VALUES FOR BLOOD GASES		
pH	7.35 7.42	[H+] 35-45 nanomol/l
PaO_2	85 - 100 mmHg	(11.0 - 13.1 kPa) while breathing air
$PaCO_2$	37 - 42 mmHg(4.9 -5.5 kPa)	
HCO_3-	22 - 25 millimol/l	

Whenever you quote the arterial PaO_2 you must state also what per cent oxygen the patient is breathing, otherwise the result is meaningless.

Alpha stat

If you need to measure the pH in a hypothermic patient, take the arterial blood and measure the blood gases as you would for a normal patient; that is at 37°C. Assess the acid/base status as you would if the patient was at a normal temperature. There is no need to try the complex calculations suggested by some of the earlier texts. As with all acidosis, be reluctant to treat it unless you can justify it; but avoid alkalosis. Remember, even in hypothermic conditions, acidosis is better tolerated than alkalosis. The oxygen dissociation curve is already moved to the left by the hypothermia and an alkalosis will make the red cells even more reluctant to release oxygen this will aggravate tissue hypoxia.

GLOSSARY

ANION GAP: The anion gap is the difference between the measured cations (Na^+, K^+) and the measured anions (HCO_3^-, Cl^-) in the blood. It is useful to detect an established alkalosis or acidosis.

BUFFER: A buffer is a substance that soaks up hydrogen ions (like a sponge), or releases them so that their concentration in the surrounding tissue fluid remains constant. Bicarbonate ion is one of the most important hydrogen ion buffers in the extracellular fluid, while haemoglobin is the major buffer in the circulation.

STANDARD BICARBONATE: This is calculated from the Henderson equation. It assumes that the carbon dioxide concentration is 40 mmHg which it would be if the there was absolutely nothing wrong with the patient's ventilation. By knowing the hydrogen ion concentration the bicarbonate level can be calculated. This bicarbonate level is called the standard bicarbonate. If the standard bicarbonate level is abnormal this indicates a metabolic disturbance.

BASE EXCESS/DEFICIT: Sometimes the laboratory will give a value for base excess/deficit. This is an indicator of the amount of sodium bicarbonate needed to correct the acid base disorder and restore the pH to normal. It is seldom used these days, although some physicians still regard it important.

To make a diagnosis in an acid base disorder you must not only analyse the blood gas results, but you need to know what has happened to the patient.

---

1. Kurz A, Sessler DL, Lenhart R: (1996) N Eng J Med, 334: 1209-15.
2. Frank SM, Beattie C, et al. (1993) Anaesthesiology, 78: 468-76.
3. Frank SM, Higgens MS, et al. (1995) Anaesthesiology, 82: 83-93.
4. Servarino FB, Johnson MD, et al. (1989) Anaesthesia and Analgesia, 68: 530-3.
5. Motamed S, Klubein K, et al. (1998) Anaesthesiology, 88: 1211-8.
6. Loning PE, (1986) Acta Anaesthesiology Scandinavia, 30: 601-13.
7. Greenberg C,(1990) Anaesthesiology Clinics, Vol 8 No 2, 377-97.
8. Ording H. (1985) Anesthesia and Analgesia, 64:700 - 704.
9. Cain AG, Bell AD, (1989) Anaesthesia and Intensive Care, 17: 500-9.

10. Physiology of Pain

In recent years enormous advances have been made in our understanding of the complex physiological, biochemical, pharmacological and psychological mechanisms involved with pain. The physiology is briefly outlined here in enough detail to enable you to manage pain more effectively. If you do not understand what a word means, then check it in the glossary at the end of the chapter.

Pain is a subjective phenomenon not easily described in words, and even less easily measured. For instance your splitting headache is not necessarily the same as my pounding headache. How can I explain to you what I am experiencing and how much it hurts? This problem mostly remains unsolved.

Pain has survival value! It is an unpleasant sensation and emotion that helps prevents further injury. A widely accepted definition of pain is: "a sensory and emotional experience from actual or potential tissue damage, or described in terms of such damage".[1] In more practical terms it is what the patients says hurts, when the patient says it hurts.

The way we perceive pain involves two inputs, the injury that hurts (*noxious stimuli*) and the anxiety or fear (*affective feelings*) associated with this. These interact in a complex way to form the sensation of pain.

If you knocked your hand against an object, then you would probably not feel very anxious about it. You know the pain will eventually go away and the consequences are unlikely to be great. This logical analysis involves: experience, memory and foresight. However if you suddenly woke in the night with a terrible pain in your abdomen, you would be alarmed, and your physiological and psychological reaction would be quite different.

Emotional response to pain can be harmful, with feelings ranging through apprehension, fear even terror. Sincere, honest reassurance and skilled nursing can reduce this factor substantially. Emotional stress activates the sympathetic nervous system; blood pressure rises, the heart beats faster and more forcibly, and the brain becomes super-aware of what is happening to the body. If pain or emotional stress remains untreated cortisol is secreted from the adrenal gland in sufficient quantities to jeopardize wound healing and predispose to infection.

Uncontrolled pain can delay healing,
and increase the risk of infection.

The sensation of pain is carried by sensory nerves to the central nervous system (spinal cord and brain) where it is integrated, and modified to produce a co-ordinated response and remembered for later analysis. This involves a series of three primary neurones. *First order neurones* have their receptors in tissues and their cell bodies in the spinal ganglion. They pass the messages through proximal extensions to the substantia gelatinosa. These link with *second order neurones* that have their cell bodies in the brain or brainstem. *Third order neurones* pass on information from second order neurones to cortical and subcortical areas.

The cortical areas analyse the conscious interpretation of pain. Where does it hurt? How much does it hurt? Have I felt it before? Am I in danger? And so on. The sub-cortical areas recruit background responses such as: increase in blood pressure, heart rate, sweating, and size of the pupils.

Nocioceptors and first order neurones

The *pain receptors* in the tissue are called *nocioceptors*. Under the microscope tissue nocioceptors are not distinctly identifiable structures, but appear as a woven network of free nerve endings distributed through the tissues and around blood vessels. Nocioceptors respond to painful stimuli caused by heat, mechanical trauma, or substances released from injured tissues (including histamine, prostaglandins, and bradykinin). What you feel depends on the type of sensory ending that is stimulated, and its connections to the spinal cord and the brain.

It takes a stimulus, such as a burn, stab, or bite of enough strength (*threshold potential*) to trigger a response; in contrast a signal of insufficient strength is said to be *subthreshold*. Mosquito bites may be subthreshold and will pass unnoticed, whereas dog bites certainly exceed the threshold potential and you will feel it.

Nocioceptors fire more easily (at a lower threshold) if they are exposed to repeated high intensity stimulation. This process is called *sensitization*. If you have ever been sunburnt you will understand sensitization.

The cell bodies of first order sensory neurones are in the dorsal root ganglion. Their axons pass peripherally to the tissues and centrally to the spinal cord.

If you have ever burnt your hand on something hot you may, with dispassionate analysis, have noticed the two sorts of pain. First, a fast pain that only lasts a short time and pricks, stabs or lances. It is carried by large myelinated A delta fibres. Second, a slow pain that occurs after the fast pain which is duller and lasts much longer. It is carried by small unmyelinated C fibres.

AN EXPERIMENT

Without having to burn yourself, you can demonstrate the fast (A delta fibres) and slow (C fibres) neuronal transmission by taking your Achilles tendon at the back of your heel between your thumb and forefinger and abrubtly squeezing it hard. You will feel the two pains: the first a sharp, well localised and brief pain, and a moment later the second; which is deep, diffuse, persistent and uncomfortable.

When a pain exceeds a threshold level the impulse is carried to the *substantia gelatinosa*. Here the quality of the pain and its intensity is analysed. If the pain is severe you will pull your limb away *(reflex withdrawal)* about 0.8 seconds before you consciously know anything has happened, and optimistically before damage has occurred. This reflex withdrawal involves principally two nerves: the sensory nerve and a motor nerve which communicate in the substantia gelatinosa.

Second order neurones

Meanwhile some of the impulses are relayed in second order neurones that spread out in the spinal cord to carry information to the brain. Some pass up to the thalamus in easily identifiable contralateral *spinothalamic tracts*. Other impulses enter the diffuse *spinoreticular tracts* that connect with the *vital centres* in the brain stem. Vital centres control innate responses such as heart rate and blood pressure, sweating, pupil size, respiratory rate and depth, and nausea and vomiting.

The *spinothalamic* tracts are the ascending *(afferent)* second order spinal pathways for pain. In the spinal cord the spinothalamic tract divides into the *neospinothalamic tract* laterally and the *paleospinothalamic tract* medially. The neospinothalamic tract passes up the spinal cord to the posterior thalamus and is associated with location, duration and intensity of pain. The paleothalamic tract sends its fibres to the medial thalamus and is associated with the autonomic and emotional aspects of pain.

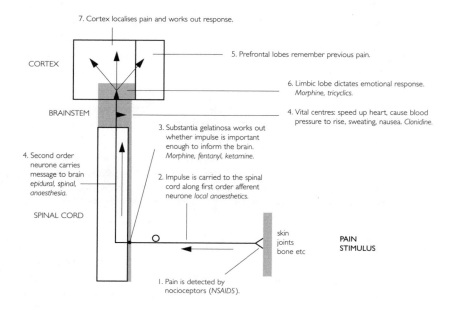

7. Cortex localises pain and works out response.

CORTEX

5. Prefrontal lobes remember previous pain.

6. Limbic lobe dictates emotional response.
Morphine, tricyclics.

BRAINSTEM

4. Vital centres: speed up heart, cause blood
pressure to rise, sweating, nausea. *Clonidine.*

3. Substantia gelatinosa works out
whether impulse is important
enough to inform the brain.
Morphine, fentanyl, ketamine.

4. Second order
neurone carries
message to brain
epidural, spinal,
anaesthesia.

2. Impulse is carried to the spinal
cord along first order afferent
neurone *local anaesthetics.*

SPINAL CORD

skin
joints
bone etc

PAIN
STIMULUS

1. Pain is detected by
nocioceptors (*NSAIDS*).

fig 10.1 Afferent pain pathways and drugs blocking them

Third order neurones

In the medial thalamus the quality of the pain touches consciousness for
the first time, and we begin to appreciate what is happening. Messages from
the medial thalamus pass on through third order neurones to the prefrontal
lobes (foresight and previous experience) and the limbic lobe (emotion)
where we analyse the memory and emotional component of the pain. In
other words "I have felt this before, it hurts - it is a burn".

Meanwhile messages from the lateral thalamus pass on to the post central
gyri in the sensory cortex where we integrate all the messages to determine
that "my left hand is on fire". Now that we know that our hand is burning,
an appropriate response can be organized.

PAIN CAN BE MODIFIED

Sometimes we need to briefly cope with, or even ignore pain. The *periaqueductal*
grey matter in the *reticular formation* of the brainstem monitors emergency

situations; and if roused inhibits pain passing to the brain. This is why men injured in war, or on the football field, often do not feel much pain until after the drama is over. In effect a life threatening event induces a shot of spinal opioid. This enables you to get away from danger without being limited by pain. This process is called *stimulation produced analgesia*.

Consider walking bare foot along a path. You would expect a number of jabs and pricks on the soles of your feet. The substantia gelatinosa distinguishes if the pain you are feeling is a small pebble, or a sharp thorn, even before you are aware of it. If the pain exceeds a threshold determined by the periaqeductal grey matter then the substantia gelatinosa will pass an impulse directly to the anterior horn initiating a reflex withdrawal. Although you are prepared for small pricks on the sole of your foot while walking along a stony path, the same intensity prick while lying in bed at night would evoke an entirely different response. It is in the spinal cord that the central nervous system adjusts the intensity of pain to which it will respond. To do this it uses inhibitory opioid receptors.

To some degree you can consciously override a response to pain. Consider the act of making a grab to pull a plug out of a sink of hot water. The pain threshold will be exceeded, but you can anticipate the degree of expected pain, and for a moment consciously override the reflex withdrawal.

Consider too, you pick up Aunty Jack's prized antique porcelain tea pot. It is hot. Your frontal lobes (foresight) integrating with your cortex (awareness) will override your reflex arcs, because it had previously, but not necessarily consciously, anticipated the awful consequences of dropping it.

All these responses which hinder the passage of pain impulses to the brain, are in part modulated through inhibitory opioid receptors in the substantia gelatinosa. Opioids given, either as part of epidural or spinal anaesthesia, mimic this process and impede the passage of pain impulses to the brain.

Plasticity and wind-up
Severe on going pain changes the shape and function of sensory nerves. The nocioceptive neurones increase the number of peripheral receptors, establish new contacts with other cells, and increase the number of receptors in the post synaptic endplates. In the central nervous system nerve cells establish new connections, allow others to lapse, and start producing peptide neurotransmitters (*glutamate, aspartate and substance P*). This adaptive process is called plasticity. With prolonged painful stimuli plasticity can induce a hyperexcitable state called *wind-up*.

How does plasticity occur? With severe pain, calcium channels in the cell membrane open, and calcium ions floods in to the cell to directly stimulate certain genes. These genes then program the microsomes to produce other neuropeptide transmitters, new receptors sites and protein pumps. With all this new equipment the cell now responds massively to impulses that previously would have passed unnoticed. One class of the ion channel that opens to allow calcium ion to pour in is called the NMDA (N-methyl D-aspartate) channels. This is blocked by ketamine, and may be the reason that this drug could be effective in preventing the onset of chronic pain.

Unrelieved long lasting uncontrolled severe pain may cause cell death of some of the dorsal horn neurones. Once this happens, pain becomes entrenched as chronic pain, and will not readily respond to analgesics. This tragedy may happen within a couple of days if the patient has severe pain that is not adequately relieved.

Uncontrolled pain
may cause problems with chronic pain.

GLOSSARY

Affective feelings are those that produce a change in the way you behave.

Afferent is an adjective than describes something to passing towards something else.

Analgesia is the absence of pain in response to stimulation that would normally be painful.

Aspartate is a aminoacid derivative used in the central nervous system as a neurotransmitter.

Calcium channels are gates in the cell membrane through which calcium ions can flow.

Efferent is an adjective that describes something passing away from something else.

Endorphins are a group of naturally occurring chemical compounds synthesized in the body that interact with opioid receptors in the central and peripheral nervous systems.

Endogenous is an adjective that describes something coming from within the body.

Exogenous is an adjective that describes something coming from outside the body.

Genes store the genetic information for the production of proteins and other substances is the cell. They contain the genetic blue print in the form of DNA.

Glutamate is a aminoacid derivative which is used in the central nervous system as a neurotransmitter.

Microsomes are the protein factories in the cells which make structural proteins and enzymes. Calcium channels are made on the microsomes and then transported to the cell membrane where they are installed.

Neo is a prefix meaning 'new'. The neospinothalamic tracts refer to the evolutionary newer form of the spinothalamic tract.

Neuropathic pain arises from damage to nerves along some part of their pathway from their origin in the periphery to their integration in the central nervous system. It is caused by nerve damage: compression, inflammation or direct trauma anywhere along the pain pathway.

Nocioceptor is a receptor preferentially sensitive to a noxious stimulus or to a stimulus which would become noxious if prolonged.

Nocioception is the ability to perceive noxious stimuli.

Nocioceptive pain is pain that arises from tissue trauma.

Nociceptors are receptors for pain.

Noxious stimulus is one that is damaging to normal tissues.

Opioid includes a diverse groups of natural and semisynthetic alkaloid derivatives of opium, and its synthetic analogues. This definition includes endogenous peptides that interact with opioid receptors.

Palaeo is a prefix meaning 'old'. The palaeospinothalamic tracts refers to the evolutionary older form of the spinothalamic tracts.

Plasticity is the ability of a nerve cell to redesign itself to adapt to new situations.

Receptor is a cell or part of a cell which is specialized to detect a stimulus or change in its environment, and to initiate the transmission of an impulse through a sensory nerve.

Reflex is an automatic response to a stimulus. It cannot be controlled by conscious effort. The same stimulus always produces the same response.

Rexed lamina are layers of nerve cell synapses found in the substantia gelatinosa of the spinal cord's dorsal horn.

Sensitization is a process that results in acute awareness of a stimulus.

Somatic pain comes from superficial structures such as muscles, and skin and is perceived through the spinal nerves. It is described as sharp, well localized, and can be usually located with one finger.

Spino-thalamic tracts are nerves passing from the spinal cord to the thalamus in the brain.

Substance P is a peptide which is released from injured tissue. The P is an abbreviation for 'pain'.

Substantia gelatinosa is part of the dorsal horn in the spinal cord where first order sensory nerve cells synapse with the second order nerve cells passing to the brain. It is divided into layers called the Rexed lamina. It works as a gate directing impulses either to the brain or to reflex arcs.

Threshold potential is a the level of stimulus at which something becomes perceivable.

Visceral pain comes from deep structures such as the gastrointestinal tract, pancreas, visceral pleura and heart. It is difficult to localize with one finger and described in terms as dull, aching, nauseating, or boring.

Wind-up is the process by which a nerve cell becomes far more sensitive to stimuli that would previously not have had much effect.

1. Merskey H, Albe-Fessard DG, *et al.* (1979). *Pain* 6:249-5.

11. PAIN MANAGEMENT

Pain in the recovery room is distressing and harmful. Emerging from anaesthesia in agony is a horrible experience. The intensity of pain can be mild, moderate or severe; but once we attempt further analysis the meanings of words begin to fail us. Enormous efforts have gone into devising various pain scales, and clever means of assessing pain, despite this, pain control is not difficult. If you want to know whether your patient is in pain, ask him; and believe what he says. Once you have established your patient is in pain then treat it until the patient says he is comfortable.

Pain is what the patient says hurts,
when the patient says it hurts.

Acute pain is easy to control, but the planning and management of the analgesic regime is frequently delegated to an inexperienced member of the surgical team. Too often doctors and nurses do not understand the properties of the analgesic drugs, and hold inaccurate, but commonly, held prejudices about their use.[1] In particular the experience, background, and biases of the staff working in recovery room determine their attitudes towards, and consequently their management of, acute pain.[2]

The recovery room is the logical place to organize a regime for postoperative analgesia, and to institute a plan for continuing pain relief in the ward. When the patient arrives in recovery room, check the notes and anaesthetic chart and ask the following questions.
• Has the patient received opioids before, or during his operation?
• Have NSAIDs been given?
• Has there been a regional technique?

Collate this information with your assessment of how much pain the patient is in. Make sure that written orders for postoperative pain relief in the ward are in line with what has already been given. Is this going to give him adequate pain relief for the rest of the day and overnight? Beware of an order for large incremental doses of an opioid in a small or elderly patient. An elderly patient who has already received large doses of opioids in theatre will not tolerate further large doses in the ward. Discuss these concerns with the prescribing doctor and have them modified if necessary.

Risks of Uncontrolled Pain

Uncontrolled pain is harmful[3] because it may:
- set up a pathway for chronic pain;
- increase the postoperative stress response, with greatly increased cortisol secretion. This delays wound healing, and predisposes to infection;[4]
- cause the patient to become restless. This increases oxygen consumption; which in turn increases cardiac work and cardiac oxygen consumption;
- demoralize the patient, disrupt sleep, and cause distressing anxiety and despair;
- increase the blood pressure, with the risk of precipitating cardiac ischaemia;
- decrease hepatic and renal blood flow, delaying the metabolism and excretion of drugs, and promoting fluid retention;
- prevent the patient from taking deep breaths and coughing, especially following thoracic, or upper abdominal operations. This increases the risk of postoperative sputum retention and pneumonia;
- discourage the patient from moving his legs. If blood flow through the legs slows the venous stasis contributes to the formation of deep vein thrombi, and pulmonary embolism;
- increase metabolic rate, protein breakdown, and the catabolic effects of injury;
- contributes to postoperative nausea and vomiting;
- delay the return of normal bowel function;
- after Caesarean section, a mother's pain may impair the bonding with her new born child.[5]

Those at greatest risk from under treated pain are: frail patients, those with heart or lung disease, those undergoing major procedures such as aortic, abdominal, or major orthopaedic surgery, the very young, and the very old.

Factors Affecting the Patient's Pain

The severity of acute pain is determined by the incision and the types of surgery. Long incisions that cut through muscles, bones and nerves, for example thoracic and abdominal surgery, are more painful than operations requiring short incisions. This is one of the reasons for laparascopic surgery becoming so popular. Orthopaedic, facio-maxillary, and perineal operations are also painful. Sites where skin has been split off for grafting are surprisingly distressing.

PERCEPTION OF PAIN

How patients perceive pain is complex and involves both physical and psychological factors. Pain is always subjective, that is – it depends on the patient's interpretation of what he is feeling. The experience of acute pain is influenced by the stimuli from tissue damage, memory of previous pain, and psychological factors, predominantly anxiety.

Individuals, also vary in their response to pain. At their core it is probable that most individuals feel pain in a equivalent way, they just react to it differently. Some patients are more stoic than others, others are less fearful. Older people often do not complain of pain as much as the young, despite being equally affected by it. There may also be complex psychosocial and environmental factors involved in how the patient interprets pain. This is determined by their expectations, what is acceptable in their social group and their willingness to tolerate pain. Some societies expect a stiff upper lip, while in others it is acceptable to scream your head off.

People vary in their response to analgesics, and young healthy patients usually require higher doses than older people, and people from Asia have been shown to require less opioids than Caucasians.[6] There is an unreasonable, but common misconception that modern surgery is absolutely pain free; and consequently patients are distressed to wake in pain if they do not expect it.

Pain is likely to be less distressing if the patient:
• expects pain;
• knows it is only temporary;
• feels it is less severe than expected;
• is not anxious about the outcome of the surgery;
• has been taught relaxation techniques before surgery.

Pain control is likely to be good if the staff:
• understand the pharmacology of the drugs they are using;
• do not consider pain to be a psychological weakness;
• use pre-emptive analgesia;
• are aware that pain tolerance varies from patient to patient;
• do not fear respiratory depression or hypotension;
• are not anxious that the patient will become addicted or dependent on opioids.

Immediate Control of Pain in the Recovery Room

A well planned postoperative analgesic regime starts before surgery during the preoperative workup. Staff should discuss with the patient:

- the amount of pain to be expected;
- how long it is likely to last;
- management options including patient controlled analgesia if that is to be offered.

Plan the patient's pain control before surgery.

Forewarning the patient instils confidence and helps eliminate unspoken fears. Do not wait to do this when the patient is admitted to the recovery room because, understandably, it is almost impossible to gain the confidence or co-operation of a patient who wakes in unexpected pain.

CONCEPTS

- Pain is easier to prevent than treat, so start the regime before the pain becomes established. This prophylactic approach is called *pre-emptive analgesia*.
- Attack the pain at more than one point in its path from the tissues to its perception in the brain. This is the basis of *multimodal analgesia*.
- Treat both the hurt (physiological) component and the fear (emotional) component of the pain.
- Uncontrolled severe *acute pain* readily progresses becoming uncontrollable *chronic pain*. This is a disaster.

THE FIVE STEPS IN PAIN MANAGEMENT ARE:

1. **C**ause of the pain?;

2. **A**ssess the amount of pain;

3. **R**eassure and comfort the patient;

4. **E**ffective and appropriate analgesia?;

5. **R**e-assess.

CAUSE OF THE PAIN

Not all postoperative pain is be due to surgery. The pain might be coming from a site well away from the operation. Ask the patient, 'Where does it hurt?'. Do not give analgesia until you are sure what is causing the pain. Consider non-surgical causes of pain such as:

- full bladder;
- bladder spasm;
- sore throat;
- headache;
- myocardial ischaemia or infarction;
- pressure on peripheral nerves during the operation;
- stretched ligaments due to poor positioning on the operating table;
- tight bandages or plasters.

ASSESS PAIN

It is useful to assess both pain and anxiety independently of each other. Subjectively, it is easy to assess pain; just ask the patient, and believe what he says. Objectively, it is difficult to measure pain because there are almost no physical signs of pain. Pain may cause the patient to complain, cry, become agitated or restless. Always exclude hypoxia as a cause of confusion, agitation and restlessness. Severe pain may cause crying, splinting, grimacing hypertension, tachycardia and increased respiratory rate. Agonizing pain can cause bradycardia, hypotension, nausea, vomiting, sweating, dilated pupils and pallor. One hopes that patients in recovery room never reach such levels of pain.

Your unit may wish to use a scoring system for measuring pain.

Patients report that the most useful way of scoring pain in an adult is the *visual analogue pain scale* (VAPS). This is a 10 cm long line drawn on a piece of paper. One end of the line is labelled "the worst possible pain" and the other end "no pain".

Various other scoring systems have been devised. Some of these are verbal and rely on a graduation of words, such as: excruciating, agonizing, intolerable, unbearable, awful, distressing, miserable, distracting, unpleasant, uncomfortable, tolerable, bearable. Using such a scale requires a good command of English, which in our experience, is not reliably attained in a patient emerging from a general anaesthetic.

Other pain scales use a 1 - 5, or even a 1 - 10 point scale. 1 = no pain, 2 = mild pain, 3 = moderate pain, 4 = severe pain, 5 = unbearable pain. In the early postoperative phase, many patients who are sedated from anaesthetic drugs, and distracted by other unfamiliar sensations, find these scales confusing to use. If you do elect to use them then aim for a pain score of 2 or less on the 1 to 5 scale; or less than 4 on the 1 to 10 scale.

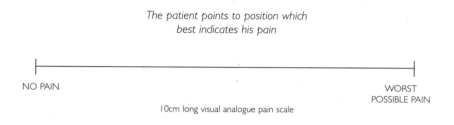

The patient points to position which best indicates his pain

NO PAIN   WORST
                                                                    POSSIBLE PAIN

10cm long visual analogue pain scale

fig 11.1 Visual Analogue Pain Scale (VAPS)

It is particularly difficult to assess pain in children, and no single test works every time. Before the age of 8 - 10 years children have difficulty with abstract thought, so even under ideal conditions numerical pain assessment scores are useless. Children over the age of seven can sometimes co-operate with visual analogues scales. Sometimes a series of five stylized faces showing increments of expressions for the increasing degree of pain are used. At one end the face is smiling and happy and at the other end agonised and crying. In some countries we have found that children from a village are unable to even recognise these drawings as faces! Furthermore it doesn't take a three year old long to realize if he points to a happy face he can avoid a feared injection, because he is unable to associate the injection with pain relief which takes effect some time later. Another way for measuring pain in older children is to use the Hester Blocks - these are five painted wooden blocks, each representing a "piece of pain". Ask the child how many pieces of pain he has.

Do not wake drowsy patients to ask them how much pain they have.

Children over the age of two will tell you it hurts and where it hurts. Toddlers express pain in more complex ways by rubbing the affected part, kicking, hitting, biting in an attempt to escape the situation. They also will cry and seek comfort from someone they trust. There is overwhelming evidence that pain is felt by, and damages neonates.[7] New born infants can mount a neurohumoral response to pain that is quantitatively greater than adults.[8] Severe stimulus, such as circumcision without anaesthesia, disturbs bonding, disrupts feeding patterns, and causes behavioural changes that persist from days to weeks.[9] Diagnosing pain in infants postoperatively is easy if they cry, but they may be too weak to do so. Look for a furrowed brow, flared nasal openings, and an open mouth.

REASSURE THE PATIENT

Anxiety is a major factor in the perception of pain. Giving patients information before their operation about what is going to happen during and after their operation substantially reduces anxiety.

A little explanation can
avoid a lot of analgesic drug.

A patient worried about whether his cancer has spread is far more likely to focus on the site of the surgery, than one who is undergoing a more benign operation.

Almost all patients, at or beyond middle age, have an understandable fear of cancer. A simple explanation of the cause of their pain, and reassurance "that everything has gone well" will often alleviate the patient's anxiety. Cuddle crying children, wrap them warmly and firmly in blankets and if possible let one of their parents come in to recovery room to be with them.

EFFECTIVE AND APPROPRIATE ANALGESIA

The two usual ways to control pain in the recovery room are:
• parenteral drugs;
• regional or local anaesthetics.

In the recovery room intravenous administration is preferable. The absorption of drugs after intramuscular injection can be unpredictable and giving analgesics by mouth requires the patient to drink and swallow. Drugs and regional techniques used for analgesia are discussed later in the chapter.

REASSESS

Do not send patients back to the ward in pain. If pain control is adequate the patient should be able to move easily about the trolley or bed, take deep breaths, cough effectively and should feel comfortable in themselves. Record your assessment of pain in the notes before the patient leaves the recovery room.

DAY SURGERY PATIENTS

In many hospitals more than half of elective surgery is done as day surgery. These patients have only a few hours before their care is handed over to their relatives. With so little time available it is essential to educate the patient, and have a plan for pain control in place before the surgery commences. They should have a prescription or a few tablets of oral analgesic to take home with them (see also chapter 11).

USING DRUGS FOR PAIN RELIEF

There are four principal groups of drugs used for pain relief:
• opioids. Including patient controlled analgesia (PCA);
• non-steroidal anti-inflammatory drugs;
• adjuvant drugs.

Since control of pain is a major objective of immediate postoperative care, the more familiar you are with these drugs, the better you will use them.

PHARMACOLOGY OF THE OPIOIDS

Opioid analgesics include: morphine, diamorphine, pethidine, fentanyl, phenoperidine, codeine, methadone, and buprenorphine.

The ones you will be most familiar with are morphine, pethidine and fentanyl. The opioids have a number of common properties, but also some important differences.

EQUIVALENT ANALGESIC DOSES

Morphine 10 mg   = pethidine 100 mg;
                                 = papaveretum 20 mg;
                                 = diamorphine 5 mg;
                                 = fentanyl 100 micrograms;
                                 = phenoperidine 2 mg;
                                 = methadone 10 mg.

Analgesia

Opioids give moderate to good analgesia. They are more effective against constant dull visceral pain, than sharp intermittent pain. Patients often say that they still feel the pain, but that it doesn't hurt any more. Anaesthetists have long known that once pain is established it takes far more opioid to relieve it, than if it is given before the pain starts. This observation is the basis for *pre-emptive analgesia*. The effective dose varies greatly from patient to patient, and may be as much as four-fold in any particular age group. This variation can be due, in part, to its effect in suppressing anxiety, rather than a simple quantitative suppression of pain.

RESPIRATORY DEPRESSION

Opioids diminish the desire to breathe. A patient affected by an opioid can hold his breath until he becomes quite cyanosed. Opioids directly suppress the CO_2 receptors in the respiratory centre in the medulla. Patients may hypoventilate, and slow their breathing to a rate of 8 breath per minute, or less. On arriving in the recovery room many patients, although rousable, seem to forget to breathe, but will take a deep breath when reminded. This phenomenon is called *Ondine's Curse**. In a patient affected this way, for a short time, you may need to remind him to take each breath. It is not usually necessary to give an opioid antagonist such as naloxone.

Respiratory depression is more likely in the following groups:

- acute drug or alcohol intoxication;
- asthmatics;
- diabetics;
- heroin addicts;
- elderly;
- frail and feeble;
- heart failure;
- intercurrent lung disease;
- liver disease;
- neonates;
- neuromuscular diseases;
- obesity.

Reduce the dose of opioid, and lengthen the interval between doses. Respiratory depression, if it is going to occur, takes place within three minutes of giving intravenous opioid. Stay with the patient and observe him closely for this period of time.

Opioids reduce the respiratory centre's response to a rising carbon dioxide level. They:

- decrease respiratory rate, or;
- decrease tidal volume, or both;
- decrease response to hypoxia;
- alter breathing patterns ranging from periodic breathing through to apnoea.

With respiratory depression, the $PaCO_2$ rises. This causes:

- raised intracranial pressure;

*Ondine's Curse
In legend, Ondine was a water nymph, who laid a curse on her wayward lover so that he would have to remember to breathe. When he eventually fell asleep, he died.

- drowsiness;
- excessive secretion of catecholamines causing sweating;
- peripheral vasodilation;
- hyperglycaemia;
- respiratory acidosis.

The rising carbon dioxide levels bubbling into the lungs displace oxygen in the alveolae. If you are using an opioid then give supplemental oxygen to keep the oximeter reading at or above 97 per cent.

If you have used an opioid for analgesia,
give supplemental oxygen.

If you have given an opioid within the last hour, send the patients back to the ward on an inspired concentration of at least 35% oxygen.

CLASSIFICATION OF OPIOIDS

Endorphins are a group of naturally occurring opioid peptides synthesized in the central nervous system. These are released in response to pain and latch onto opioid receptors on nerves in the spinal cord and brain, to modify the awareness, and response to pain. The opioids also interact with the opioid receptors, and mimic the effects of the endorphins. In the brain opioid receptors can be found in the periaqueductal grey matter, the limbic system, medial thalamic nuclei, and the area postrema. In the spinal cord they are found in the sustantia gelatinosa. They are also found in peripheral nerve ganglia, adrenal medulla, and throughout the gut.

The opioids can be classified in a long series depending on how they act on the opioid receptors. There are three main groups: mu, delta and kappa. The following are generally accepted: mu_1, mu_2, $delta_1$, $delta_2$, $kappa_1$, $kappa_2$. It is the mu (μ) receptor or morphine receptor which is the main mediator of pain relief. Unfortunately this is also one of the receptors involved in respiratory depression. The delta receptor in the chemotrigger receptor zone in the medulla that is involved with vomiting.

Cardiovascular effects

Opioids do not significantly alter a stable, well perfused patient's blood pressure. If they do, then look for another reason. It may be simply because the opioids have reduced the sympathetic response to pain; but if there is a large fall in blood pressure then look for other causes such as: hypovolaemia, hypoxia, cardiac failure, septicaemia or interaction with other drugs. Sometimes opioid analgesia is withheld because of the fear that it will drop the blood pressure. Even sick patients tolerate small doses of morphine given slowly intravenously.

The opioids do not cause hypotension
in stable adult patients.

Pethidine is more likely to cause vasodilation, impair cardiac contractility, and cause tachycardia and hypotension than most other opioids. This is especially likely to occur if the patient is already hypovolaemic. Neonates and infants may drop their blood pressure with morphine and almost certainly will with pethidine. The short acting opioids, fentanyl, (and its son alfentanil, and daughter sufentanil) cause bradycardia and profound respiratory depression. Do not use them in the recovery room.

SEDATION
Opioids cause drowsiness. Patients lie quietly, and do not move unless prompted. When asked what they are thinking about, they report a non-dreaming, sleep like state, but they are aware of their surroundings. This inability to structure thoughts, anticipate or plan; and the disinclination to move is called *psychomotor retardation*. An interesting phenomenon, is lid lag where the upper eyelid blinks down fast, but comes up more slowly than a normal person. The same effect is seen after administration of a benzodiazepine (the so-called *benzo-blink*). Do not give any more opioid once the patient becomes sleepy. He has had enough.

AMNESIA AND TIME COMPRESSION. Do not tell the patients important information while they are under the influence of opioids including any instructions about their care after surgery. They will almost invariably forget it. Patients must not sign legal documents, such as consent or release forms, while under the influence of opioids. Opioids make it difficult for the patient to judge the passing of time; it appears to pass more quickly.

Nausea and vomiting
Opioids used during the operation, or in the recovery room cause postoperative nausea and vomiting in 20 - 30 per cent of patients. All opioids are roughly equivalent in their ability to trigger nausea and vomiting. Opioids make patients susceptible to motion sickness, increasing the sensitivity to input from the vestibular apparatus in the inner ear.

Euphoria

Two factors contribute to a patient's perception of his pain; one is hurt, and the other is fear. Opioids promote an overwhelming feeling of well-being. They make it difficult to worry about anything, and anxiety melts away. As

---

MORE ABOUT THE OPIOIDS

The properties of the Asian poppy, *Papaver somniferum*, have been known for thousands of years, and are detailed in the writings of ancient Egypt, Babylonia, Greece. The sticky brown gum extracted from the opium poppy contains about 21 alkaloids including: morphine, codeine, thebaine, narcoteine, papaverine. Not all have analgesic properties for instance papaverine is a vasodilator that led the way to the development of the calcium channel blocking drugs.

Over the years the terminology of the opioids has evolved. *Opioid* includes all natural and semisynthetic alkaloid derivatives of opium, and its synthetic analogues. *Opiates*, an outdated term, usually just to the refers to alkaloids derived from the opium poppy but excludes their synthetic cousins. Although commonly used narcotic is a vague term implying the ability to cause a stupor or deep sleep. *Alkaloids* are a group of alkaline (hence their name) nitrogenous compounds derived from plants containing a *pyridine ring*. Many of the synthetic opioids are based around the piperidine ring.

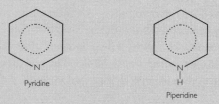

Pyridine

Piperidine

fig 11.2 Synthetic opioids

Agonists are drugs that strongly bind to and stimulate receptors. *Antagonists* are drugs that strongly bind to, but block receptors. Partial agonists are drugs that partially stimulate receptors but cannot produce a maximal response. *Opioid agonists* include morphine, pethidine, fentanyl, codeine and phenoperidine. Opioid antagonists include naloxone, and nalorphine. *Partial opioid agonists* include nalbuphine, pentazocine, and buprenorphine; however these drugs are not used routinely.

---

the threatening feelings of alarm and fright dissolve, so does the activity of the sympathetic nervous system. Tachycardia, hypertension, and other metabolic effects resolve. Pain becomes less threatening, and although often still present, does not concern the patient as much.

Tolerance and addiction

With frequent administration, opioids gradually lose their effect, and higher and higher doses are required to achieve the same response. This phenomenon is called tolerance, and takes a few days to develop. Then if the drug is suddenly stopped a *withdrawal syndrome* occurs. This is characterized by sweating, shaking, shivering, runny nose, abdominal cramps, headache, nausea, dilated pupils - and is most unpleasant, but (unlike alcohol withdrawal) is rarely fatal.

A patient with cancer pain presenting for surgery and who routinely taking oral opioids, such a slow release morphine (MS Contin®) may need up to ten times as much opioid as a normal patient to control his pain postoperatively. Consult with the oncology staff about his opioid requirements.

Patients in pain almost never get psychologically dependent (*addicted*) to the opioids. It is wrong to withold opioid analgesia from a patient, because of the fear of addiction. A drug addict finds opioids seductive, they enable him to escape from anxiety and feelings he would rather not have. Opioids hijack the addict's judgement, and once tolerance occurs the consequences are well known. Tolerance occurs over days or weeks, with higher and higher doses needed to achieve the same level of analgesia. The type of patient at risk is one coming for repeated procedures like debridment and change of dressings. His wound is getting better every day but his complaints of pain are getting louder. Wean him off opioids and onto NSAIDs.

Itch

Opioids cause itchy nose; and the patients sometimes rub them vigorously. If this becomes a problem after eye, or plastic surgery on the face or nose, then give a small dose of promethazine (Phenergan®) 0.25 mg/kg. If this fails, naloxone will relieve the itch, but will probably precipitate pain.

Opioids, particularly morphine, used in spinal or epidural anaesthesia commonly cause troublesome itching and sometimes an urticarial rash.

Urinary retention

Opioids reduce the desire to pass urine, and cause the vesical sphincter to tighten, while relaxing the detrusor muscle. This particularly affects older men. Patience, encouragement, privacy, and the sound of running water help overcome the problem. It may be necessary to pass a catheter.

PUPILLARY CONSTRICTION

Pupillary constriction causing pin-point pupils (*meiosis*) is greatest with fentanyl and least with pethidine. It does not abate as tolerance develops.

Other problems

True allergic response are rare, more commonly idiosyncratic responses occur such as blurred vision, dizziness and injected conjunctiva. In theory morphine

---

ADVERSE EFFECTS OF THE OPIOIDS

Common adverse effects:
- nausea, vomiting;
- respiratory depression;
- drowsiness;
- dry mouth;
- constricted pupils;
- orthostatic hypotension if patient is volume deplete.

Infrequent adverse effects:
- confusion is almost invariably secondary to hypoxia;
- vivid dreams;
- itching and urticaria;
- biliary spasm causing biliary pain;
- increased intracranial pressure - secondary to a rising PCO_2;
- urinary retention.

Rare:
- irritability, confusion, convulsions, coma;
- true allergic response.

---

should be avoided in asthmatics, because of the risk of precipitating bronchospasm, but in practice this is not a problem. Ethnicity can affect drug metabolism. Asians metabolise opioids more slowly than Caucasians [10].

PRACTICAL POINTS IN THE USE OF OPIOIDS

MULTIMODAL ANALGESIA is the practice of combining several different analgesic drugs or techniques to interupt the pain pathways at different points: for example a patient who has had a radical nephrectomy might have intercostal blocks to treat with the *somatic pain* from muscle and skin, morphine to control the *visceral pain* from the peritoneum and an NSAID to quieten the inflammatory reponse due to tissue trauma.

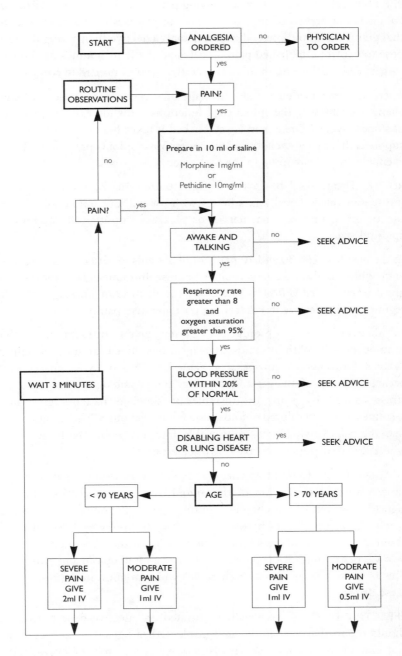

fig 11.3 Plan for treating pain

PRE-EMPTIVE ANALGESIA means giving pain relief before the pain occurs. Pain is better prevented than relieved. Clinical anaesthetists have observed that giving an opioid premedication is more effective than giving the same dose to control established pain. Local anaesthetic techniques used during surgery reduce the amount of postoperative opioids needed to control pain.

There is some evidence that the pain of surgery may cause prolonged changes in the way the spinal cord functions. This increases the pain felt postoperatively.[11] Once pain is established it takes high doses of opioid to suppress this hyper excitable state. Pre-emptive opioids prevent the hyper-excitable state developing in the first place.

ROUTE: Drugs may be given orally, intramuscularly, intravenously, or transcutaneously. Local anaesthetics with, or without opioid supplement can be given into regional nerves or plexuses, intrathecally or into the epidural space.

In the past between 30 and 70 per cent of patients experienced severe acute pain while in the recovery room[12] because intramuscular opioids were given *when needed* (*PRN*) as judged by the medical or nursing staff. This regime was ineffective in controlling postoperative pain.[13]

In recovery room opioids are better given intravenously than intramuscularly. With intramuscular injections there is an up to 30 minute delay before effective analgesia is achieved. This delay is unacceptable because the aim of analgesia is to reduce the physiological and emotional stress caused by pain. In unstable or shocked patients give small increments of well diluted opioids, slowly intravenously. This is much safer than the risk of giving large, irretrievable doses into poorly perfused muscle where the absorption and uptake will be erratic.

LOADING DOSE. To build up adequate blood levels, load the patient with a slow intravenous injection of the opioid over 5 minutes. Use the pain algorithm set out in this chapter. Continue giving the opioid until the pain is relieved or the patient becomes drowsy with droopy eyelids and pupils about 2 - 3 mm in diameter. Stop the titration if the respiratory rate falls below 8 per minute. Some patients will need a lot of opioid and others less. This is to be expected because there is a wide variation in the response to these drugs.

EFFECTIVE DOSE. When you have titrated an effective dose the patient should report that his pain is manageable. Other signs that the patient has had enough opioid include: drowsiness where the patient dozes, but is rousable, pupils less than or or equal to 2 mm in diameter, a respiratory rate of 8 - 10 breaths per minute.

Reduce the dose of the opioid if the drug elimination is likely to be delayed such as with renal or hepatic impairment, in the elderly or in young children. If you are in doubt then give half the calculated dose twice as slowly as recommended. You can always give more later if necessary, but once given you can't get it back.

Give half the dose,
twice as slowly.

RENAL IMPAIRMENT. Doses must be reduced in renal impairment because of the risk of accumulation of active or toxic metabolites.

See Cockcroft and Gault Formula for estimation of creatinine clearance on page 135.

HEPATIC IMPAIRMENT. It is necessary to titrate the dose carefully because the respiratory depression and coma may occur.

ELDERLY. Patients over 65 years of age metabolize and excrete the opioids more slowly than younger people. Start with a lower dose and increase the increments slowly. Opioid requirements can vary by up to 10 fold in older people.

CHILDREN (see also page 395). Neonates,[14] especially premature babies up to the gestational age of 22 months, or those with neurological or pulmonary abnormalities are at risk of respiratory depression and apnoea if given systemic opioids. Their blood brain barrier is more permeable and the drugs easily reach the respiratory centres to depress their drive to breathe. Apnoea and respiratory depression are dose related. Babies require lower doses, and longer dosing intervals. Start with a small dose and increase it incrementally.

For infants under the age of 3 months the initial opioid dose should be a quarter of the dose recommended for older infants or children. If their pain is not relieved it is easy to give another incremental dose.

Metabolism and excretion of opioids is at least three times slower in the neonate than an older child. The clearance of opioids increases rapidly with age, and approaches adult rates by the age of 3 months (370 post conceptual days). Despite this an infant under the age of 22 gestational months is at higher risk of respiratory depression from systemic opioids. Monitor them careful for at least 24 hours.

Paracetamol suppositories reduce the amount of opioid required to relieve pain in babies. Stroking and massaging the baby's limbs and back also calms him.

PREGNANCY. Safe to use in pregnant patients. Be cautious in labour because they may cause respiratory depression in the newborn.

LACTATION. Pethidine is preferable to morphine.

HYPOTHERMIA. Patients with temperatures less than 35.5°C on admission to recovery room are susceptible to opioid respiratory depression, because their liver metabolises the drug slowly, and their kidneys excrete it. Use small doses with great caution if you need to use them at all.

Reduce the dose or if possible avoid opoids in: chronic obstructive airways disease, asthma, following neurosurgery, suspected raised intracranial pressure, cor-pulmonale, infants under three months.

Patients recovering from nasopharyngeal surgery are at risk because of sleep apnoea or silent airway obstruction.

Morphine and pethidine are the two most commonly used opioids for postoperative pain relief. You need to understand the properties of these drugs to use them effectively.

MORPHINE

Given intravenously it works slowly with the patient reporting a 'light feeling' in the head within 2 - 5 minutes . In patients who are not in pain it may cause a distressing sense of uneasiness called *dysphoria*. Sedation is gradual. Onset of nausea occurs in about 20 per cent of patients 5 - 10 minutes after injection. Respiratory depression occurs slowly with the patients respiratory rate falling below 12 breaths per minute after about 10 minutes. The tidal volume seems to be affected more than the respiratory rate. Morphine may produce a transient erythematous flair along the vein that is itchy and last for about 10 minutes.

Useful properties
Good analgesic, safe, unlikely to cause hypotension or tachycardia, less sedating than pethidine, supresses cough reflex, unlikely to interact dangerously with other drugs, safer in patient with cardiac disease than

pethidine. Said to cause more smooth muscle spasm (such as biliary pain) than pethidine. Morphine 1 - 5 mg into intra-articular space following arthroscopy gives analgesia for up to 48 hours.

Indications
Moderate to severe perioperative pain, and control of pulmonary oedema.

Dose
Titrate to patient needs. The limiting factors are adverse reactions of respiratory depression, sedation and drowsiness. In some cases maximum doses can be high especially if the patient has been preoperatively on opioids for a relief of chronic or cancer pain.

Neonate:	Morphine	10 - 20 microgram/kg loading dose
	Infusion	10 - 20 microgram/kg/hr in 5% dextrose
Child:	Morphine	100 - 200 microgram/kg loading dose
	Infusion	20 - 50 microgram/kg/hr in 5% dextrose

Make up the infusion with 500 microgram/kg morphine in 50 mls of 5% dextrose. (1 ml/hour = 10 microgram/kg per hour.)

| Adult: | Morphine | 30 - 150 microgram/kg loading dose |
| | Infusion | 20 - 50 microgram/kg/hr in 5% dextrose. |

Make up the infusion with 0.5 mg/kg morphine in 50 mls of 5% dextrose. (1 ml hour = 10 microgram/kg per hour.)

Normal dose requirements are 2 - 10 microgram/kg/hr.

- For an adult patient (over 20 years) the average 24 hourly intravenous morphine requirements = (100 - age) in milligram.
- The single dose = average 24 hourly requirement divided by 8 and given 2 hourly.
- Thus for a 56 year old patient the average 24 hourly dose would be 56 - 8 = 48 mg; and the intravenous dose would be 48/8 = 6 mg every 2 hours.
- Far less optimally the daily dose can be divided by 6 and given 3 - 4 hourly intramuscularly.

Pharmacokinetics
Onset of action after intravenous loading dose IV: 10 - 15 minutes.
Peak action: 45 minutes. Duration: 3 - 4 + hours
Respiratory depression may last longer than analgesia.

Hepatic impairment

Reduce the dose by 50 - 75 per cent. Increase the interval between dose by 50 per cent.

Renal impairment

If the creatinine clearance is less than 30 ml/minute give 50 - 75 per cent calculated required dose. To estimate creatinine clearance see page 135.

Acute pulmonary oedema

1- 5 mg IV slowly over 5 minutes. Use the low end of the dose range in the elderly.

Compatible fluids

5% dextrose, 0.9% saline, Ringer's lactate, Hartmann's solution.

PETHIDINE

Meperidine (Demerol®) in the USA. Given intravenously it works quickly with the patient reporting a 'swimming feeling' in the head after 1 - 2 circulation times. Sedation is rapid and the patient may close their eyes, or even become obtunded. About 30 per cent of patients feel abruptly nauseated and may vomit. Respiratory depression occurs quickly with the patients respiratory rate falling to less than 10 breaths per minute. The patient may develop an initial tachycardia. Pethidine may produce a transient erythematous flair along the vein which resolves within a few minutes.

Useful properties

Good analgesic, quick acting, not as safe as morphine because of very toxic metabolites, likely to cause hypotension or tachycardia especially in volume depleted patients or those with insipient heart failure, more sedating than morphine, does not supresses cough reflex, may interact dangerously with other drugs, not so safe in patient with cardiac disease as morphine, said to be better for smooth muscle spasm (such as biliary pain) than morphine. Less well tolerated in elderly than morphine.

Indications

Moderate to severe perioperative pain

Metabolism

Hydrolyzed in liver to 6 norpethidine which is not analgesic, is toxic and has to be excreted by the kidneys. Continuing norpethidine accummulation cause a progression of jitters, irritability, disorientation, confusion, convulsions, coma, death.

Problems

Do not use pethidine to treat pulmonary oedema, because the already compromised cardiac ouput will drop catastrophically.

Do not use in renal failure or impairment, because of risk of norpethidine toxicity. Do not use naloxone (Narcan®) for norpethidine toxicity because it antagonises the sedation, but not the excitatory effects and will therefore make the problem worse.

Do not use pethidine in patients who are on the monoamine oxidase inhibitors (MAOIs) because of toxic reaction: restlessness, hypertension, cardiac arrhythmias, convulsions, coma and possibly death. MAOIs (type A) include phenelzine (Nardil®) and tranylcypromine (Parnate®). These MAOIs (type A) should be stopped 14 days before surgery if pethidine or vasopressors are to be used. MAOIs (type B) include moclobemide (Aurorix®) should be stopped a clear 24 hours before surgery to avoid problems.

Dose

Titrate to patient needs. This drug has a low therapeutic index. This means the toxic dose and the therapeutic dose are close together. The limiting factors are hypotension, and excitability.

Adult: Intramuscular: 0.75 - 1.5 mg/kg or
            Intravenously: 0.5 - 1.0 mg/kg loading dose.
            Infusion: 100 - 300 microgram/kg/hr in 5% dextrose.

Make up the infusion with 5 mg/kg pethidine in 50 mls of 5% dextrose. (1 ml hour = 100 microgram/kg/hr in 5% dextrose.) See also appendix I.

Normal dose requirements are 0.2 - 1.0 mg/kg/hr.

Neonate: Because of its toxicity we do not recommend pethidine for use in the neonate.

Child: Pethidine: 0.5 - 1.0 mg/kg loading dose.
            Infusion: 50 microgram/kg/hr in 5% dextrose.

Make up the infusion with 0.5 mg/kg morphine in 50 mls of 5% dextrose. (1 ml/hour = 10 microgram/kg/hr.)

The average intravenous requirements for patients between 18 - 65 years is 15 - 35 mg/hr.

Use intravenous pethidine infusions cautiously.

The maximum average daily intramuscular requirements for patients between 18 - 65 years is 600 mg.

The intravenous dose is between 15 - 50 mg intravenous 2 - 3 hourly. If giving intermittently divide the daily dose by 12 and give 2 hourly IV, or far less optimally divide by 8 and give 3 - 4 hourly intramuscularly.

COMPARISON OF MORPHINE AND PETHIDINE		
	Morphine	**Pethidine**
Dose* (intravenous)	0.03 – 0.15 mg/kg	0.5 – 0.75 mg/kg
Dose* (intramuscular)	0.15 mg/kg	0.75 – 1.5 mg/kg
Basal infusion rate*	0.03 mg/kg/hr	0.3 mg/kg/hr
Onset (intravenously)	5 – 10 min	1 – 2 min
Onset (intramuscularly)	10 – 20 min	5 – 10 min
Peak action (intravenously)	45 min	20 min
Duration of action	3 – 4 hr	2 – 3 hr
Toxicity in overdose	low	high
Metabolism	conjugated in liver	hydrolysed in liver
Excretion	biliary and renal	renal
Metabolites	active respiratory depressant	toxic (CNS irritability)
Respiratory depression	Equal, but dose dependent	Equal, but dose dependent
Cough suppression	Yes	No
Hypotension after IV injection	Possible	Probable
Interactions with other psycho-active drugs	Possible	Probable
Spasm of sphincters	Big effect	Smaller effect
Shaking and shivering	Not useful treatment	Most effective treatment

*These recommended doses of opioids do not apply to patients with renal or hepatic disease, or other conditions that may increase their effect, or delay their metabolism.

Pharmacokinetics

Onset of action after intravenous loading dose IV: 5 minutes.
Peak action: 20 minutes. Duration: 2 - 3 hours.
Respiratory depression lasts longer than analgesia.

Hepatic impairment

Reduce dose by 50 - 75 per cent.

Renal impairment

Use with extreme caution. Loading dose well tolerated, but subsequent doses inadvisable. If creatinine clearance less than 30 ml/min then reduce dose by 50 per cent and dosing interval by 50 per cent.

Acute pulmonary oedema

Absolutely contraindicated.

Compatible fluids

5% dextrose, 0.9% saline, Ringer's lactate, Hartmann's solution.

FENTANYL (SUBLIMAZE®)

Fentanyl is not recommended for use in recovery room because of its ability to cause profound respiratory depression. Furthermore the respiratory depression of fentanyl can be delayed for several hours after the patient returns to the ward, especially in the elderly. Fentanyl is sequestered in muscle vascular beds, and released back into the circulation when the patient begins to move around. The effect of this is unpredicatable, respiratory depression.

*Do not use fentanyl for postoperative pain relief
- its action is brief, and it causes respiratory depression.*

Given intravenously, the younger patient rarely reports any feelings of sedation or swimming in the head, however they may become drowsy. Their respiratory rate drops to less than 8 breaths a minute within a couple of minutes (the patient may even stop breathing). Fentanyl is commonly used as an adjuvant to epidural infusions. If this is so, be wary of giving an opioid intravenously.

Properties
Good analgesic, quick acting, not as safe as morphine because of tendency of the patient to stop breathing without necessarily becoming overly sedated, cardiac stable and unlikely to cause hypotension or tachycardia even in volume depleted patients or those with insipient heart failure. Fentanyl is much less sedating than morphine, does not supress cough reflex, safe in patients with cardiac disease provided they continue to breathe, not effective for smooth muscle spasm (such as biliary pain). This is a drug to be used with great caution in unintubated patients.

Problems
Fentanyl can cause bradycardia. Delayed respiratory depression may occur, especially in the elderly, up to 3 - 6 hour after the last dose. Because of its respiratory depression, it is not recommended as an postoperative analgesic. With higher doses in some patients truncal rigidity makes it difficult to inflate their lungs. It may be reversed with naloxone and is overcome with muscle relaxants.

Contraindications
Do not use for management of pulmonary oedema. Fentanyl is safe to use in patients who are on the monoamine oxidase inhibitors (MAOIs)

Infusions
These are only suitable for ventilated patients.

Pharmacokinetics
Onset of action after intravenous loading dose IV: 5 minutes.
Peak action: 6 minutes. Duration: 30 - 40 minutes
Respiratory depression lasts longer than analgesia. Late respiratory depression may occur especially in the elderly. There are reported cases of respiratory arrest up to 6 hours after a single IV loading dose.

Hepatic impairment
Reduce dose by 25 - 50 percent. Once loaded reduce dosing interval by half.

Renal impairment
Fentanyl is well tolerated in patients with renal impairment with little risk of toxicity.

Acute pulmonary oedema
Absolutely contraindicated.

OTHER OPIOID ANALGESICS

DIAMORPHINE (Heroin). Its use is illegal in Australia, New Zealand, Canada and the USA. Diamorphine is reputed to have a quicker onset, causing less nausea and vomiting than morphine. It is highly lipid soluble and penetrates the blood brain rapidly accounting for the 'rush' experienced by addicts. Dose 0.015 mg/kg intravenously or intramuscularly. It is metabolized in the liver to morphine-6-glucuronide which is a powerful analgesic. Its onset of action is within 5 - 10 minutes, and it is unlikely to cause hypotension.

HYDROMORPHONE (Dilaudid®) is a synthetic derivative of morphine. It is 7 - 10 times more potent than morphine. It is popular in some parts of the USA, because it is believed to be less likely to cause hypotension than morphine. Dose 0.02 mg/kg. Typical adult dose 1.5 mg. Duration of action 4 - 5 hours.

METHADONE (Physeptone®) is a long acting opioid, which is equipotent with morphine, but has a clinical effect for about 20 - 30 hours. This means a 10 mg dose of morphine given every 4 hours is equivalent to 10 mg methadone given daily. Although it has been used as a postoperative analgesic its long action does not allow for flexible dosing.

PHENOPERIDINE (Operidine®) is a synthetic analgesic 275 times as potent as pethidine and 75 times as potent as morphine. An undervalued drug - probably quite useful.

Onset of action is about 1 minute. Duration of analgesia 40 - 60 minutes. It is less sedating than morphine or pethidine but more so than fentanyl. In a fit adult 1 - 2 mg IV gives about 2 - 5 minutes sedation. Minimal effect on blood pressure, but may cause bradycardia. Respiratory depression last longer than fentanyl and respiratory effort may cease after about 2 mg - useful in for gaining quick control of coughing patient. Has been reported to cause the extrapyramidal syndrome with rigidity and nystagmus. Effects easily reversed with naloxone or nalorphine.

Compatible fluids

5% dextrose, 0.9% saline, Ringer's lactate, Hartmann's solution.

NEW OPIOID DRUGS

Opioid drugs are introduced every few years; initially they have enthusiastic support, but then fall by the wayside. They appear to have little advantage over older ones, and in many cases are neither as effective or safe as morphine or pethidine. The objective of these new arrivals is provide good analgesia, without the risks of respiratory depression or addiction. These newer drugs include buprenorphine, dipipanone, meptazinol, nalbuphine, pentazocine, phenazocine, and tramadol. None of these selective opioid drugs have successfully uncoupled strong analgesia from unwanted side-effects. Although morphine has unpleasant, and annoying side effects, inconvenient pharmacokinetics and is a bad drug from many points of view; all the others are worse. The drugs we already have are probably better than we are likely to get in the near future.

Opioid Antagonists

Naloxone (Narcan®) is a potent antagonist to the opioid drugs. It is used to reverse opioid induced respiratory depression, but it completely reverses all the actions of the opioid (and the patient's own endorphins too). This may suddenly plunge the patient into severe pain, causing severe hypertension, myocardial ischaemia, and even acute pulmonary oedema[15]. It is a difficult drug to titrate, and tends to work in an all-or-nothing way.

Useful properties
Naloxone acts rapidly. It totally reverses respiratory depression for about 35 minutes after an intravenous dose, but may wear off before the opioid, allowing the patient to become re-narcotised.

Indications
Respiratory depression secondary to opioid overdose.

Metabolism
In conjugated to glucorinic acid in liver and its metabolites are excreted in the urine over the next 48 hours.

Dose
The initial dose is naloxone 0.01 mg IV and wait 2 minutes before repeating up to a total of 0.04 mg over 8 minutes.

Pharmacokinetics
Onset of action after IV dose is about 90 seconds and 3 - 5 minutes after IM dose.
Peak action: about 5 minutes after IV dose and 10 minutes after IM dose
Duration: about 20 - 40 minutes after IV dose and 35 - 60 minutes after IM dose.
Plasma half life: 60 - 90 minutes in adult, but 2.5 - 3.5 hours in the neonate.

Limitations

Naloxone is not effective against the respiratory depression caused by buprenorphine, use doxapram, or if this fails the patient may need ventilation. Higher doses will be needed to reverse the respiratory depression due to pentazocine. Naloxone does not reverse other toxic effects of the opioids such as cardiac arrhythmias due to propoxyophene, myocardial depression due to pethidine, bradycardias due to the fentanyls or seizures due to norpethidine. Failure to respond to a 2 mg IV dose within 2 minutes suggests some other cause of unconsciousness apart from opioid overdose.

Hepatic impairment

There is no need to reduce single dose, but naloxone clearance is reduced six fold.

Renal impairment

No need to single reduce dose. Safety not yet determined.

Acute postoperative reversal of opioid activity

Use naloxone cautiously in patients with cardiac disease because abrupt reversal of opioid analgesia may cause cardiac arrhythmias and myocardial ischaemia. Other signs include: nausea and vomiting, sweating, tremors, tachycardia, hypertension. If a patient is suddenly catapulted into severe pain, catastrophic sympathetic discharge can cause acute pulmonary oedema,ventricular arrhythmias including ventricular tachycardia, ventricular fibrillation. Deaths have been reported.

NALORPHINE (LETHIDRONE®)

Nalorphine is a partial opioid antagonist. It has been withdrawn from sale in some countries because the more efficacious and popular naloxone has replaced it. It is a most useful drug, because it is far more easily titrated than naloxone to partly reverse the respiratory depressant effects of the opioids and is unlikely to abruptly jolt the patient into pain. Start with nalorphine 1 mg IV bolus, and repeat at 2 minute intervals up to a total of 10 mg. Its duration of action is about 4 hours.

WITHDRAWAL SYNDROME

An opioid antagonist may precipitate withdrawal syndrome in a pharmacologically dependent patient in recovery room. For this reason, do not give an opioid antagonist or partial agonist (naloxone, pentazocine, buprenorphine) to using heroin addicts unless absolutely necessary.

Signs and symptoms of acute opioid withdrawal include: abdominal cramps, diarrhoea, tachycardia, hypertension, fever, sneezing, runny nose, goose bumps (piloerection), yawning, sweating, nausea and vomiting, nervousness, shivering and dysphoria, and rarely depressed conscious state and convuslsions.

Signs in the neonate include: convulsions, excessive crying, and hyperactive reflexes.

PATIENT CONTROLLED ANALGESIA[16]

Since the patient is the only one who really knows how much pain he has, it seems reasonable to allow him to give enough analgesia to control his pain. Patient controlled analgesia (PCA) is an effective way to administer opioids. It is safe, effective, and has fewer complications than intermittent intramuscular injections.[17] PCA is efficient because it achieves adequate pain relief with the minimum dose of opioid.

There are a number of infusion devices controlled by microprocessors, such as the Graseby® and Abbott Lifecare® that give a bolus dose of opioid when the patient presses a button. This is followed by a *lock-out time* where no further drug is given, no matter how often the button is pressed. If the patient is not in pain, or is drowsy, he will not press the button.

Some devices give a background maintenance infusion. We firmly believe that background infusions should not be used in adults. There is no evidence that they are helpful, and may lead to overdose. They create a high risk of respiratory depression.[18] It is better to have small doses, and a short lock-out time, than to use a background maintenance infusion and longer lock-out times. A constant background infusion does not reduce the night time demands for analgesia, nor ensure a better sleep.[19] If you do decide to use them, the hourly basal infusion rate should not exceed the amount of a single bolus dose.

PCA devices are expensive and cannot be expected to be available for every patient; however the principals of analgesia on demand can still be applied[20], even though this involves more nursing care than if the patient delivers his own dose.

Advantages of PCA:
- patients like it because they feel in control of their pain;
- good safe pain relief;
- hypoxaemia is less common than with intramuscular opioids;[21]
- readily adapts to changes in the diurnal need for analgesic;
- few sleep disturbances;
- decrease in length of hospital stay;[22]
- analgesia is prompt and given only when needed;
- frees up nursing staff;
- lower total doses of narcotics are used;
- can be used in children over the age of about 6 years.

Disadvantages of PCA:
- considerable incidence of drowsiness, nausea, vomiting[23] and itching;
- costs include equipment, nursing and patient training. PCA only really works well if it is being used regularly and there is constant teaching;
- written protocols have to be precisely worded, easily understood and strictly followed;
- respiratory depression must always be watched for, especially in the elderly;
- it ties the patient to the bed.

In many hospitals, patient controlled analgesia is started in the recovery room. Here the staff give the first dose of postoperative analgesia, gauge its effect, and then set up a regime that suits the patient. This does increase the work load on the recovery room staff, but has been shown to be cost effective in terms of patient stay in hospital and reducing demands on busy ward staff.

Protocols should include details of the:
- drug dose and dilution;
- dose increment, which is the dose given when the patient presses the button;
- allowable number of doses per hour;
- lock-out time;
- maximum amount of drug given in a 4 hour period;
- volume remaining in the syringe;
- options to change settings;
- nursing observations and frequency;
- limits of respiratory rate;
- disposal of unused solutions;

- treatment of common side-effects;
- details of where to find medical support (preferably a pager number to call).

Reduce the chance of mishaps

Accidents and mishaps have been frequently reported with PCA devices. They should never be regarded as absolutely fail safe. You will need to monitor your patients carefully.

There are many different makes of PCA devices on the market, so you must make sure that you are totally familiar with the devices used in your hospital. Check the features on each device before you use it. Most errors occur when setting up the infusion. Problems occur with prescription errors, administration errors and patient factors.

PRESCRIPTION ERRORS
These include: wrong dose, wrong lock-out time, wrong infusion rates. Make up a standard PCA order form; and set it out so that times and decimal points are clear, and errors difficult to make.

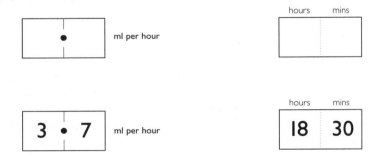

fig 11.4 Setting time and decimal points on PCA device.

ADMINISTRATION ERRORS
These include: wrong concentration prepared, wrong interpretation of instructions, equipment wrongly set up, and accidental injection when replacing the syringe. To prevent these errors, check through all the instructions carefully when you hand over. Ideally infusions should have their own separate intravenous line, and nothing else should run through it. If a line cannot be dedicated to the infusion make sure there is an non-reflux valve correctly fitted into the branch line, so that the opioid will not run backwards up into the other line should the cannula become blocked.

Doses can be either written as milligrams, or millilitres; this is a common source of confusion. The PCA form should be designed to eliminated the chance of error. Orders should be written exactly as they are to be programmed into the machine.

Patient factors

Confusion or hypoxia make it impossible for the patient to control PCA. Intentional abuse; accidental administration and intercurrent haemorrhage may cause the patient's response to alter. Visitors or staff can, and sometimes do, press the button. If the patient has been given a benzodiazepine, or phenothiazine, this increases the risk of respiratory depression. Some patients, especially those with a passive dependent personality, do not like PCA so respect their wishes.[24] Some patients think pressing the button will summon the nurse !

Opioids for PCA

If you decide to use pethidine, then do so with care. Morphine is safer. There have been numerous reports of norpethidine toxicity causing myoclonic jerks, agitation, restlessness and seizures. Pethidine should not be used when it is anticipated that the requirements for analgesia will be high.[25] Recent reports suggest that pethidine is best avoided in both children and adults.[26,27] For the first 24 hours, age is the best predictor for opioid requirements,[28] with older patients requiring smaller bolus doses.

The use of background infusions is considered safe and effective in children.[29]

Adults' doses for PCA (see appendix I)

Children's doses for PCA (see appendix I)

CONTINUOUS OPIOID INFUSIONS (SEE ALSO APPENDIX 1)

Opioid infusions remain an undeservedly popular means of giving pain relief to adults. In our experience they are not as safe as PCA. It is important to have disciplined, strict and carefully planned protocols for continuous infusions. They are really only suitable for ICU, as they require constant, skilled nursing supervision to be safe and effective. In a busy surgical ward this is usually not possible, in which case, do not use them. The biggest risk is respiratory depression. The danger is that a patient may quietly slip from sleep into an opioid induced coma. This can easily pass unnoticed, especially at night. The patients head may flop into a position that obstructs their airway causing a respiratory arrest and death follows shortly after.

Opioid infusions are not suitable for the elderly because their tolerance to opioids is reduced and the correct dose may be difficult to gauge.

Opioid infusions do appear to be safer in children. Unlike adults, oxygen desaturation at night is uncommon in infants and children receiving opioid infusions.[30] The usual doses are:

Morphine	Loading dose:	0.1 - 0.2 mg/kg IV
	Make up an infusion:	0.5 mg/kg in 50 mls of 5% dextrose
	Rate:	1 - 5 ml/hr (= 10 - 15 µg/kg/hr).
Pethidine	Loading dose:	0.5 - 1 mg/kg IV
	Make up infusion:	5 mg/kg in 50 mls of 5% dextrose
	Rate:	1 - 3 ml/hr (= 100 - 300 µg/kg/hr).

NON-STEROIDAL ANTI-INFLAMMATORY DRUGS

Non-steroidal anti-inflammatory drugs (NSAIDs, pronounced en-saids) are a group of compounds with anti-inflammatory and analgesic action. They are useful in the management of mild to moderate postoperative pain, because they do not cause respiratory depression, sedation and tolerance.[31]

NSAIDs have a number of adverse actions limiting their usefulness. They:
• aggravate asthma;
• jeopardize renal function in hypoxic or hypoperfusion states;
• cause bleeding tendencies;
• cause peptic ulceration in the stomach;
• cause hypersensitivity phenomena including urticaria, angioedema, and rhinitis.

They also interact with, and increase the activity of antihypertensive diuretics (such as the thiazides and frusemide), ß-blockers, and angiotensin-converting enzyme inhibitors.[32]

Pharmacology

Prostaglandins form part of the chemical soup that causes pain in injured tissue. NSAIDs block the synthesis of prostaglandins, suppressing the inflammatory response, and its effect on generating pain. This action is (with exception of aspirin) temporary, and is reversible by simply withdrawing the NSAID concerned. For some of the longer acting NSAIDs it can take up to a week for the effects to wear off.

CYCLO-OXYGENASES ENZYME SYSTEMS:

When cells are damaged by infection or trauma arachidonic acid is released from the phospholipids in the cell membrane. A group of enzymes called cyclo-oxygenases (COX) oxidize arachidonic acid as the first step in the formation of a variety of prostaglandins.

COX 1. (The "protective COX") This enzyme system is present in most cells and produces prostaglandins for normal bodily functions such as blood clotting, bronchodilation, maintaining renal medullary flow, and gastrointestinal mucosal integrity (especially in the stomach). Prostaglandin F_2 (PGF_2) and PGI_2 are two of these important protective prostaglandins.

COX 2. (The "inflammatory cox") This is an inducible enzyme system that produces prostaglandins which help produce an inflammatory and pain response. They are an ingredient in the chemical soup bathing the tissues which stimulates peripheral nerve receptors. Prostaglandin E_2 (PGE_2) is one of these important inflammatory prostaglandins.

NSAIDs acetylate both COX 1 and COX 2 and inhibit the production of all prostaglandins.

By inhibiting COX 2 they inhibit the inflammatory response and usefully reduce pain. But they also inhibit COX 1 and its beneficial effects. Recently the selective COX 2 inhibiting NSAIDs, rofocoxib and celecoxib, have been introduced.

Prostaglandins have many physiological actions in other parts of the body. Inhibition of their action causes a variety of adverse effects including bronchoconstriction, peptic ulceration and inteference platelet aggregation and blood clotting.

Adverse effects of the NSAIDs[33]

ASTHMA

Some prostaglandins are bronchodilators. Inhibition of their function in patients with asthma or allergies can precipitate an acute asthma attack. Be particularly careful of aspirin in these patients. Paracetamol, on the other hand, does not cause a problem.

KIDNEY EFFECTS[34]

Prostaglandins have little function in a normal kidney. In a kidney whose blood supply is jeopardized they become important renal vasodilators improving the blood flow and oxygenation of the nephrons. The use of NSAIDs in the elderly, especially if they are dehydrated, hypotensive or hypoxic, impairs renal blood flow and predisposes to renal failure. It is wise to avoid them in heavy smokers or those with vascular disease or hypertension. None of the available NSAIDs are safe in patients with renal dysfunction.

BLEEDING TENDENCY

Platelets are vital for blood clotting. Platelets need prostaglandins to function properly. Platelet function should return to normal within 4 to 5 half-lives of the last dose of NSAIDs. Aspirin however, permanently destroys the function of cyclo-oxygenase, and it takes 12 - 15 days for a new batch of platelets to be produced by the bone marrow. A platelet transfusion is the only way to reverse this if it becomes a problem; fresh frozen plasma will not help.

PEPTIC ULCERATION

All NSAIDs cause chronic mucosal damage especially in the stomach and can trigger peptic ulceration. Even in the short term they can cause upper abdominal discomfort or pain (dyspepsia). Gastric irritation is more likely with aspirin, napoxen and piroxicam. Less likely with ibuprofen, indomethacin and diclofenac. Do not use NSAIDs in any patient who has had a peptic ulcer or a patient who is taking oral steroids for chronic inflammatory disorders. Patients over the age of 65 years are more at risk.

LIVER

Aspirin can cause a transient rise in liver enzymes, but other NSAIDs also do this especially diclofenac and sulindac. It resolves rapidly on withdrawal.

HYPERSENSITIVITY

Urticaria, angioedema, and rhinitis occur in some people. These responses are not true allergic reactions, but due to the pharmacological action of the NSAID. Apart from the synthesis of prostaglandins, arachidonic acid is also used for synthesis of lipoxygenase compounds, one of which is the slow-reacting substance of anaphylaxis. If the cyclo-oxygenase pathway is blocked there is an overproduction of lipoxygenases which cause the allergic-like response.

DRUG INTERACTIONS

NSAIDS are a commonly prescribed class of drugs and adverse interactions with other drugs can be a problem, especially in the elderly on multiple medication. NSAIDs are tightly bound to proteins in the blood, and by displacing other drugs bound to the same proteins , can increase their effect or toxicity. These drugs include: anticoagulants, digoxin, phenytoin, and valproate. NSAIDs reduce the antihypertensive effects of thiazides, loop-diuretics, beta blockers, and angiotensin-converting enzyme inhibitors.

HEADACHE

A common, but not often recognised problem. Indomethacin can cause severe headache. Others NSAIDs can cause drowsiness or subtle personality or thought-processing changes.

Practical points

1. Ibruprofen is probably the drug with least side effects.

2. Try combinations of pain relief (multi-modal therapy). Use NSAIDs and opioids for moderate pain, and add local or regional analgesia for more severe pain.

3. NSAIDs take time to work. They are more effective if they are given before the pain is expected. This allows sufficient time for the drugs to interfere with prostaglandin synthesis. The onset of their analgesic effect occurs after one hour, but they need up to 5 hours to start working, and the analgesia becomes even more pronounced over the next 48 hours. This time lag is a major disadvantage for their use in the recovery room.

4. Patients who have had laproscopic cholecystectomies benefit from NSAID pain relief.

5. NSAIDs are effective as suppositories and are well tolerated. They are useful for all forms of pelvic surgery which include most minor gynaecological procedures.

6. Do not use NSAIDs in pregnancy, or to breast feeding women.

7. They appear to be effective in the treatment of ureteric or renal colic.[35]

8. Bleeding times are prolonged with NSAIDs, but apart from aspirin taken pre-operatively, it is rarely a problem.

9. When combined with an opioid, NSAIDs reduce the dose of opioid needed, and reduce its side effects. This opioid sparing effect means the dose of opioid can be reduced by 25 - 50 per cent. This is useful after painful orthopaedic arthroscopic procedures.[36]

10. Avoid NSAIDs especially ketarolac in patients whom you suspect have poor renal perfusion; eg diabetics, vascular disease, the elderly; or those with heart failure especially if there is peripheral oedema.

11. Asthma may be precipitated by any of the NSAIDs, but aspirin, naproxen, indomethacin and ibuprofen are particularly bad offenders.

Paracetamol

Paracetamol (acetominophen) is the drug to choose first for minor pain. It is an effective, safe drug if given in the correct dose. Combined with codeine or propoxyphene it enhances the analgesia. The advantages are that it does not aggravate bleeding, cause peptic ulcers or damage the kidney. Use it cautiously in alcoholics, or patients with liver disease because it can cause liver damage. The dose is 500 mg 4 - 6 hourly. The ceiling dose is 500 mg, and increasing the dose does not increase its effect. To get better analgesia increase the dosing frequency rather than the dose. The maximum daily dose for an adult is 8 tablets of 500 mg (4000 mg). In overdose (more than 15 tablets) it may cause fulminating irreversible hepatic failure.

Paracetamol is available in suspensions of 120 mg/5 ml for children. For analgesia, the oral dose is higher than that recommended for controlling fever. For pain control, the oral dose for children is 20 mg/kg 4 hourly lean body weight. Be careful when you prescribe paracetamol, because a number of different strength formulations are available (24, 48, and 60 mg/ml). This may cause confusion, both for staff and parents. The current recommended maximum daily dose is 100 mg/kg. Paracetamol is safe to use for 2 - 3 days in children. Suppositories give unreliable plasma levels, but 20 to 30 mg/kg seems to be effective. Use the smaller dose range in infants.

Paracetamol and codeine

Paracetamol and codeine is a good analgesic combination having few side effects. There are many combinations available, a useful one is paracetamol 500 mg with codeine 15 mg.

Ketorolac

Ketorolac gives moderate to good pain relief. It is popular analgesic for day surgery because it does not cause the problems of the opioids (nausea, vomiting, sedation, or respiratory depression). It is inadvisable to give repeated doses if bleeding could complicate surgical integrity. Aim to use the minimum dose for the shortest period eg. ketorolac 0.2 - 0.5 mg/kg every 6 hours. It is unnecessary to use a loading dose. Do not use ketorolac if there is any doubt about the patient's renal function such as with hypovolaemia or pre-existing renal disease. Avoid using it postoperatively in patients older than 65 years or children. Avoid its use in patients with coagulopathy, hypovolaemia, renal disease, diabetes, or peptic ulcers. Anaphylaxis can occur with ketorolac, and it should never be used in patients who are sensitive to aspirin or other NSAIDs.

Tramadol

Tramadol can be used for moderate to severe pain. Tramadol 250 mg given over 24 hours in divided doses is said to be equivalent to five doses of paracetamol 300mg with codeine 30mg. It is less likely than the NSAIDs to cause gastrointestinal side effects, but it does have many of the disadvantages of opioids especially nausea and vomiting.

Ibuprofen

Ibuprofen has the lowest side effects of any of the NSAIDs, but its anti-inflammatory properties are weaker. It is rapidly cleared and has a half life of 1 - 2 hours. It is useful for the pain following dental extractions. Give it pre-operatively to allow time for it to work. The oral dose of ibuprofen is 200 - 400 mg 6 hourly. It has caused asceptic meningitis in patients with systemic lupus erythematosis

Diclofenac

Diclofenac is useful for the control of ureteric colic and pain after insertion of ureteric stents. It is rapidly absorbed from the gut and has a half life of 1 - 2 hours. The dose of diclofenac is 25 - 50 mg orally three times daily. Suppositories of 100 mg are available. It is sometimes used as eye drops after eye surgery to supress inflammation.

REYE'S SYNDROME

Reye's syndrome is a fulminating encephalopathy associated with liver failure that occurs in children. It occurs after an acute viral illness, and is thought to be aggravated by aspirin. The child becomes drowsy, confused, ataxic, starts to vomit and may develop a coagulopathy. It has a high mortality rate.

Aspirin

Aspirin (sodium salicylate) is used for mild to moderate pain, and often combined with codeine, or paracetamol to increase analgesia. It is not a drug that is routinely used in recovery rooms. Use a dispersable (soluble) form. The oral dose is 300 - 900 mg every 4 - 6 hours. It will probably exacerbate asthma, and must not be used in patients who have reported an allergic response to any of the NSAIDs. It is contra-indicated in children under the age of 14 years, and in breast feeding mothers because of the risk of Reye's syndrome. Remind parents that aspirin is not a drug for children. Aspirin is irreversibly bound to COX enzymes and inteferes with platelet function.

Adjuvants

Clonidine [37]

Clonidine has been used to treat hypertension, but it is a useful adjuvant for controlling pain when combined with other analgesics. It is a highly lipid soluble, centrally acting alpha 2 agonist with analgesic properties. It causes sedation and lessens anxiety in doses of 3 microgramg/kg IV. It potentiates all analgesics, and reduces the incidence of postoperative shivering, nausea and vomiting, but may predispose to hypotension. It reduces the dose of analgesia required for PCA.[38,39] It has been used to supplement epidural analgesia [40] in doses of 2 microgram/kg. It is potentially a useful drug although the onset of action is slow. It is available in tablets and transdermal patches, as well as by injection.

Ketamine

Given by infusion ketamine is extremely useful for controlling agonizingly severe postoperative pain.[41] This sort of pain is encountered where there has been a severe injury in the past, and the pain had not been effectively treated. An example is *phantom limb pain* which can reappear during, or after, spinal or epidural anaesthetic, or with severe metabolic stress. It is due to neuronal *wind-up* in the dorsal horn of the spinal cord where synapses become hyperexcitable and the slightest stimuli will trigger a massive response. It is also useful for severely burned patients who are extremely emotionally distressed. The addition of ketamine to their opioid gives a better balance of pain relief. Use a loading dose of ketamine of 0.1 mg per kilogram and follow this with a continuous ketamine infusion of 0.14 mg/kg/hr. This should achieve plasma concentrations of ketamine between 100 - 150 microgram/litre. The analgesic effect takes about an hour to become effective and reaches its peak in 48 hours. At this level of infusion hallucinations and dysphoria should not be a problem.

1. Weis OF, Sriwatanakul K, et al. (1983) Anesthesia and Analgesia, 62:70-4.
2. Sullivan LM (1994). Journal of Post Anesthesia Nursing, 9:83-90.
3. Editorial Lancet (1985) 1. 1018-9.
4. Kehlet H. (1989). British Journal of Anaesthesia, 63:189-95.
5. Hughes SC. (1989). Current Opinion in Anesthesiology, 2: 295-302.
6. Aun C, Houghton T, et al. (1988). Anaesthesia and Intensive Care, 16:396-404.
7. Anesthesiology Clinics of North America (1991) Vol 9. No. 4.
8. Anand KJ, Hickey PR. (1987). New England Journal of Medicine, 317:1321-9.
9. Williams N., Kapla L. (1993). British Journal of Surgery 80: 1231-6.
10. Aun C, Houghton T, et al. (1988). Anaesthesia and Intensive Care, 16:396-404.
11. Katz J, Kavanagh B. (1992). Anesthesiology, 77:439-46.
12. Harmer M, (1991). Anaesthesia, 46: 167-8.
13. Donovan M , Dillon P, et al. (1987). Pain, 30:69-78.
14. Koetntop D, Redman J, et al. (1986). Anesthesia and Analgesia, 65:227-32.
15. Wride SR, Smith RE. (1989). Anaesthesia and Intensive Care, 17:374-7.
16. Norcutt WG, Morgan RJM. (1990). Anaesthesia, 45: 401-6.
17. Mather LE, Owen H. (1986). Anaesthesia and Intensive Care, 16:427-47.
18. Schug SA, Torrie JJ, (1993). Pain, 55: 387-91.
19. Parker RK, Holtman B, et al. (1992). Anesthesiology, 76:362-7.
20. Rawal N, Berggren L. (1994), Pain, 57:117-123.
21. Wheatley RG, (1990). British Journal of Anaesthesia, 64: 267-75.
22. Thomas VJ, Record KE, et al. (1995) British Journal of Anaesthesia, 74:271-6.
23. McIndoe AK, Warwick P, et al. (1996) Anaesthesia, 51:333-337.
24. Johnson LR, Ferrante FM et al. (1988), Anaesthesia, 13:525.
25. Stone PA, McIntyre PE (1993), British Journal of Anaesthesia, 71:738-740.
26. Plummer JL, Owen H. (1997) Anesthesia and Analgesia, 84:794 -99.
27. Kussman BD, Sethna NF (1998), Paediatric Anaesthesia, 8:349-52.
28. McIntyre PE, Jarvis DA (1996), Pain, 64:347-364.
29. Gaukroger P. Australian Anaesthesia, (1992), (ed D.Kerr, J.Thirlwell) pp. 11-14, Australian and New Zealand College of Anaesthetists, Melbourne.
30. Tyler DC, Woodham M. et al. (1995) Anesthesia and Analgesia, 80:14-19.
31. Dahl JB, Kehlet H. (1991). British Journal of Anaesthesia, 66:703-12.
32. Tonkin AL, Wing LMH. (1988). Clinics of Rheumatology, 2:455-83.
33. T. Lehmann, R. O'Day et al. (1997). MJA 166: 378-83.
34. Murray MD, Brater DC. (1990). Annals of Internal Medicine, 112:559-60.
35. Sommer P, Kromann-Andersen B, et al. (1989) British Journal of Urology, 63:4-6.
36. McGlew IC, Angliss DB, et al. (1991) Anaesthesia and Intensive Care, 19:40-5.
37. Maze M, Tranquilli W. (1991). Anesthesiology, 74:581-605.
38. De Cock M, Lavandhomme P. (1994). Anaesthesia and Intensive Care, 22:15-21.
39. Park J, Forrest J et al. (1996). Canadian Journal of Anaesthesia, 43:900-906.
40. Bennet F, Boico O, et al. (1990). Anesthesiology, 72:423-7.
41. Knox DJ, McLeod BJ. (1995) Anaesthesia and Intensive Care, 23,: 620-2.

12. REGIONAL TECHNIQUES FOR PAIN CONTROL

EPIDURAL ANALGESIA

Abdominal, thoracic operations and perineal are very painful. To control postoperative pain the anaesthetist may insert a fine catheter into the epidural space to give, either local anaesthetic drugs, or opioids, or sometimes both.

Epidural blocks can be sited in the lumbar region, caudal or thoracic region. A thoracic epidural is useful for upper abdominal and thoracic incisions such as a radical nephrectomy; the lumbar route is used for lower abdominal and upper limb operations, such as abdomino-perineal resections and hip replacements, and the caudal route for operations around the perineum such as haemorrhoids.

In the recovery room epidurals are sometimes inserted for pain therapy.

Inserting an epidural is strictly a sterile procedure requiring, gloves, gown, drapes and a mask. Position the patient comfortably on his side with his legs tucked up. It is not usual to sit patients up to insert epidurals in the recovery room.

Graduated Tuohy's needles are used. They usually come with an epidural kit such as those manufactured by Portex®, which contain everything to perform the procedure. The epidural needles are 8 cm long, sized either 16 gauge or 18 gauge, embossed in 1 cm graduations and have a Huber tip that guides the catheter along the axis of the epidural space. A 10 or 20 ml syringe containing air or normal saline is attached to the needle which is then slowly advanced between the vertebrae to locate the epidural space. With each incremental advancement the anaesthetist gentle presses the plunger on the syringe. The pressure in the epidural space, being in communication with the pleural space, is below atmospheric pressure. This enables the anaesthetist to locate the space. When the tip of the needle enters the space there is a sudden loss of resisitance to the pressure he applies to the plunger. If the tip of the needle is advanced too far, it will piece the dura mater and cerebrospinal fluid will gush back into the syringe. This unwanted complication is called a *dural tap*.

If the dural tap is not recognized, and a large volume of local anaesthetic is accidentally injected into the cerebrospinal fluid it causes *total spinal anaesthesia*. The patient collapses, loses consciousness and becomes hypotensive. He will need intubation, ventilation and ionotropic support with dopamine to maintain his blood pressure. With suitable care the patient usually recovers uneventfully, but he needs support in intensive care for up to 24 hours. Fortunately total spinal anaesthesia is rare, and at the worst most dural taps cause a post dural puncture headache.

> *The recovery room must be equipped*
> *to handle complications of regional anaesthesia.*

Sometimes the needle penetrates an epidural vein with blood coming back into the syringe. In either case the needle is withdrawn and the epidural re-attempted in an adjacent space.

Once in the epidural space the anaesthetist may wish to insert a fine graduated catheter. Local anaesthetics and other drugs can be injected into the catheter to give continuing pain relief. The drugs can be given at intervals or continuously infused.

The catheter may be left in place for some days. Local anaesthetic agents such as bupivacaine anaesthetize the somatic nerves as they leave the spinal cord, while the opioids interrupt the transmission of pain impulses in the spinal cord itself. This provides analgesia for the incision, the nearby skin, and muscle, and will almost completely relieve postoperative pain. Ill-defined deep visceral pain from the underlying organs may persist, because these impulses are transmitted through the vagus nerve, and do not travel in the spinal cord. If deep visceral pain becomes distressing, a small dose of opioid will relieve it.

Advantages of epidural analgesia
1. The patient should have only minor discomfort from their wound, with little need for opioids.
2. Postoperative drug induced nausea and vomiting is minimal.
3. Epidural blockade reduces the bad effects of postoperative stress syndrome helping wounds to heal faster, reducing wound infection and lowering the metabolic insults caused by surgery.

4. The incidence of deep vein thromboses and pulmonary emboli is reduced because blood flow through the lower body and legs is increased. This helps prevent the formation of clots.

5. Epidurals reduce postoperative myocardial ischaemia by reducing cardiac preload and afterload, and reducing adrenergic effects.[1]

Disadvantages of epidural analgesia

1. An intravenous infusion is essential to treat hypotension that can occur after the initial injection or subsequent *top-ups*.

2. Regional blockade in a patient who has received substantial doses of opioids may cause respiratory depression. This occurs because the opioid induced respiratory depression was antagonized by the pain. Once pain is gone, respiratory depression becomes active.

3. Sometimes, for reasons that are not clear, epidural analgesia skips segments so that an area may not be anaesthetised yet everything around it will be pain free. *Skipped areas* are more common in patients who have previously had an epidural anaesthetic, probably due to scarring in the epidural space preventing the anaesthetic solution from spreading evenly.

4. The patient must have his bladder catheterised, which has its own set of complications.

5. Extra care is required with thoracic epidurals. If the patient feels nauseated when sitting up, it means that the block is too high and the rate of infusion.

6. If the patient feels that he is choking when he lies flat, the block is also too high and reaching the respiratory centres.

Never give intravenous and
epidural opioids at the same time.

Risks of epidural anaesthesia

The main risks arising during the insertion of epidural injections are:
- toxicity;
- accidental dural puncture;
- hypotension;
- respiratory depression if opioids are used;
- epidural haematoma.

TOXICITY OF THE LOCAL ANAESTHETIC

Before injecting any local anaesthetic into the epidural space it is essential to be absolutely sure that the injection will not go into a vein, or the sub-arachnoid space. If you have doubts about the location of the catheter tip, disconnect the syringe and leave the catheter to lie open for a couple of minutes below the level of the spine. Do not aspirate back on the catheter. If blood comes back then resite the catheter. If clear fluid returns this may be either local anaesthetic or cerebrospinal fluid (CSF). If you are in doubt then test the fluid for glucose, which is normally present in CSF.

Give a small test dose of lignocaine 30 - 50 mg with 1:200 000 adrenaline and wait for 2 minutes. If the epidural inside the sub-arachnoid space the patient will report the onset of block; and if it has found its way into an epidural vein then the pulse rate will rise by 30 - 40 beats per minute.

ACCIDENTAL DURAL PUNCTURE (DURAL TAP)

If the epidural needle is advanced too far it will puncture the dural membrane and allow cerebrospinal fluid to escape into the epidural space. This results in severe headache, the so called post-spinal headache. If the headache does not resolve with simple measures such as hydration and analgesia,[2] then stop the leak with a blood patch.

BLOOD PATCH FOR CONTROL OF SPINAL HEADACHES [3]

Although dural puncture during epidural anaesthesia is rare in experienced hands there is an overall incidence of 1 - 4 per cent. When it occurs cerebrospinal fluid leaks into the epidural space causing a severe headache. This sometimes develops in the recovery room. The anaesthetist may decide to place a *blood patch* over the hole in the dura. Two operators are needed to carry out the procedure, one takes blood from the patient's arm, while the other locates the epidural space. Ten to twenty millilitres of blood is taken from the patient's arm and injected into the epidural space at the level of the hole. Lie the patient flat for 2 hours. Ideally the blood will clot over the hole to block the leak. In most cases the headache eases almost immediately.

It is essential that the procedure is carried out with strict sterile precautions. If the clot becomes infected in the epidural space, an abscess will develop and irreversible paraplegia may follow.

LOW MOLECULAR WEIGHT HEPARINS AND SPINAL HAEMATOMA

In the past five years *low molecular weight heparins* (LMWH) have become deservedly popular as effective and life saving prophylaxis against deep vein thrombosis and pulmonary embolism particularly after major hip and knee surgery.[4] The two most frequently used low molecular weight heparins are daltaparin (Fragmin®) and enoxaparin (Clexane®). Since their introduction there has been a steep rise in the previously very uncommon problem of bleeding into the epidural or subdural space causing haematomas.[5]

Recommendations on using LMWH in conjunction with spinal or epidural anaesthesia.

- Avoid using LMWH if the patient is on antiplatelet drugs such as aspirin or ticlopidine.
- Use the smallest needle practicable for the procedure.
- Do not use epidural catheters unless you need to. Single shot technique is safer.
- Patients with renal impairment and those who are on long term NSAIDs may excrete LMWH more slowly.
- Use postoperative infusion regimes that do not cause motor blockade.
- The once daily dosing schedule used in Australia, UK and Europe, rather than the twice daily dose used in the USA, appears to reduce the risk of haematoma.[6]

Commencing LMWH pre-operatively.

- Do not use an epidural or spinal techniques if the patient has had prophylactic LMWH (ie. Enoxaparin 40 mg) within the preceding 12 hours.
- If the patient is on therapeutic LMWH ie. Enoxaparin 1.5 mg/kg daily or enoxaparin 1 mg/kg bd. then wait 24 hours before inserting either spinal or epidural.
- If the patient has had pre-operative LMWH, and your have waited the 12 hours and to place an epidural catheter or do a spinal, then wait a further 12 hours before the next dose of LMWH.

Commencing post-operative LMWH

- Delay the initial dose of LMWH 12 hours after catheter insertion.
- If there is a traumatic tap then delay the initial dose of enoxaparin for 24 hours.

Removing the epidural catheter

- Perform catheter manipulation during a trough in LMWH activity.
- Remove the catheter 2 hours before the first dose of LMWH.
- If the catheter is already in situ do not remove or manipulate it until 12 hours after last dose of LMWH.
- Remove catheters in the morning so that the patient can be monitored for signs of a developing haematoma during daylight hours.

HYPOTENSION

Sympathetic blockade occurs with hypotension and bradycardia if the block extends to T4 or above. Vasodilation in the lower body causes hypotension. This can happen up to an hour after the initial procedure, it responds to a colloid load, or to a small dose of ephedrine (10 - 30 mg) intravenously. Take care not to give more than a litre of colloid to an elderly person. If you need to treat the hypotension, monitor the blood pressure every quarter hour for the next four hours.

RESPIRATORY DEPRESSION IF OPIOIDS ARE USED

There have been many reports of profound respiratory depression, occurring up to 2 hours after a single dose of epidural opioid. This is discussed more fully on page 223.

SPINAL HAEMATOMA

An spinal haematoma is a medical emergency. You will need to act fast to prevent permanent damage and probable paraplegia. It is far more likely to occur in those patients who have received low molecular weight heparins or who are taking anticoagulants preoperatively including warfarin, aspirin or ticlopidine, or who receive heparin or dextrans intraoperatively, or who may have any clotting defect. Elderly women having knee or hip surgery are most susceptible.

Signs that a spinal haematoma is developing include:
- numbness or weakness in the lower limbs;
- pain referrable to the nerve roots at the site of the injection, pain occurs in less than half the patients;
- incontinence of bladder or bowel;
- urinary retention.

All these may develop in the recovery room.

Care of epidural lines

Measure the vital signs, blood pressure, pulse respiratory rate, and oxygen saturation every ten minutes for the first hour. Watch carefully for trends in the patient's respiratory rate especially if epidural opioids have been used. Once the patient is pain free, encourage him to deep breath and cough. Record the neurological signs of pupil size and reactivity, and level of consciousness.

Motor function of the lower limbs is particularly important because any loss of motor function may be a sign that an epidural haematoma is developing. This is a surgical emergency. Unless detected early this can result in permanent nerve damage with probable paralysis of the lower limbs. Other signs of cord compression include urinary or faecal incontinence. Haematomas are more likely to occur in elderly women undergoing major hip and knee surgery, but in particular if the patient has been given a low molecular weight heparin such as daltaparin or enoxaparin as prophylaxis against deep vein thrombosis. If you see any of these signs inform the surgeon and anaesthetist immediately.

As with all surgical patients record fluid intake and urine output. This will help detect urinary retention and the patient's blood volume status. Observe the surgical incision site. Is it tense or hard? Is the surgical dressing dry or soaked? The epidural removes the warning signs of pain.

Routinely keep an ampoule of naloxone and a syringe at the bedside in case you need them in a hurry.

Problems that need immediate attention include:
• respiratory rate less than 10 breaths per minute;
• oxygen saturation of less than 92 per cent;
• bleeding from the surgical site;
• persistent nausea or vomiting;
• decrease in motor or sensory function;
• inability to void;
• urinary or faecal incontinence;
• itch.

Precautions with epidural lines
Once established, epidural catheters rarely cause any problems. However haematoma and infection are possible, though fortunately rare complications. To help prevent infection in the epidural space a small bacterial filter is fitted to the end of the catheters. Do not disconnect this for any reason. Protect the catheter and filter as a neat package in a sterile plastic bag, wrapped in a sterile drape. Label it clearly so that nothing will be inadvertently injected into it. Do not disturb the dressings because of the danger of dislodging the catheter.

Top-ups
Intermittent administration of drugs through the epidural catheter are called *top-ups*. Only specifically instructed staff should top-up the epidural catheter with local anaesthetic. Hypotension is common after top-ups. It occurs within 10 - 15 minutes and may require treatment. Lie the patient flat, give oxygen and infuse 250 - 500 mls of colloid such as polygeline. If the blood pressure does not rise give ephedrine. Dilute ephedrine 30 mg in

10 mls of sterile saline and give 1 ml (3 mg) increments every 2 minutes until the blood pressure returns to a safe level. Monitor the blood pressure frequently to ensure the hypotension does not recur. An automated non-invasive blood pressure machine is a useful monitor in these patients.

Local anaesthesia wears off abruptly,
be ready to top it up.

Continuous infusion

To avoid the inconvenience of continually having to top up the epidural use a volumetric pump to infuse epidural opioids when the patient returns to the ward. This can be set up in recovery room. Record the rate of the infusion, the volume infused, and the patient's vital signs status as laid down in your hospital's protocol. Never purge a pump that is connected to an epidural catheter.

Removal of the catheters

Ease the catheters out gently. If you meet resistance, then call for skilled assistance. Rarely these fine catheters break off in the epidural space while being removed. For this reason carefully inspect them after removal to make sure the catheter is intact, and record this fact in the patient's notes. Usually the piece left behind causes no problems, but the patient must be warned in writing of the danger of it becoming a focus for infection.

AGENTS USED IN EPIDURAL ANAESTHESIA

Bupivacaine and epidural opioids are the agents most frequently used for epidural analgesia. Lignocaine is sometimes used, but it is too short acting for postoperative analgesia.

BUPIVACAINE (MARCAIN®)

Epidural bupivacaine is the most commonly used drug.

Useful facts

1. Bupivacaine takes 10 - 20 minutes to work and its effect lasts 3 - 6 hours.
2. Some anaesthetists speed the onset and prolong the duration of bupivacaine by alkalinizing the solution. We do not encourage this practice because the manufacturers of the local anaesthetic have spent a

great deal of effort in ensuring the stability of the drug, and modifications may upset this. The dose usually used is 0.05 ml of 8.4% sodium bicarbonate for every 10 mls of bupivacaine.

3. Weaker concentrations are more suitable in elderly patients, where it is important to keep the total dose low.

EFFECTS OF EPIDURAL BUPIVACAINE		
	Motor effects	Analgesia
Bupivacaine 0.5%	blocks all movement	deep analgesia
Bupivacaine 0.375%	weak motor function	good analgesia
Bupivacaine 0.25%	moderate motor function	good analgesia
Bupivacaine 0.2%	moving, no weight bearing	moderate analgesia

4. Bupivacaine with commercially added adrenaline does not have a significantly longer duration of action than the plain solution, but it does reduce the incidence of toxic symptoms by retarding absorption, and it does warn of accidental intravascular injection. If you add fresh adrenaline to the solution it will greatly increase not only the duration and intensity of the block, but also its spread. A typical dose of adrenaline would be 0.1 ml of 1:1000 adrenaline added to 20 mls of bupivacaine.

5. The toxic dose of bupivacaine is about 2 mg/kg of lean body mass. 20 mls of 0.5 per cent bupivacaine contains 100 mg of bupivacaine. Do not exceed this dose in any given top-up period as it may produce convulsions, ventricular arrhythmias and cardiac failure.

6. Age is one of the most important factors influencing the spread of the block. Minimal spread occurs in 20 year olds, and only half the volume is needed for 70 - 80 year olds. From 20 - 40 years about 1 ml of local anaesthetic is needed to block each dermatome. Taller patients need about 10 per cent more solution.

7. The dose of bupivacaine required for effective analgesia depends on the level of the tip of the epidural catheter, normally between 8 - 12 ml for a catheter inserted in the lumbar region and between 3 - 8 ml for a catheter inserted in the thoracic region. A rapid injection will extend the spread of the block, but this is difficult to achieve through a fine catheter and bacterial microporous filter. Always use the same technique and you will soon discover the optimal dose and spread of the drugs. If you

continually change your catheter size, needles gauge and solutions strength, you will become confused.

8. A common problem with epidural anaesthesia is an inadvertent block of the sympathetic supply to the heart (T_1 - T_4) reducing the cardiac output and cause the blood pressure to fall.

Ropivicaine is similar to bupivacaine but less potent. It causes less cardiotoxicity, and a less reliable motor block. It is also slightly shorter acting.[7]

EPIDURAL OPIOIDS

Epidural opioids do not interfere with motor function or cause as much hypotension as local anaesthetics agents. However opioids do cause:
• respiratory depression;
• itching;
• urinary retention.

Fentanyl
Fentanyl works quickly and lasts 2 - 4 hours. Draw up 100 micrograms of fentanyl in a 10 ml syringe and make up to 10 ml with saline. Use a volume of 0.1 ml/kg of estimated lean body mass.

Fentanyl provides good analgesia by blocking pain pathways in the spinal cord without affecting the sensations of touch or pressure. Motor pathways are left intact, in contrast to the local anaesthetics, this allows the patient to move about. Fentanyl will not cause sympathetic blockade, or peripheral vasodilation, and so the blood pressure should remain unaffected.

If the blood pressure falls after epidural fentanyl
- the patient may be hypovolaemic.

Pethidine
Epidural pethidine crosses the dura and enters the cerebrospinal fluid in 5 - 8 minutes and reaches peak analgesic effect in 15 - 30 minutes. Its analgesic effect lasts for 1 - 4 hours. Draw up 100 mg of pethidine in a 10 ml syringe and make up to 10 mls with saline. Use a volume of 0.1 ml/kg of estimated lean body mass. The incidence of respiratory depression is less than morphine.

Morphine

Epidural morphine crosses the dura and enters the cerebrospinal fluid in effective concentrations in 20 - 40 minutes and its effect lasts up to 18 hours. Draw up 10 mg of morphine in a 10 ml syringe and make up to 10 mls with saline. Use a volume of 0.1 ml/kg of estimated lean body mass. An unsettling and irritating itch can be a problem. Try promethazine 0.25 mg/kg (Phenergan®). If this doesn't work, naloxone will but it will also reverse the analgesia. The incidence of respiratory depression is about 0.25 per cent.

Mixtures of opioids and local anaesthetic agents

Mixtures of opioids and local anaesthetic agents are clearly superior to either agent used alone. The advantages are a low incidence of motor blockade, shivering, and urinary retention.[8] Some infusion packs containing fentanyl and bupivacaine are available commercially. They contain 0.1 per cent bupivacaine and fentanyl 100 micrograms in 100 mls of saline with a usual rate of infusion of 10 - 20 mls/hour. For larger volumes take a bag of 500 mls of saline, and withdraw 120 mls of the saline. Then add 100 mls of 0.5 per cent bupivacaine and 200 microgram of fentanyl. For a thoracic epidural start with 4 - 6 mls and hour, and a lumbar epidural 8-16 mls per hour. Titrate an initial loading dose until the pain is relieved. Morphine and bupivacaine are sometimes used, Bupivacaine 0.1 per cent at 3 - 4 ml per hour with morphine 0.3 - 0.4 mg per hour. Pethidine and bupivacaine are also effective, and have the advantage of not causing an itch,[9] but the incidence of vomiting and urinary retention is higher.

Patient Controlled Epidural Analgesia (PCEA)

PCEA is gaining popularity. The principle is similar to the patient controlled analgesia used for intravenous opioid infusions. We have found that a basal background infusion is necessary.

PRECAUTIONS WITH EPIDURAL AND INTRATHECAL OPIOIDS

Respiratory depression

There have been a number of reports of profound respiratory depression, occurring up to 2 hours after a single dose of epidural fentanyl.[10] Patients should be kept under close observation for at least 3 hours after epidural fentanyl.

Respiratory depression can occur from any time from 30 minutes to 18 hours after commencing an epidural opioid infusion.[11] The onset of respiratory depression is not sudden. Typically the respiratory rate falls slowly to 6 - 8 breaths a minute (or even less) over an hour or more. The patient becomes drowsy, sweaty, and even cyanosed. Severe respiratory depression occurs if any additional systemic opioids are given (either intramuscularly, subcutaneously, or intravenously) in conjunction with the epidural opioids. Respiratory depression typically outlasts the analgesia. Put a warning sign DO NOT GIVE OPIOIDS on the patient's drug sheet, and bed head.

Epidural opioids exclude the use of systemic opioids.

Respiratory depression can be reversed with small doses of naloxone 0.1 mg IV at intervals of one minute up to a total dose of 0.8 mg. Keep syringes and ampoules of naloxone at the bedside. If respiratory depression is not relieved by this dose, then it is unlikely to be due to the opioids, so consider other causes. For established opioid induced respiratory depression use a naloxone infusion of about 10 microgram/kg/hr intravenously. This dose reverses the analgesic effects of morphine, but not necessarily the analgesia of epidural fentanyl.[12] A stat order for naloxone must always be written in the drug sheet in case it is needed for emergency use.

Give naloxone intravenously
if the respiratory rate is less than 8 breaths per minute,
OR
the patient is sweaty and drowsy in the absence of pain.

Before returning to the ward record the following in the patient's notes:
• the site of the infusion;
• the total volume of the infusion;
• the concentration of the drug;
• time of commencement;
• the rate of infusion in millilitres an hour;
• instructions about what to do if set limits of respiratory rate and blood; pressure changes are exceeded;
• orders for an antidote and the doses needed;
• name and signature of the doctor supervising the infusion;
• where and how the doctor can be contacted.

Epidural opioids require a stat order for naloxone
and provision for an infusion.

INTRATHECAL OPIOIDS

Small doses of a variety of drugs have been introduced into the cerebrospinal fluid in conjunction with spinal anaesthesia. The major risk with opioids used in this way is respiratory depression, which has been reported to occur from 30 - 45 minutes after injection, to peak at 3 - 6 hours, but may be delayed as late as 18 hours. This event can be catastrophic if not noticed in the ward. If the patient has received an intrathecal opioid, warn the ward about this. Continuous infusion of intraspinal drugs is not advised, because of the risk of nerve damage.

1. Breslow MJ, Jordan DA. (1989). *Journal of the American Medical Association*, 261: 3577.
2. Stride PC, Cooper GM. (1993). *Anaesthesia*, 48: 247-55.
3. Carrie LES. (1993). *British Journal of Anaesthesia*, 71:177-81.
4. Nurmohamed MT, Rosendaal FR *et al.* (1992). Lancet 340:152-6.
5. Berqvist D (1992). *Acta Anaesthesiol Scandanavia* 36:605-9.
6. Horlocker TT *et al.* (1994), *Regional Anesthesia and Pain Management* 79:1165-77.
7. Katz JA, *et al.* (1990) *Anesthesia and Analgesia* 70:16.
8. Westmore MD. (1990). *Anaesthesia and Intensive Care*, 18:292.
9. Periss BW, Latham BV. (1990). *British Journal of Anaesthesia*, 64:355-7.
10. Brockway MS, Noble DW, *et al.* (1990). *British Journal of Anaesthesia*, 64:243-5.
11. Knill R, Clement J, *et al.* (1981). *Canadian Anaesthetic Society Journal*, 28:537-41.
12. Gueneron JP, Ecoffey C. (1988). *Anesthesia and Analgesia*, 67:35-41.

13. POSTOPERATIVE NAUSEA AND VOMITING

Postoperative nausea and vomiting (especially after day surgery) can turn an otherwise successful operation into a disaster. In many cases patients fear postoperative nausea and vomiting (PONV) more than pain. The severity ranges from mild queasiness through to a distressing, prolonged, life threatening illness needing resuscitation with intravenous fluids. The incidence ranges roughly from 10 - 45 per cent (or even more) of patients having a general anaesthetic. It is probable that patients are willing to accept drowsiness, increased pain, increased cost, and even dysphoria (feeling agitated), to avoid postoperative nausea and vomiting.[1]

Postoperative nausea and vomiting delays the patient's discharge from the recovery room, and increases the nurses' work load. Just under one per cent of day surgery patients have to stay in hospital overnight because of uncontrollable nausea and vomiting, making it an expensive complication.

VOMITING

Vomiting (*emesis*) is an involuntary protective reflex for evicting injested toxins from the body. In contrast to regurgitation it is an active process producing either solid or liquid matter. The patient usually realises a few seconds beforehand that they are about to vomit. They both begin with a deep inspiration. The glottis closes, the diaphragm and abdominal muscles contract violently ejecting the stomach contents.

NAUSEA

Nausea is an unpleasant feeling of the need to vomit. It is accompanied by sweating, pallor, bradycardia, and salivation. If a patient is nauseated, it means that he feels as though he wants to vomit. On the other hand if a patient is nauseous, it means the patient is so vile and repulsive that he makes you feel sick. On the whole, patients are nauseated, and rarely nauseous. It is easy to remember! Consider the statement "people are poisoned, and rarely poisonous".

Vomiting is hazardous because it can cause:
• aspiration into the lungs with fulminating chemical pneumonitis;
• damage to the cornea if it gets into the eyes;

- damage to facial skin flaps;
- raised intraocular pressure;
- physical exertion that may tear suture lines;
- bradycardia in patients with ischaemic heart disease;
- hypotension in patients with peripheral vascular disease;
- if prolonged, it leads to hypokalaemia and saline depletion;
- tearing and rupture of the oesophagus in a few susceptible individuals.

Mendleson's syndrome (see page 379)

Mendleson's syndrome is a peculiarly vicious, and sometimes fatal, aspiration pneumonitis of pregnancy. The term is occasionally used for all aspiration pneumonitis.

PHYSIOLOGY OF VOMITING

Nausea and vomiting is an adaptive reflex to protect against ingested toxins. There are three components to the vomiting reflex: emetic detectors, co-ordinating centres, and motor outputs.

Emetic detectors are stretch receptors in the gut wall that respond to distension; and polymodal chemoreceptors in the mucosa of the stomach and duodenum that monitor the intraluminal environment. The stimulus is carried by the afferent fibres of the vagus nerve to the brain stem.

Co-ordinating centres. The centres co-ordinating vomiting in the brainstem have neural inputs from the stomach, the vestibular apparatus in the ear, emotional centres, in the cortex and from direct stimuli by toxins carried in the blood.

The *vomiting centre* lies inside the blood brain barrier in the lateral reticular formation of the medulla. It co-ordinates the control of the complex vomiting reflex. Rich in cholinergic receptors, it receives incoming signals from the pharynx, gastrointestinal tract and mediastinum via the vagus nerve; and from the vestibular portion of the eighth cranial nerve and the chemotrigger receptor zone. It is interconnected with other centres that control various aspects of the autonomic nervous system, such as salivation, sweating, bradycardia and blood pressure control.

The *chemotrigger receptor zone* (CTZ), on the other hand, lies outside the blood brain barrier in the medulla where it is exposed to circulating toxins. It is rich in dopaminergic, opioid and 5-HT$_3$ receptors. Stimulation of the chemotrigger receptor zone triggers the vomiting centre to co-ordinate vomiting.

Motor output. Sweating, skin vasoconstriction, pupillary dilation, and tachycardia are mediated by sympathetic nerves; while salivation is mediated by parasympathetic nerves. The ejection phase consisting of retching and vomiting, involves vilent contractions of the abdominal wall and diaphram. The effort may be strong enough to fracture ribs in the elderly.

Regurgitation

Regurgitation is a passive process where fluid matter refluxes up the oesophagus from the stomach. It occurs without warning, and can cause aspiration pneumonitis in a comatose or obtunded patient. Regurgitation is likely to occur in a patient with:

- hiatus hernia;
- distended abdomen;
- intestinal obstruction;
- ascites;
- pregnancy.

CAUSES OF NAUSEA AND VOMITING

Postoperative nausea and vomiting occurs in all types of patients, and with all types of operations and anaesthetics.[2] There are, however certain groups of people, and certain types of procedures where vomiting is more likely.[3]

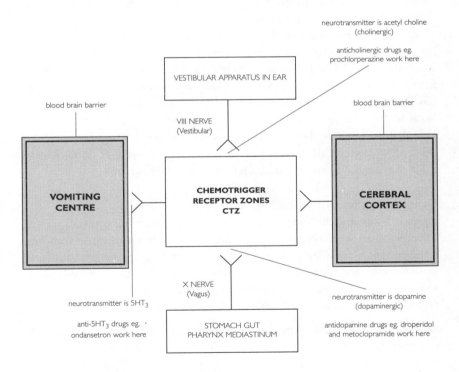

fig 13.1 Simplified diagram showing inputs that cause nausea and vomiting

Surgical factors[4]

- intra-abdominal operations where the peritoneum is stretched;
- hypotension during the operation;
- prolonged surgery;
- biliary surgery;
- thyroid surgery;
- gynaecological surgery;
- ophthalmic operations, especially squint surgery (up to 85 per cent of children vomit without prophylaxis);
- ENT surgery, especially tonsillectomy, adenoidectomy, and middle ear surgery;
- urological surgery, especially if the spermatic cord is involved;
- emergency surgery, especially for fractures;
- laparoscopy.

Patient factors

Children are more likely to vomit than adults. The incidence is low in infants (about 5 per cent) and increases through childhood reaching a peak of 30 - 50 per cent in the 6 - 16 year age group[5]. Women, especially during the last half of their menstrual cycle[6], are two to four times more likely to vomit than men[7]. Elderly patients, over 70 years, do not often vomit. Obese patients are often thought to be more likely to vomit than thin patients, but the evidence is slim. Obese patients have a high risk of regurgitation, because they often have hiatus hernias. Patients who get motion sickness are at high risk. There is also a strong psychological factor; those patients who think that they are likely to vomit, or who have a history of doing so, are three times more likely to vomit after subsequent operations.

Drugs as a cause of vomiting

Opioid drugs are the most potent cause of nausea and vomiting. They directly act on the brainstem centres; and are more likely to cause vomiting if the patient is ambulant. They sensitize the vomiting centres to input from the vestibular apparatus; in effect opioids make one sea-sick. Opioids given as premedication, and during operations more than double the incidence of vomiting. All opioids are approximately equivalent in this respect.

All the inhalational anaesthetic agents; and many induction agents such as thiopentone, methohexitone, ketamine, and particularly etomidate, cause nausea and vomiting. Propofol is the least likely of the induction agents to cause nausea and vomiting. Benzodiazepines, and muscle relaxants have no effect on the incidence of nausea and vomiting.[8]

Anaesthetic technique

Patients who breath spontaneously during the anaesthetic are less at risk, than those who are ventilated, but this could be related to the increased use of opioids in the ventilated group. The way in which patients are ventilated before intubation also plays a part. An experienced anaesthetist is unlikely to put air into the stomach to cause gastric distention. Neostigmine, given at the end of surgery, contracts the stomach and may cause vomiting on waking. Patients who have been hypotensive during their anaesthetic tend to vomit, but the reason for this is unknown.

Spinal and epidural anaesthesia cause less vomiting than general anaesthesia, providing the block does not cause hypotension.

Factors in the recovery room

In the recovery room nausea and vomiting may be induced by:

- pain which tends to produce nausea rather than vomiting;
- hypotension;
- hypoxia;
- hypovolaemia;
- anxiety;
- early mobilisation;
- swallowed blood;
- acute water intoxication.

Nausea or vomiting after epidural, or spinal anaesthesia may be a sign of hypotension that needs immediate treatment.

MANAGEMENT OF NAUSEA AND VOMITING

Conscious patients will often dry retch before vomiting. They become pale and sweaty with a weak pulse, and their blood pressure falls. They find it easier to vomit while sitting up.

If the patient is fully conscious
and about to vomit - help him sit up.

IMMEDIATE MANAGEMENT

1. In a semiconscious patient; roll him onto his side, take his pillow away, and suck out his mouth and pharynx with a wide bore sucker. Be gentle, or you will stimulate further vomiting.

2. Patients who are expected to be susceptible to either regurgitation, or vomiting usually leave the theatre with a nasogastric tube draining freely. Be aware that a nasogastric tube will not prevent regurgitation, nor reduce the risk of aspiration pneumonia.

3. Most children only vomit once or twice following anaesthetics, and recover quickly. Side effects from the anti-emetic drugs are severe in children, and it is better to withold drug therapy and wait.

4. Moving patients around after giving an opioid is a potent cause of nausea and vomiting postoperatively.[9] Sit your patients up, and face them forward when transporting them on their trolleys. Turn the trolley from the foot end, so as not to swing the head in a wide arc when turning corners. We have found these simple measures reduce vomiting in the first hour after returning to the ward by about half.[10]

5. Try to work out the cause of the vomiting and select the appropriate antiemetic drug. Postoperative nausea and vomiting has so many causes that a multimodal approach using several different drugs sequentially may be necessary

ANTI-EMETICS GROUPS			
GROUP	**DRUG**	**DOSE**	**MAIN SITE OF ACTION**
Antihistamines	Cyclizine	0.75 – 1 mg/kg	vestibular input + central action
	Promethazine	0.2 – 0.4 mg/kg	central action
Phenothiazines	Prochlorperazine	0.1 – 0.2 mg/kg	vestibular input
	Trifluperazine	0.05 – 0.1 mg/kg	vestibular input + central action
	Perphenazine	0.1 mg/kg	vestibular input + central action
Benzamides	Metoclopramide	0.15 mg/kg	vagal input + gut receptors
Butyrephenones	Droperidol	10 – 20 µg/kg	vagal input + central action
5-HT antagonists	Ondansetron	60 µg/kg	central action + gut receptors
Catecholamine	Ephedrine	0.5 mg/kg I/M	? central action ? antihypertensive

ANTIEMETIC THERAPY [11]

There are many controlled studies of the efficacy of antiemetic drugs, but they often contradict each other. It is difficult to compare these studies to arrive at valid conclusions.

The following facts emerge:
- Antidopaminergic antiemetics seem to work best against inputs from the vagus nerve;
- Anticholinergic drugs appear to work best against cholinergic input from the labyrinth (vestibular apparatus) in the ear;
- Antiseritonin (5-HT$_3$) antagonists work well against both;
- Antiemetic drugs are often sedating and delay discharge from the recovery room.

If the drug you have given is not effective,
try one from another group.

Anticholinergic drugs

Anticholinergic drugs block the cholinergic muscarinic receptors in the brain, and in the periphery. Centrally acting anticholinergic drugs block input from the vestibular apparatus in the ear to the chemotrigger receptor zone; so they are effective against motion sickness.

SCOPOLAMINE is an anticholinergic drug, used in premedication of children and young adults. Its antiemetic effects last about an hour, which is not long enough to cover the postoperative period. It gives patients a dry mouth and prevents them sweating; this is not a good thing in a hot climate. Other side effects include drowsiness, blurred vision, and urinary retention. Scopolamine causes disorientation, and confusion in the elderly. Treat this with physotigmine.

Antihistamines

Antihistamines block H$_1$ receptors, in the brain and periphery. Their antiemetic effect is probably due to their anticholinergic muscarinic blocking activity. Although they are less effective than scopolamine in alleviating motion sickness, they are also less sedating. The cyclizine and promethazine are two phenothiazines without significant antidopaminergic activity.

CYCLIZINE (Valoid®, Marezine®), a piperazine phenothiazine, is an effective antiemetic against opioid induced vomiting. It is less sedating than other phenothiazines, and deserves to be more popular. The adult dose is 50 mg I/M and it works for about 4 hours.

PROMETHAZINE (Phenergan®), an aliphatic phenothiazine, is sometimes used, but makes patients drowsy, delays emergence, and can drop their blood pressure by causing peripheral vasodilation. It works mainly through its antimuscarinic action on the chemotrigger receptor zone. The adult dose is 12.5 - 25 mg I/M, 4 - 6 hourly.

Phenothiazines

Phenothiazines work primarily because they are dopaminergic D_2 antagonists acting on the chemotrigger receptor zone. Because of their slow total body clearance, they are all long acting with a half life of more than 30 hours. In elderly or debilitated patients they are prone to cause hypotension, agitation, apprehension, and sleep disturbance.

EXTRAPYRAMIDAL SYNDROME

Children, young adults, and debilitated elderly patients are susceptible to *extrapyramidal syndrome* (dystonia and nystagmus). This is frightening for the patient, who develops a syndrome of muscle rigidity, and marked oscillations of the eyes (nystagmus) known as an *oculogyric crisis*. With phenothiazines the incidence is about 0.3 per cent, but a quarter of these reactions occur after a single parenteral dose. Treat this with benztropine (Cogentin®) 1 mg IV, and repeat in 10 minutes if necessary.

PROCHLORPERAZINE (Stemetil®) is a widely prescribed for postoperative nausea and vomiting, and morphine induced symptoms, particularly if the input is coming from the vestibular apparatus in the ear. The dose is 0.1 - 0.2 mg/kg I/M, because of its long action, do not repeat the dose in less than 6 hours. Thiethylperazine (Torecan®), and perphenazine (Fentazin®) are similar, but longer acting drugs. They both delay emergence from anaesthesia.

Benzamides

Metoclopramide and dromperidone are dopamine D_2 antagonists that have a peripheral action on the gut, as well as a central action similar to the phenothiazines. They are superior to the phenothiazines if the stimulus to vomit is coming from the gut. They are useless against motion sickness that is triggered by the vestibular apparatus in the ear, and are not as effective against opioid induced vomiting as the phenothiazines.

METOCLOPRAMIDE (Maxolon®, Reglan®) seems more useful for symptoms induced by handling of the bowel, or uterus and ovaries, or swallowed blood. It is often prescribed for the wrong reasons. Surprisingly 50 per cent of studies have found metoclopramide to be no more effective than placebo in the treatment of postoperative nausea and vomiting [12]. It is ineffective against opioid induced vomiting, and is useless against motion sickness. The dose is 0.15 mg/kg I/M 4 - 6 hourly as needed. Higher doses are more effective, but are more likely to cause side effects. Severe bradycardia can occur with intravenous metoclopramide, so give it slowly over one minute. Metoclopramide can cause an unpredictable *extrapyramidal syndrome*, particularly in children and young women. Keep the dose below 0.5 mg/kg/day.

Since it is a dopamine antagonist, do not give metoclopramide to a patient whose blood pressure is being supported by a dopamine infusion.

Butyrephenones
The butyrephenones have strong antidopaminergic activity, and work in a similar manner to the phenothiazines and benzamines on the chemoreceptor trigger zone. They are also alpha blockers, and in larger doses cause postural hypotension.

DROPERIDOL (Droleptan®, Inapsine®), a potent neuroleptic agent, is certainly effective, but the side effects of agitation, anxiety, and sometimes severe dysphoria are unpleasant if higher doses are used. The patient outwardly appears calm and tranquil, and inwardly feels miserable, and fearful. It is not a drug to use in day case surgery.[13] It is more effective in smaller, rather than larger doses, with the most effective dose being about 10 - 20 microgram/kg[14]. Doses of up to 75 - 100 microgram/kg IV are sometimes given during the anaesthetic. In this dose range, it is a long acting drug, and may cause sedation or dysphoria for more than 6 hours, postoperatively.

5-Hydroxytryptamine (serotonin) antagonist
ONDANSETRON (Zofran®) is a specific antagonist of the $5HT_3$ receptor in the vomiting centre, and is effective in controlling nausea and vomiting. $5HT_3$ is a neurotransmitter involved in activating vagal afferent pathways. Give 4 mg IV over 90 seconds. Apart from an annoying headache, flushing, and arrythmias, it has few side effects, and does not cause extrapyramidal syndrome. It is an expensive drug, and about twice as effective as metoclopramide for prophylaxis of postoperative nausea and vomiting in

gynaecological surgery[15]. The optimal dose is 50 microgram/kg. Doubling the dose does not increase efficacy.

Catecholamines

EPHEDRINE: In day case surgery ephedrine 0.5 mg/kg I/M is thought to be as effective as droperidol, but without the side effects. It is the preferred antiemetic in many day surgery centres, It probably acts by preventing postural hypotension in ambulant patients, but there may be a central mechanism.

Benzodiazepines [16]

MIDAZOLAM: A low dose infusion is effective treatment for persistant nausea and vomiting.

Acupressure and acupuncture

Acupuncture and acupressure have been advocated for the control of postoperative vomiting.[17] It is sometimes effective, and worth trying. The pressure point (P6 or *Neiguan point*) is in the midline on the anterior aspect of the left forearm about a Chinese inch above the proximal skin crease of the wrist. A Chinese inch is the length of the interphalangeal joint of the thumb. Probe about with your thumb until you find a point of deep ache. (It has to cause an ache to be effective.) Press firmly here and the nausea may abate, let go and it will return. Instruct the patient to find his own pressure point.

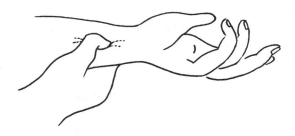

fig 13.2 Acupressure at point P6

If acupressure is successful in relieving the nausea a more prolonged effect can be obtained by acupuncture. Insert a fine 26 gauge needle at the point directing it straight down at right angles to the skin to a depth of 1.5 cm.

Twist the needle about its axis several times and then leave it for 5 minutes before withdrawing it. Stimulation of the of the P6 point by transcutaneous electrical stimulation is ineffective.[18]

HINTS

- Some patients will be nauseated and vomit, and often there is not much you can do about it.
- Nausea after a spinal or epidural anaesthetic is a warning sign of worryingly low blood pressure. Use ephedrine or phenylepherine to restore the blood pressure.
- When the input for nausea or vomiting is coming from the abdomen, or mediastinum via the vagus nerve then try metoclopramide. Ondansetron is better, but expensive.
- When the input is coming from the vestibular apparatus, or is opioid induced, try prochlorperazine.
- Metoclopramide is ineffective against opioid induced vomiting.
- Patients do not like the butyrephenones, and find their side effects unpleasant.
- If one of a group of anti-emetic drugs does not work, try a drug from a different group.
- Acupressure is noninvasive, and many patients favour it. We have not found it useful once vomiting has started. Acupuncture is better, but transcutaneous electrical stimulation is ineffective.
- Transport your patients sitting up, and facing forward.
- Children are likely to get dystonic side effects from the anti-emetic drugs. As children usually only vomit once or twice, it is best to avoid these drugs. If it is necessary to use an antiemetic in children; try droperidol 20 microgram/kg I/M, This often stops vomiting, and will not cause prolonged sedation.
- Lignocaine 2 mg/kg IV used in place of succinylcholine for intubation in children undergoing strabismus surgery, reduces postoperative vomiting[19].
- Hunger is a good sign of a functioning gut, but thirst is not. If a patient is hungry he will probably tolerate fluids and food without vomiting. Usually this occurs about an hour or so after day case surgery, and 4 – 6 hours after non-abdominal surgery. If it is safe, and the patient feels hungry, feed the patient a small sandwich, and a glass of clear fluid. This often reduces nausea and vomiting.
- In hot weather, start intravenous fluids and keep the patient fasting until he feels up to tolerating 60 ml of cold clear fluid. Wait 15 – 30 minutes to see what happens, then gradually increase the oral fluids.
- Prolonged preoperative fasting aggravates postoperative vomiting.
- It is easier to prevent nausea and vomiting, than to treat it. Preoperatively, teach your patient about acupressure, give prophylactic anti emetics in the operating theatre, control his pain, do not move him roughly, and sit him up as soon as possible after he has regained consciousness.

1. Orkin FK. (1992). *Anesthesia and Analgesia*, (Suppl) 74:S225.
2. Watcha MF, White PF. (1992). *Anesthesiology*, 77:162-84.
3. Rabey PG, Smith G. (1992). *British Journal of Anaesthesia*, 69:(Suppl.1) 40S-5.
4. Lerman J (1992) *British Journal of Anaesthesia* supplement 24-32.
5. Cohen MM, Cameron CB, *et al.* (1990). *Anesthesia and Analgesia*, 70:160-7.
6. Kenny GN. (1994). *Anaesthesia*, 49:(Suppl) 6-10.
7. Lerman J. (1992). *British Journal of Anaesthesia*, 69: (Suppl. 1) 24S-32S.
8. Forrest JB, Beatties WS, *et al.* (1990). *Canadian Journal of Anaesthetists*, 37 (Suppl.): S90.
9. Muir JJ, Warner MA, *et al.* (1987). *Anesthesiology*, 66:513-8.
10. Tronson M. Unpublished data.
11. Rowbotham DJ. (1992). *British Journal of Anaesthesia*, 69: (Suppl.1) 46S-59.
12. Rowbotham DJ. (1992). *British Journal of Anaesthesia*, 69: (Suppl.1) 46S-59.
13. Melnick B, Sawer R, *et al.* (1989). *Anesthesia and Analgesia*, 69:748-751.
14. Pandit S, Kothary S. (1989). *Anesthesia and Analgesia*, 68:798-802.
15. Malins AF, Field JM, *et al.* (1994). *British Journal of Anaesthesia*, 72:231-33.
16. Di Florio T, Goucke C R, (1999) *Anaesthesia and Intensive Care* 27: 38-40.
17. Dundee JW, Young J, *et al.* Lancet, (1990). (i) 541.
18. Ho RT, Jarwan B, *et al.* (1989). *Anaesthesia*, 45: 327-9.
19. Warner LO, Rogers GL, *et al.* (1988). *Anesthesiology*, 68:618-621.

14. THE CARDIO-VASCULAR SYSTEM

This chapter contains an outline of the important points in the physiology of the heart and circulation that you need to understand if you are to successfully manage the first few postoperative hours.

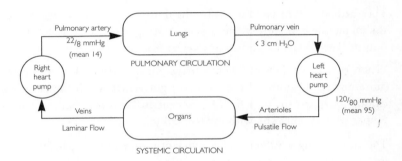

1. By convention arterial blood pressures are measured in millilitres of mercury (mmHg) and venous pressures in centimetres of water (cm H_2O).
2. The systemic arterial circulation is a high pressure system, and the pulmonary circulation is a low pressure system.
3. Arterioles are resistance vessels which control the blood flow to the organs.
4. Veins are capacitance vessels which store up to 3 litres of blood.

fig 14.1 The basic organization of the circulation

The circulatory system consists of the heart and the blood vessels. Its function is to supply a blood flow to the organs. This flow must be sufficient to deliver the required oxygen and nutrients, and remove the waste products of metabolism.

CARDIAC OUTPUT

The heart is made up of two demand volume pumps set in series. The two pumps are:

- the right side of the heart, which works at low pressures to pump blood through the pulmonary circulation to the lungs;

- the left side of the heart, which works at higher pressures to pump blood to the organs.

The output of each ventricle must be identical otherwise blood would rapidly bank up in either the lungs or the organs.

The normal heart at rest ejects a *cardiac output* of about 5000 mls of blood a minute. Each beat of the heart ejects a *stroke volume* of about 70 mls from each ventricle and the heart rate is about 72 beats per minute.

$$\text{Cardiac output} = \text{heart rate} \times \text{stroke volume}$$
$$5000 \text{ ml/min} \cong 72 \text{ bpm} \times 70 \text{ mls.}$$

The cardiac output is adjusted by the autonomic nervous system to meet the metabolic demands of the tissues. During exercise or stress the cardiac output rises to ensure sufficient oxygen reaches the tissues.

When the heart's left and right atria contract they kick-start (*prime*) the more powerful pumps of the left and right ventricles. If the atria fail then cardiac output can drop by 25 per cent in a normal patient, and up to 50 per cent in someone with cardiac failure.

The heart being a *volume pump* efficiently maintains organ blood flow at low pressures. It is not a *pressure pump*, and if forced to pump at high pressures it will eventually fail causing *cardiac failure*.

Starling's law of the heart

Starling's law of the heart describes how cardiac muscle behaves: "The more the myocardial fibres are stretched during diastole, the more forcibly they will contract during subsequent systole, and therefore the more blood will be expelled."

Variables affecting cardiac output include:
- heart rate;
- preload;
- mocardial contractility;
- afterload.

Just like a piece of elastic the more heart muscle is stretched, then the harder it will contract. Obviously the health of the myocardial fibres will determine their ability to contract (*contractility*). Patients with some forms of cardiac failure have poor *myocardial contractility* with floppy flabby muscle fibres.

When the atria contract they drive blood into the ventricles. This pressure forcing blood into the ventricles, and stretching the myocardial fibres, is called *preload*.

If, the myocardial fibres have to strain against something resisting their ability to eject blood from the heart, such as high blood pressure or narrowed valves, this raises the *afterload* on the fibres.

HOMEOSTASIS AND THE AUTONOMIC NERVOUS SYSTEM

The autonomic nervous system helps maintain cardiac output and control blood pressure. The processor is the *vasomotor centre* in the medulla which signals the controller in the hypothalamus. The autonomic response is affected by many anaesthetic agents and can be manipulated by certain drugs.

For more about the autonomic nervous system see appendix IV.

Control of blood pressure

Blood pressure control is a homeostatic mechanism. Blood pressure is quickly and tightly controlled to ensure the tissues are getting sufficient blood flow to provide oxygen and foodstuffs, and to remove the waste products of metabolism.

Mean arterial blood pressure is maintained by a balance between cardiac output and the resistance to blood flow through the systemic vascular bed.

NEURAL REGULATION

The arterial blood pressure is maintained by increasing cardiac output, or by increasing the systemic resistance to blood flow. This physiological feedback is achieved by quick acting sympathetic nerves, and backed up by slow acting humoral factors.

Sympathetic nerves have a background (or base line) discharge rate that maintains smooth muscle tone. Once the sympathetic nervous system is activated some organs are affected more than others, so that blood is diverted from skin, muscle and gut, to where it is needed in the brain, heart and kidney. This helps protect these *vital organs* during severe hypovolaemia, or life-threatening haemorrhage.

The neurotransmitter is *noradrenaline*. It acts through alpha receptors to stimulate arteriolar smooth muscle to contract. This action can be blocked with alpha antagonist drugs such as phentolamine

Baroreceptors are specialized stretch receptors in the arch of the aorta and carotid sinus in the neck. They detect changes in arterial blood pressure and adjust the autonomic nervous system to realign the blood pressure.

Baroreceptor responses may be blunted in patients where the autonomic nerves are damaged by diabetes or vascular disease; or in those receiving vasodilator drugs, or recovering from general anaesthesia. In the recovery room sitting these patients up abruptly may drop their blood pressure so sharply that their cerebral perfusion will fall and they will become nauseated, or may even lose consciousness and fit.

Chemoreceptors located in the aortic and carotid bodies respond to hypoxia, and also stimulate the autonomic nervous system. Even tiny amounts of volatile anaesthetic agents blunt this response, so the patient in recovery room may not be able to increase his rate and depth of breathing if he becomes hypoxic.

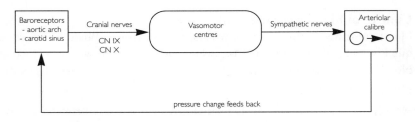

SEQUENCE

1. Blood pressure falls.
2. Arterial baroreceptors detect fall in blood pressure.
3. Message sent to vasomotor centre.
4. Vasomotor centres trigger sympathetic nerves to fire.
5. Sympathetic nerves release noradrenaline:
   – Arterioles constrict impending blood flow:
   – heart musle contracts more forcibly.
6. Blood pressure rises.
7. Baroreceptors detect rise in blood pressure and stop sending signals to the vasomotor centre.

fig 14.2 Feedback in response to a fall in blood pressure

HUMERAL REGULATION

If the blood pressure remains low then other slower acting hormonal mechanisms come into action to increase the force and rate of contraction of cardiac muscle (adrenaline); to increase vasoconstriction (angiotensin II), and to prevent the loss of isotonic fluid from the kidney cortisone and aldosterone. These mechanisms are not involved in acute stress lasting a few moments, such as standing up, but are far more active in prolonged stress such as bleeding or other fluid loss.

ELECTROPHYSIOLOGY OF THE HEART

The pumping action of the heart is initiated by *pacemakers* and coordinated by an electrical *conducting* system. Disease disturbing the function of the conducting system causes *cardiac arrhythmias*.

As a myocardial muscle cell contracts, sodium and calcium ions flood into the cells through special channels in the cell membrane and potassium leaves. This ion *flux* is called depolarization. As the muscle fibre relaxes the ion flux is reversed, this called *repolarization*. These ion exchanges generate a small wave of electrical current (called an *action potential*) that spreads from cell to cell stimulating each of them to contract.

In the normal heart there are two *pacemakers*. The *sinoatrial* (SA) *node* high in the right atrium near the entrance of the vena cava is the dominant pacemaker setting the heart rate. At rest it discharges about 70 times per minute. If it fails the *atrioventricular* (AV) node will take over at an intrinsic rate of about 40 discharges per minute. Sympathetic (adrenergic) nerve stimulate the SA node to fire faster, and parasympathetic vagal (cholinergic) nerves slow it down.

When the SA node discharges the action potentials spread from cell to cell in the atrial muscle stimulating it to contract. The wave of contraction propels blood through the atrioventricular valves into the ventricles. On reaching the AV node the impulse is delayed slightly, before fizzing like a fast burning fuse through the specialized conducting tissues of the bundle of His down to the apex of the heart. The bundle of His divides into two main branches going to the right and left ventricles respectively. Once in the ventricles the impulse ignites a wave of contraction (*systole*) in the cardiac muscle that starts at the apex and spreads up towards the base of the heart squeezing blood up through the semilunar valves into the arteries. For about 200 milliseconds after the myocardial cell has contracted and while it is recovering it cannot contract again. This is called the *refractory period*. The ventricles then relax (*diastole*). The aortic and pulmonary valves close to prevent blood reflux back into the heart from the arteries. Then, the SA node fires to initiate atrial contraction, and the cycle starts all over again.

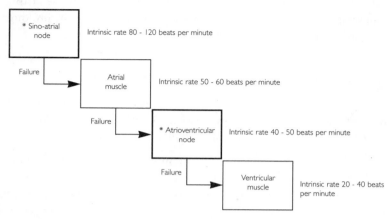

* these pacemakers initiate normal drive

1. There are two principle pacemakers in the body, the SA and AV nodes which normally control heart rhythm.
2. Electrical impulses pass from one pacemaker to the next in a sequential cascade.
3. Should the SA node fail then the AV node will take over as the driving pacemaker.
4. Both atrial and ventricular muscle have their own intrinsic rate of firing.
5. Background tonic impulses from the vagus nerve slows the rate of the sino-atrial node to about 70 bpm.

fig 14.3 Hierarchy of pacemakers in various parts of the heart.

Arrhythmias

All myocardial muscle cells can spontaneously generate their own action potential, but normally they do not do so. This is because their *intrinsic rate* is so slow that before the cells get a chance to spontaneously depolarize they are triggered by an impulse arriving from elsewhere.

MECHANISM OF ARRHYTHMIAS

There are two mechanisms that cause arrhythmias, abnormal impulse generation, and abnormal impulse propagation.

1. Abnormal impulse generation

The cardiac impulse originates in the SA node and proceeds to the ventricles, but irritable cells anywhere can start up their own rhythm. Irritability is caused by:
• drugs such as digoxin;
• electrolyte imbalance especially Mg^{++} and K^+;
• hormones such as thyroxine.

Ischaemic, irritated or inflamed myocardial cells will discharge spontaneously. These stray *ectopic beats* may arise anywhere in the heart to set off uncoordinated, inefficient contraction, such as atrial fibrillation, premature atrial or ventricular contractions. Tachycardia, or bradycardia can arise in the SA node. The SA node can be driven faster by sympathetic impulses, or slowed down by parasympathetic discharges.

Normally the SA node and the AV node pacemakers fire frequently enough to trigger the myocardial cells before they have a chance to discharge spontaneously. However if an impulse from a pacemaker fails to arrive in time, the myocardial cells will, as if becoming impatient, spontaneously discharge to become an *ectopic pacemaker*. If the SA node stops firing, the AV node will become the heart's pacemaker, and having escaped the influence of the SA node it sets an intrinsic rate of 35 - 40 beats per minute - a phenomenon known as *AV nodal escape*.

If not stimulated by an impulse arriving from elsewhere, the ventricles will adopt their own intrinsic rate of about 25 - 30 beats per minute.

If ectopic beats arise from a single source (*unifocal ectopics*) the danger is not as great as when a large part of the myocardium is abnormal, and impulses are arising all over the place (*multifocal ectopics*).

2. Abnormal propagation
Impulses can be blocked, delayed or go the wrong way. Arrhythmias may arise at any point in the impulse's journey from the SA node to its final extinction in the ventricles. If a group of myocardial cells becomes severely hypoxic, or part of the heart muscle dies, impulses are diverted from their usual path. This upsets the normal sequence of cardiac contraction. Impulses blocked or delayed while passing through the AV node cause heart blocks. Impulses blocked in one of the major branches of the bundle of His cause right or left bundle branch blocks. Damage to the minor branches of the bundle of His cause right or left hemiblocks.

Electrocardiograph (ECG)
The ECG records the millivolt electrical activity of the heart, and displays it on a screen. It warns of cardiac ischaemia and disturbance of cardiac rhythm. Some monitors have arrhythmia detection, and ST segment analysis built into them. These monitors are better at detecting abnormalities than trained staff who just glance at the monitor screens now and again.

COMPONENTS OF AN ECG TRACE

Feature	Coincides with	Duration	Remarks
P wave	Atrial contraction	0.06 – 0.10 sec	Disappears in atrial fibrillation.
			Saw tooth pattern in atrial flutter.
			Typically upside down in nodal rhythms.
PR interval	Atrial relaxation	0.12 – 0.20 sec	Prolonged in heart block.
			Shortened in WPW syndrome.
QRS complex	Reveals the path the impulse takes as it passes down the bundle of His	0.08 – 0.12 sec	Abnormal patterns or broadened complexes suggest conduction abnormalities such as the various types of heart block.
ST segment	Continuous contraction of ventricular muscle	0.08 – 0.12 sec	If it is raised, depressed, or sloping, it indicates serious problems in the ventricular muscle such as ischaemia.
QT interval	Contraction and relaxation of ventricular muscle	0.35 – 0.42 sec	Prolonged in hypocalcaemia, and patients at risk of developing Torsades de pointes.
			Shortened in hyperkalaemia.
T-wave	Cardiac muscle recovery phase following contraction.		Narrow peaked T-waves suggest hyperkalaemia.
			Flattened T-waves may be hypokalaemia, but also may be non-specific.
			Inverted T-waves may indicate endocardial irritation, such as ischaemia or inflammation.
U-wave	Small, but often absent		Prominent U-waves occur in hypocalcaemia.

The heart rate can be calculated by counting the number of large squares on the ECG paper that come between consecutive R waves, and dividing this into 300.

$$\text{Heart rate} = \frac{300}{\text{number of large squares between R waves}}$$

If you have a print out on a paper trace then look along the edge of the paper and you will find little marks which are three seconds apart. To find the heart rate count the number of complexes that fall between two successive marks (that is 6 seconds) and multiply by ten.

PR interval   0.12 – 0.20s
QRS complex 0.08 – 0.12s
QT interval   0.35 – 0.42s

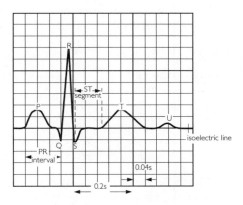

fig 14.4 Normal ECG complex

HOW TO DETECT SERIOUS ECG CHANGES

Start by answering the following five questions:
1. What is the heart rate?
2. Look at lead II. Is the rhythm regular?
3. Is there a P-wave?
4. Is the QRS wave normal in form and width?
5. Are there ST changes?

Consider treatment if the:

- heart rate is < 60 or > 100 bpm;
- P-waves are absent;
- rhythm is irregular;
- QRS complex is wider than normal;
- ST segments are elevated, depressed or sloping;
- the patient has a poor perfusion status.

ECG TERMINOLOGY

Asystole means the heart has stopped (cardiac arrest). The ECG shows a straight or gently undulating line with no electrical activity.

Atrial ectopics occur when the impulse arises in odd places within the atria and not in the SA node.

Atrial fibrillation (AF) occurs where the atrial excitation wave is uncoordinated and atria ceases to contract. No P-waves can be seen on the ECG and the ventricles contract irregularly. If you could see the atria they would appear to be shivering.

Atrial flutter occurs where the atria are contracting ineffectively fast. It is seen as a saw-toothed picture between the QRS complexes.

Bradycardia is a heart rate less than 50 beats per minute.

Complete heart block is where no P waves can be seen and the ventricles beat at their intrinsic rate of about 25 - 35/min.

Ectopic beats arise where they should not. They are "out-of-place" beats.

Electromechanical dissociation (EMD) occurs where a formed wave can be seen on the ECG, but there is no detectable peripheral pulse. This is usually fatal.

Heart block is where the P-waves are further away from the QRS complex than normal. They might be a constant distance from the QRS complex (serious) or they may vary (dangerous).

Idioventricular rhythm occurs when all the higher pacemakers are suppressed, and the ventricle contracts at its intrinsic rate of 25 - 35/min.

Multifocal premature beats (MPBS) are signs of a very irritable myocardium. Premature excitations are ectopic beats arising from many different sites in the ventricles. It needs urgent treatment.

Nodal rhythms occur where the AV node triggers the beat instead of the SA node. The P-waves are either absent (hidden in the QRS) or upside down.

Premature atrial contraction (PAC) occurs when the atrial beat does not arise in the SA node, but somewhere else in the atria. Sometimes it is the result of a wave in the AV node taking a U-turn.

Pro-arrhythmias are drug induced arrhythmias. They occur in about 10% of patients on antiarrhythmic agents.

R-on-T Phenomenon with the R wave snuggles right up next to, or even inside the T-wave. This is a dangerous sign as the patient may flip into ventricular fibrillation, or a ventricular tachycardia. Treat this urgently.

Sick sinus syndrome is a condition of sinus bradycardia or even sinus arrest, following a supraventricular tachycardia. Sometimes this is known as the tachycardia-bradycardia syndrome.

Sinus rhythm occurs when the sinoatrial node dictates the heart rate at a regular rhythm between 50 - 100/min.

Sinus bradycardia is a bradycardia where the P-waves are a normal distance from the QRS complex.

Sinus tachycardia is where the heart rate is greater than 100/min. The P-waves and QRS waves are normal.

Supraventricular arrhythmias arise in the atria.

Supraventricular tachycardia (SVT) is a heart rate of 150 - 250/min. The P-waves are usually, but not always, still visible. There are a number of causes.

Tachycardia is a heart rate greater than 100/minute.

Tachycardia bradycardia syndrome - see Sick sinus syndrome

Torsades de pointes (twisting of the points) is a very fine ventricular tachycardia with rapidly changing QRS shapes. It looks as though they are rotating about a baseline.

Ventricular Fibrillation (VF). If the chest is open the heart muscle is seen to be writhing like a bag full of earthworms, and there is no cardiac output.

Ventricular Premature Beats (VPBs) are wide, bizarre QRS complexes with a down sloping ST segment, and not preceded by a P-wave. They indicate an irritable myocardium, where the ventricle has contracted without a normal triggering sequence. Sometimes these are known as ventricular ectopics, or ventricular extrasystoles (VEs), or even premature ventricular contractions (PVCs). Suspect myocardial ischaemia.

Ventricular Tachycardia (VT) occurs when there are runs of more than three VPBs together.

Wolff-Parkinson-White (WPW) Syndrome is one of the pre-excitation syndromes heart, where the ventricle is prematurely activated because the impulse has taken a shortcut through an accessory pathway. Usually the PR interval is short (0.1 - 0.2 seconds), and there is a wider QRS complex.

PATHOPHYSIOLOGY OF CARDIAC FAILURE

Cardiac failure can be usefully classified into two types: *systolic dysfunction* and *diastolic dysfunction*.[1]

SYSTOLIC DYSFUNCTION is characterized by poor left ventricular contractility, a ventricular *ejection fraction* of less than 40 per cent, and a dilated large heart displacing the apex beat laterally. The myocardial fibres in this large heart have difficulty generating enough tension in the walls to eject an adequate stroke volume. In effect the heart is large and floppy, and uses more oxygen than a smaller heart.

Systolic dysfunction is usually due to a previous myocardial infarction, and associated coronary artery disease; but it also may be due to alcoholic cardiomyopathy or hypertension.

HEART SOUNDS IN CARDIAC FAILURE

Listen to the chest over the apex beat, you may hear a *triple rhythm* (sometimes called a *gallop rhythm*). A triple rhythm is caused by an added heart sound. An extra sound in diastole may be *physiological* in pregnancy, or in children and young people. In older people it is usually *pathological*, and a useful sign of heart failure. Beware of drawing conclusions from an isolated sign. Look for further evidence, such as hypertension, fluid overload, dyspnoea, and so on.

Normally you will hear two heart sounds, the first heart and second heart sounds. Together they sound like "LUB DUB". It helps to say it while you listen, "LUB DUB". If a gallop rhythm starts it will probably be either a *third*, or a *fourth heart sound*. A third heart sound occurs with a floppy, dilated ventricle, and sounds like "LUB DUBBA". A fourth heart sound occurs when the atria are contracting forcefully, and sounds like "daLUB DUB". Occasionally you may even hear both. If you are having difficulty telling if the extra sound comes before, or after, the first and second heart sound, time the rhythm by feeling the carotid pulse. If there is a tachycardia it is difficult, or impossible to time the sounds; this is called a summation gallop. Practise actually singing the gallops to yourself until they are familiar.

DIASTOLIC DYSFUNCTION is characterized by normal left ventricular contractility, the left ventricular ejection fraction may be greater than 40 per cent and the heart a normal size. The ventricle is stiff and incompliant. In effect the myocardial fibres have been remodelled so that they cannot stretch enough to adequately contract as described by Starling's law.

Diastolic dysfunction can be due to intermittent ischaemia, or hypertensive, or hypertrophic cardiomyopathy. Other causes include thyrotoxicosis, myxoedema and Paget's disease. Since the myocardium is contracting adequately, inotropes are of no use.

There is some overlap between the two. A history of myocardial infarction, Q-waves on the ECG and a third heart sound (S_3 *gallop*) favour systolic dysfunction. A history of hypertension, a fourth heart sound (S_4 *gallop*) and normal cardiac size favour diastolic dysfunction.

Pulmonary oedema can occur in either group.

Pulmonary oedema

Pulmonary oedema is a feature of low output left ventricular failure and occurs when fluid enters lung tissue. There is a progression of symptoms starting with a rise in respiratory rate and a dry cough, then the patient starts to wheeze and finally become cyanosed, and extremely distressed coughing up frothy pink sputum.

Listening to the chest you will hear showers of crackling *crepitations* at first in the bases of the lungs, and then all over the chest. A chest X-ray will reveal the classic white *bat's wing* appearance of the lung fields, which later may progress to a generalized white infiltrate as though someone had thrown a handful of snow on to the chest film.

The pulmonary artery wedge pressure (PAWP) measures the blood pressure in the pulmonary capillaries. If this pressure rises beyond the colloid osmotic pressure of plasma (about 25 - 30 cm H_2O) fluid seeps from the circulation into the lung tissue (*interstitial pulmonary oedema*) and finally into the alveoli (*alveolar oedema*). These are two forms of *high pressure* pulmonary oedema. Interstitial pulmonary oedema presents with wheeze, cough and breathlessness, and alveolar oedema causes frothy pink sputum. For the oedema to resolve the pressure in the pulmonary capillaries must fall below the colloid osmotic pressure.

Low pressure pulmonary oedema occurs when lung tissue is damaged, such as in septicaemia, pneumonia, or adult respiratory distress syndrome.

Fluid in the interstitium of the lung, or in the alveolar, quickly impedes the uptake of relatively insoluble oxygen, but only in the late stages interferes with the transfer of carbon dioxide. Arterial oxygen pressures fall swiftly, but carbon dioxide does not accumulate until the patient is moribund.

CARDIAC ISCHAEMIA

Emergence from anaesthesia is characterized by physiological turmoil. The resultant adrenergic stress contributes to cardiac ischaemia by:

- changing calibre of myocardial vessels, so called *spasm*;
- changing blood viscosity;
- increased blood coagulability.

The heart muscle has its own blood supply. Coronary blood flow is about 250 ml/min and the heart uses about 40 ml/min of oxygen. Coronary artery disease cause cardiac ischaemia. Some drugs and circulating hormones will dilate while others will constrict the coronary arteries.

You can diagnose myocardial ischaemia with two criteria: chest pain and ECG changes. It is unfortunate, but either or both these cardinal signs may be absent in some patients (especially diabetics) with acute severe ischaemia; phenomena known respectively as *silent angina* or *silent ischaemia*.

If myocardial ischaemia is not quickly relieved it may progress to acute myocardial infarction with death of heart muscle. There is clear evidence that repeated episodes of ischaemia cause myocardial infarction[4].

Supply and demand induced ischaemia[5]

Heart muscle can become hypoxic in two main ways. Firstly, not enough oxygen reaches the heart, because the patient is hypoxic, anaemic, hypotensive, or the coronary arteries are blocked. This is sometimes called *supply induced ischaemia*. Secondly the heart may be working so hard that its oxygen requirements outstrip its oxygen supply. This is called *demand induced ischaemia*.

If the heart muscle does not receive enough oxygen, it may: fail to contract hard enough to maintain an adequate cardiac output; become irritable and contract prematurely causing ectopic beats; give rise to ischaemic pain; infarct and die.

Four factors determine cardiac work, and therefore the amount of oxygen it needs: heart rate, pre-load, after-load, and heart size.

HEART RATE is important, because the heart is only perfused when it is not contracting; that is, during diastole. During systole blood flow to the myocardium almost ceases. As the heart rate increases during a tachycardia, diastole gets shorter, leaving less time for perfusion of the heart muscle.

Bradycardia too, can be dangerous, particularly in the elderly. It is common following an anaesthetic where propofol and fentanyl have been used.

PRE-LOAD is the pressure needed to fill the ventricle. It is measured by the pulmonary artery wedge pressure. A high pre-load may be associated with pulmonary oedema, and may be a sign of *diastolic dysfunction*.

HIGH AFTERLOAD causes myocardial ischaemia by making the heart work harder to eject blood through a tight valve, or against a high systemic blood pressure. Hypertensive patients are at high risk from cardiac ischaemia, particularly if they develop a tachycardia or arrhythmia. A high afterload causes endocardial ischaemia by partially squashing the blood vessels impeding the flow of blood carrying oxygen to the myocardial tissues lining the ventricles. This can be detected by T-wave flattening or even inversion on the anterior leads of the ECG.

HEART SIZE is a factor, because the harder the heart works, the more oxygen it consumes. Big hearts need more oxygen than little hearts, because the myocardium has to contract more strongly to achieve the same pressure within the ventricle. Hearts can enlarge because the myocardium is damaged by infarction and the ventricular walls become thin, dilated and floppy; or the myocardium can hypertrophy because of the extra effort needed to pump blood through a tight valve, or with hypertension.

Cardiogenic shock (see page 286)

Cardiac arrest (see page 287)

1. Goldsmith SR, Candace D. (1993). American Journal of Medicine, 95:645-55.
2. Roy WL, Edelist G. (1979) Anesthesiology, 51: 393-7.
3. Ashton CM, Petersen NJ, et al. (1993). Annals of Internal Medicine, 118:504-10.
4. Braunwauld E, Kloner RA. (1982). Circulation, 66:1146-9.
5. Cutfield G. (1992). Australian Anaesthesia 1992, pp 216-22, published by the Australian and New Zealand College of Anaesthetists, Melbourne, Australia.

15. MANAGEMENT OF CARDIAC PROBLEMS

MONITORING HEART FUNCTION AND BLOOD PRESSURE

Adequate perfusion to all vital organs depends on both blood pressure and cardiac output. Cardiac output is not easily measured, but its adequacy can be deduced from other parameters such as peripheral perfusion, acid base status, and urine output. Blood pressure is easy to measure and we learn most from the diastolic and mean pressures. Coronary vessel perfusion depends on diastolic pressure. A mean blood pressure not more than 25 per cent below the preoperative value is essential for an adequate blood supply to the brain and kidneys.

Perfusion status

The assessment of the perfusion status of a patient is the clinical core of cardiovascular monitoring.

PERFUSION STATUS			
Observation	**Adequate**	**Poor**	**No perfusion**
Conscious state	Alert, oriented in time and place	Obtunded, confused, anxious or agitated	Unconscious
Skin	Warm, pink, dry	Cool, pale, clammy sweating	Cool/cold, pale +/- sweating
Pulse	60 – 100/min	Either < 60/min or > 100/min	Absent or feeble pulse
Blood pressure	> 100 mmHg	< 100 mmHg	Unrecordable

Example: John Smith,
Conscious state: alert
Skin: cool
Radial pulse: 76 bpm
Blood pressure: 135/95

Further signs of poor perfusion are:
- dyspnoea;
- chest pain;

- poor capillary return in fingernail beds;
- peripheral or central cyanosis;
- acidosis;
- ECG signs of ischaemia with ST and T wave changes, or the onset of arrhythmias or bundle branch blocks;
- abdominal pain.

Other ways of gaining information about the functioning of the heart and the circulation are pulse oximeters, blood pressure monitors, the ECG, and if you have it available, the CVP.

Pulse oximeters measure skin perfusion by registering changes in capillary blood flow (*plethsymography*). The skin blood flow is exquisitely sensitive to the activity of the sympathetic nervous system. Cold hands, poor perfusion or sweating, are excellent indicators that the body's alarm mechanisms are responding to stress. Do not ignore these signs.

CALCULATION OF MEAN BLOOD PRESSURE

The mean arterial blood pressure (MAP) can be roughly calculated viz:

$$MAP = \text{diastolic blood pressure} + \frac{\text{pulse pressure}}{3}$$

where the pulse pressure = systolic pressure - diastolic pressure

---

*Cold hands are a warning sign
that something is wrong.*

With an intra-arterial cannula and a transducer you can display the pulse form on a monitor screen. Two important wave forms are *pulsus alternans* and *pulsus paradoxus*. Pulsus alternans occurs where a bigger pulse wave alternates with a smaller pulse wave. It is a sign of heart failure. Pulsus paradoxus is a sign that the patient may be volume deplete. The height of the pulse wave rises on expiration. If the patient is on a ventilator, the reverse occurs, and the pulse wave rises on inspiration (reverse paradox).

Pulsus Alternans   Pulsus Parodoxus

fig 15.1 Pulse forms

The electrocardiograph (ECG) is also sometimes known as a EKG out of deference to its German origins. The ECG records the millivolt electrical activity of the heart and displays it on a screen. It warns of cardiac ischaemia and disturbance of cardiac rhythm but does not provide direct information about how powerfully the heart muscle is contracting. Some recovery room and anaesthetic monitors have arrhythmia detection and ST segment analysis built into them. These monitors are better at detecting abnormalities than trained staff who just glance at the monitor screens now and again. See page 33 for hints on how to use your monitor.

A catheter placed in a central vein, usually the subclavian vein, allows you to measure the central venous pressure (*right atrial filling pressure*).

INTERPRETATION OF CENTRAL VENOUS PRESSURE		
Central venous pressure	Blood pressure	Causes
Low (hypovolaemia)	Low	hypovolaemia shock
High (normovolaemia)	Low	low cardiac output cardiac failure cardiac tamponade pulmonary embolism vasodilation
High	High	fluid overload

HYPOTENSION

Hypotension is a serious and common complication in recovery room. Patients with vascular disease may suffer cerebral or cardiac ischaemia if their blood pressure falls more than 20 per cent. Hypotension may also cause renal damage or strokes if the patient suffers from chronic hypertension.

Causes of hypotension

Hypotension occurs if there is an inadequate cardiac output, or the blood volume is insufficient to completely fill the capacity of the circulation. Either one, or both, of these factors will cause hypotension.

When to worry about hypotension

THERE IS NO NEED TO WORRY ABOUT HYPOTENSION:

• until the mean pressure falls to less than 20 per cent below the baseline preoperative blood pressure, or the mean blood pressure falls below 100 mmHg;

• unless the pulse rate is less than 60 in a baby or an elderly person, or less than 55 in a young person.

WORRY IF:

• the ST segments rise above, or fall below the iso-electric line by more than 0.5 mm;

• the patient complains of chest discomfort, angina or finds it "difficult to get his breath";

• the patient complains of nausea or visual disturbances; or his conscious state deteriorates;

• the patient's oxygen saturation falls below 93 per cent;

• the patient's perfusion state deteriorates.

If the patients perfusion state is poor or critical the patient will be, clinically, in shock (see page 461).

Failure in cardiac output

Factors affecting the cardiac output are the heart rate and rhythm, its contractility, and the preload and afterload.

HEART RATE AND RHYTHM PROBLEMS

Too slow:

• sinus bradycardia (see page 539);

• heart blocks (see page 547);

• drugs, such as neostigmine and ß-blockers.

Too fast:

• sinus tachycardia (see page 538);

• atrial flutter or atrial fibrillation (AF) (see page 545);

• paroxysmal supraventricular tachycardias (PSVT) (see page 542);

• drugs, such as adrenaline and atropine.

CONTRACTILITY PROBLEMS

In the recovery room factors affecting cardiac contractility include:

• *negative ionotropic drugs* such as ß-blockers, pethidine, and residual effects of the volatile anaesthetics;

• myocardial ischaemia or infarction (see page 278);

• heart failure (see page 250);

• valvular heart disease (see page 285);

• cardiac tamponade (see page 286);

• pulmonary, or air embolism (see page 336).

BLOOD VOLUME PROBLEMS

ABSOLUTE LOSS OF BLOOD VOLUME:
- haemorrhage and hypovolaemia;
- extracellular fluid loss, as seen in burns (see page 57);

These cause insufficient preload on the heart. They are treated by giving plasma expanders to increase circulating blood volume.

RELATIVE LOSS OF BLOOD VOLUME
- sepsis - use noradrenaline infusion (see page 524);
- epidural or spinal anaesthesia - use intravenous colloids and short acting vasopressors such as ephedrine (see page 000);
- adrenal insufficiency (decreased aldosterone or cortisone) - use hydrocortisone;
- residual effects of antihypertensive drugs (ACE inhibitors, calcium channel blockers) that dilate the peripheral blood vessels;
- anaphylaxis - use adrenaline.

These cause insufficient afterload on the heart. They are treated by giving drugs that increase arteriolar resistance which raises the blood pressure.

The blood pressure does not fall initially
in young patients who are bleeding.

Treatment of absolute loss of blood volume

The first signs of absolute loss of blood volume (*absolute hypovolaemia*) is tachycardia. (Be wary in patients on ß-blockers, they will not have this response). Hands and feet become cool, and later the skin becomes clammy. Urine output falls, and will soon be less 0.5 ml/kg /hr. If the patient progresses to shock the urine output will probably cease completely. Shock is a life threatening event.

Tachycardia is the earliest sign of haemorrhage.

MONITOR: Perfusion status, pulse, blood pressure, oximetery, ECG including ST analysis, and jugular venous pressure (or central venous pressure). Prepare to measure blood gases, haemoglobin and haematocrit, and serum electrolytes and urea, and clotting screen.

IMMEDIATELY:

- call for help;
- give high flow oxygen by mask;
- lay the patient flat and raise his legs on pillows;
- look for a source of haemorrhage, and if possible apply direct pressure to the bleeding site. If there is bleeding from a limb, consider applying an arterial tourniquet at least 50 mmHg higher than the blood pressure while you summon help;
- make sure the intravenous line is running freely, and prepare to set up an infusion with a large wide bore cannula (see page 354).

Treatment of relative loss of blood volume (additional notes)

The commonest cause of relative loss of blood volume (*relative hypovolaemia*) is spinal or epidural anaesthesia. The patient may not be pale but will often feel nauseated and faint unless he is lying flat. He may have a tachycardia. His legs and feet will be warm with easily visible veins; in contrast the veins on the back of his hands may be empty, and barely visible. His hands will be cool.

MONITOR: Perfusion status pulse, blood pressure, oximetery, ECG including ST analysis, and jugular venous pressure (or central venous pressure). Check the perfusion status, and record it in the patient's notes.

IMMEDIATELY:

- Raise the patient's legs on pillows;
- give oxygen by mask;
- give 200 - 500 mls of polygeline (Haemaccel®) rapidly.

THEN IF NECESSARY:

- Dilute 30 mg of ephedrine in 10 mls of saline, and slowly over 30 seconds inject 1 ml increments intravenously;
- wait 2 minutes and repeat the dose of ephedrine until the blood pressure rises, some patients respond more readily to ephedrine than others. The effect lasts 10 - 15 minutes, and may be repeated;
- Consider adrenal (cortisone) deficiency if the blood pressure does not rise with ephedrine. Give hydrocortisone 100 mg intravenously.

Hints

1. The blood pressure does not always fall in haemorrhagic shock. Young people can compensate initially for a depleted blood volume by extreme vasoconstriction; however they will have a tachycardia, and other signs of poor perfusion, such as cold hands and low urine output.

2. Most opioids (apart from pethidine) do not cause a fall in blood pressure in otherwise stable patients. If the blood pressure drops after you have given an opioid analgesic, then look for haemorrhage, vascular fluid depletion or heart failure.

3. Severe hypotension is likely if the vasodilatory effects of spinal or epidural anaesthesia are combined with drugs that depress the heart.

4. If a patient complains of nausea, feels dizzy, or shows signs of ST changes on his ECG monitor, then treat the hypotension urgently.

5 If there has been surgery in the chest, or near the diaphragm; or the patient has asthma or emphysema consider the possibility of tension pneumothorax. Unless quickly relieved this may be fatal (see page 334).

6. The aim of treatment is always to improve tissue perfusion.

7. If the patient's perfusion, blood pressure and urine output is not restored with fluids or blood then suspect either continuing concealed blood loss or cardiac failure as a cause of the problem. Look at the drains, and under the blankets for blood loss.

8. Pain tends to keep the blood pressure up. The usual causes of hypotension in the recovery room are the residual effect of general anaesthesia, or the vasodilation caused by spinal or epidural blocks.

9. Do not tip the hypotensive patient head down, because it impairs oxygen transfer in the lungs, and is very uncomfortable. The blood pressure will come up just as effectively if you simply raise his legs up on a pillow.

Hypotension is a common cause of nausea
in a patient with an epidural or spinal anaesthetic.

HYPERTENSION

Hypertension is common in the recovery room. It occurs in previously normotensive as well as hypertensive patients. Postoperative hypertension may lead to bleeding at the operative site, myocardial ischaemia, cardiac arrhythmias, cardiac failure, and intracerebral haemorrhage. Hypertension is usually the result of activation of the alarm system of the body (the sympathetic nervous system), or secondary to drugs or an overfilled circulation. Patients with poorly controlled preoperative hypertension are likely to have roller-coaster changes in blood pressure in recovery room.

Causes of hypertension

- Pain;
- hypoxia;
- CO_2 retention;
- obstructed airways;
- shivering;
- full bladder;
- over transfusion;

- vasopressors;
- carotid artery surgery;
- ketamine anaesthesia;
- hypoglycaemia;
- phaeochromocytoma;
- tetanus;
- carcinoid syndrome.

Worry about hypertension if:

- the systolic blood pressure remains greater than 180 mmHg for more than 5 minutes;
- the diastolic blood pressure remains greater than 110 mmHg for more than 5 minutes;
- the mean blood pressure is 20 per cent higher than the preoperative baseline blood pressure;
- the patient develops symptoms including: angina or chest discomfort, sweating, headache, visual disturbances, ST depression on the ECG or arrhythmias (usually ventricular ectopic beats).

The patient with a tachycardia and hypertension
is at high risk of myocardial ischaemia.

Management of hypertension

The aim of management is to restore the patient's blood pressure to within 20 per cent of its preoperative level.

MONITOR: Blood pressure, pulse, respiration, ECG (look for signs of ST depression) pulse oximetery, blood glucose, conscious state and perfusion status.

IMMEDIATELY:

- Reassure the patient, give high flow oxygen;
- sit him up if he wishes it;
- it is important to detect angina signalling myocardial ischaemia. Ask about pain or discomfort which is away from the operation particularly in the chest, arm or neck;
- apply a glyceryl trinitrate (GTN) patch.

> **WARNING**
>
> Peripheral vasodilation to reduce blood pressure can cause severe hypotension in patients who are unable to increase their cardiac output. Do not vasodilate patients with:
>
> - aortic or mitral stenosis;
> - hypertrophic obstructive cardiomyopathies;
> - cardiac tamponade;
> - restrictive pericarditis;
> - head trauma;
> - hypovolaemia;
> - epidural or spinal anaesthesia;
> - closed angle glaucoma.

Malignant hypertension

Fulminating *malignant hypertension* can occur if the blood pressure rises acutely beyond 220/120 mmHg. Control the blood pressure urgently if the patient shows signs of developing cerebral oedema, such as:

- headache;
- deterioration in mental state;
- an up-going plantar response;
- drowsiness;
- disorientation;
- nystagmus;
- muscle weakness.

Hints about antihypertensive drugs

- Myocardial oxygen supply is improved with oxygen and glyceryl trinitrate;
- peripheral vasodilation is achieved with glyceryl trinitrate, hydralazine, or nitroprusside;
- pain causing excessive sympathetic drive is best relieved with morphine;
- if there is cardiac ischaemia with persistent extrasystoles or ST changes, then consider ß-blockers such as esmolol;
- eclamptic and pre-eclamptic hypertension is treated with magnesium infusions and hydralazine;
- phaeochromocytoma responds to phentolamine, but you will need to control the tachycardia with a ß-blocker.

USEFUL ANTIHYPERTENSIVE DRUGS

Be careful with drug therapy. Elderly patients with long standing hypertension tend to be exquisitely sensitive to antihypertensive drugs, so start with half the usual dose, and give it twice as slowly .

GLYCERYL TRINITRATE (GTN) Also called nitroglycerine, is a short acting drug that dilates vascular smooth muscle and improves myocardial oxygenation. It is a better drug than sodium nitroprusside in those with ischaemic heart disease, or where you wish to dilate the pulmonary vasculature. If possible, give it through a central line with intra-arterial monitoring and an ECG. Tachyphylaxis will occur. If the patient is initially hypertensive but does not have a tachycardia, try a sublingual glyceryl trinitrate (Anginine®). This works for about 10 minutes, and will give you time to set up a GTN infusion. Use glass or polyethylene containers, because GTN loses potency if it comes in contact with polyvinyl chloride (PVC). Large doses of nitroglycerine will cause methaemoglobinaemia. Start the GTN infusion with an initial drip rate of 10 microgram/min, but you may need to increase in steps of up to as much as 200 microgram/min . The onset of hypotensive takes 3 - 4 minutes, and it wears off in about 8 - 10 minutes. Headaches are a problem with GTN but they are not as unpleasant as with nitroprusside.

HYDRALAZINE is a direct acting peripheral arteriolar vasodilator. It causes a reflex tachycardia, with increased cardiac contractility, so it may cause cardiac ischaemia. The diastolic blood pressure responds to a greater extent than the systolic pressure. Hydralazine has a slow onset over 10 - 20 minutes and lasts about 3 - 8 hours. It is useful to treat pre-eclampsia. The dose is 10 - 20 mg IV. As its effects are unpredictable, dilute it and give it in 5 mg increments every 5 minutes. If necessary treat reflex tachycardia with a small dose of esmolol. You may need to repeat the hydralazine within 4 - 5 hours, in which case use about two-thirds of the original dose.

BETA BLOCKERS should not be used as first line therapy of hypertension in the recovery room. They diminish cardiac contractility, but since they do not dilate the arterioles, tissue perfusion will decrease. Apart from causing tissue hypoxia this may jeopardize the perfusion of suture lines and promote disruption.

PHENTOLAMINE is a short acting α_1 blocker that causes arteriolar vasodilation. The initial dose is 0.1 mg/kg IV followed by an infusion 5 - 50 microgram/min. It causes a pronounced reflex tachycardia, and its effects wear off after about 6 - 10 minutes. It is normally reserved for the treatment of phaeochromocytoma.

LABETALOL is a combined selective α_1 blocker and a non-selective ß-blocker. It has a greater ß-effect than alpha effect so bradycardia or even heart block may become a problem with larger doses. It is an adrenergic inhibitor and reduces blood pressure by reducing cardiac output and heart rate, and decreasing the peripheral vascular resistance. The adult dose is 20 - 80 mg given intravenously over at least one minute, repeat it 5 minutes later if necessary.

The onset of action is 5 - 10 minutes. The half life is between 3.5 and 6.5 hours depending on the dose given. The blood pressure can drop precipitously with labetalol. Use it carefully, because it is difficult to raise the blood pressure again if it drops too much.

SODIUM NITROPRUSSIDE (SNP) (Nipride®) is a potent ultra-short acting vasodilating drug. It is the best drug for the control of fulminating hypertension where the blood pressure is greater than 220/120 mmHg, but it will cause a reflex tachycardia. It dilates cerebral vessels and so raises intracranial pressure. It must be given as an infusion and preferably through a central line, (or at least through a dedicated drip with no other drugs added). It is so potent and so effective that you must have an arterial line to monitor blood pressure continuously. The dose is 0.5 - 10 microgram/kg/min. An initial response should be seen in 30 seconds and a maximum effect in 3 minutes. Aim for a diastolic pressure of 90 - 110 mmHg. The blood pressure will return within 2 - 4 minutes of turning off the SNP.

SNP decomposes rapidly to release cyanide if exposed to bright light or heat. Protect the infusion; cover the diluted SNP with light proof black paper once it is diluted. If the solution starts to turn a bluish colour, it means it is breaking down and you should discard it.

To prevent cyanide toxicity keep the infusion rate below 10 microgram/kg/min. The maximum total dose should not exceed 70 mg/kg in a patient with normal renal function. Nausea, sweating, apprehension, headache and muscle twitching are side effects.

Hints

1. Hypertension combined with a tachycardia will cause cardiac ischaemia in patients with coronary artery disease. Aim to keep the blood pressure lower and the pulse rate slower.

2. Pain is the commonest cause of acute hypertension in the recovery room. Treat it with intravenous analgesia.

3. If elderly patients, or those with long standing hypertension, receive too much fluid while in the operating theatre, they may be hypertensive in the recovery room. An overfilled vascular system usually responds to a glyceryl trinitrate (GTN) patch, or a small dose of frusemide.

4. The symptoms of angina are often sneakily obscure. They include retrosternal chest discomfort or heaviness, pain in the arm or shoulder, neck or jaw or even the top of the head. A wise approach is to regard any pain above the umbilicus, which is relieved by sublingual GTN, as cardiac ischaemia.

5. Patients with essential hypertension are often hypovolaemic because of chronic vasoconstriction and diuretic therapy. It is very important to carefully record the fluid intake and losses in these patients.

6. Hypertensive patients treated preoperatively with ACE inhibitors or calcium channel blockers may have an almost fully dilated circulation, and not be able to vasoconstrict readily. These patients become hypotensive with small fluid losses.

7. Sometimes the residual effects of ionotropes or vasopressors given in theatre cause the blood pressure to remain elevated in the recovery room. This usually resolves spontaneously with a GTN patch, or tablet sublingually. It is unwise to actively counteract their effects with vasodilators or ß-blockers.

8. The TURP syndrome will cause hypertension (see page 81).

9. Rare causes of fulminating hypertension are undiagnosed phaeo-chromocytoma, tetanus, carcinoid syndrome, and spinal cord damage.

ARRHYTHMIAS

Arrhythmias are common in the recovery room, however identifying them on the monitor screen is not always simple.

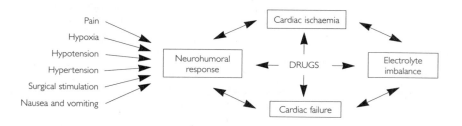

fig 15.2 Priniciple causes of arrhythmias in the recovery room

Causes of arrhythmias

1. Patient factors:
   • pain;
   • hypoxia;
   • cardiac ischaemia;
   • hypercarbia;
   • hypertension or hypotension;
   • electrolyte imbalance, especially of potassium and magnesium;
   • drugs, such as tricyclic antidepressants, and digoxin.

2. Surgical factors:
   - thoracic operations, especially if the pericardium has been damaged;
   - unrelieved pain, particularly from upper abdominal surgery;
   - operations on the eyes, ears, and upper jaw;
   - drugs, such as adrenaline, or cocaine, used to reduce bleeding;
   - the onset of shock.

3. Anaesthetic factors:
   - residual effects of drugs, such as fentanyl, or neostigmine causing bradycardias; or atropine causing tachycardias;
   - hypothermia;
   - adrenaline used with local anaesthetics (especially if halothane is used).

Patients complain of one or more of the following: palpitations, chest pain, nausea, light headedness, or shortness of breath. You may feel a slow, fast or irregular, or even absent pulse.

Types of arrhythmias
Innocent arrhythmias usually have a rate less than 120 beats per minute, the ECG monitor shows narrow QRS complexes, the blood pressure is within 20 percent of preoperative levels, and the oxygen saturation is greater than 95 percent;

More serious tachycardias can be divided into *broad complex tachycardias*, and *narrow complex tachycardias*. If there is a wide QRS complex call for help, and bring the cardiac resuscitation trolley (including the defibrillator) to the bedside.

If the patient becomes hypotensive you will have use *cardioversion* ("defibrillate") to restore the cardiac output (see below).

BRADYCARDIAS
The most common bradycardia is *sinus bradycardia*. Sinus bradycardia occurs when the heart rate falls below 60 per minute; and the ECG complexes are normal in form and the rhythm is regular. If the patient is stable and the heart rate is above 50 per minute it does not require treatment. If the heart rate is less than 50 then a small dose of atropine 0.4 - 0.6 mg usually solves the problem. Give atropine slowly and use the smallest effective dose.

Other bradycardias including heart blocks (see page 547).

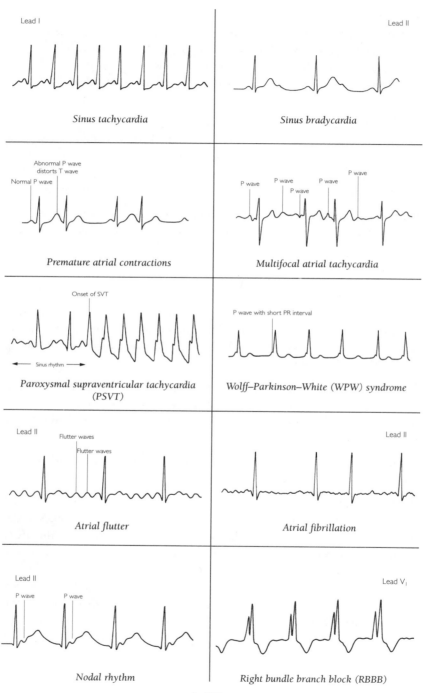

fig 15.3a

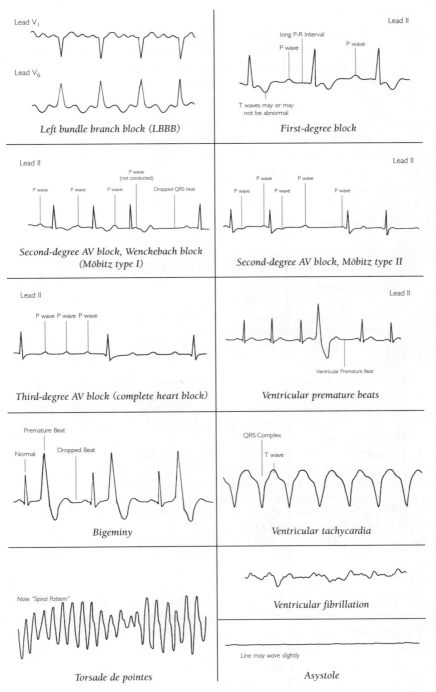

fig 15.3b

TACHYCARDIAS

The most common arrhythmia is a simple *sinus tachycardia*. Sinus tachycardia occurs when the heart rate rises beyond 100 per minute; the ECG complexes are normal in form, and the rhythm is regular. Find the cause and treat it. The tachycardia will usually resolve.

ATRIAL (SUPRAVENTRICULAR) ARRHYTHMIAS

- atrial arrhythmias usually have a narrow QRS (less than 0.12 sec);
- you can usually see a P wave in lead II;
- a regular rate of above 150 beats/minute suggests an atrial flutter;
- a very fast rate of 200 beats/minute suggests Wolf-Parkinson-White syndrome;
- if the rhythm is irregular and you can not see P-waves then it is probably atrial fibrillation.

WHY ARRHYTHMIAS CAUSE HEART FAILURE

BRADYCARDIAS

If the myocardial muscle is abnormal the compensatory increase in stroke volume that occurs at slow pulse rates is limited in the presence of bradycardia, and this reduces the cardiac output.

TACHYCARDIAS

- Reduce diastolic filling time;
- reduce perfusion of the myocardium - perfusion only happens in diastole;
- increases myocardial work load and myocardial oxygen demand;
- if they are chronic and the rate is not adequately controlled they lead to ventricular dilation and impaired ventricular contractility (*tachycardia induced cardiomyopathy*).

ABNORMAL ATRIAL AND VENTRICULAR CONTRACTION

- Loss of atrial systole in atrial fibrillation or flutter prevents atrial push and there is no active ventricular filling. This lowers the cardiac output and raises atrial pressures (you may see atrial dilation);
- if the atria and ventricle do not act in harmony the diastolic filling is impaired, particularly when there is a tachycardia.

VENTRICULAR ARRHYTHMIAS

- a wide QRS complex (greater than 0.12 sec) suggests the arrhythmia is arising the ventricle.[1] Treat wide complex arrhythmias immediately;
- a supraventricular arrhythmia superimposed on a bundle branch block will also give a wide complex. Check the patient's preoperative ECG, this will usually show a bundle branch block. If a new bundle branch block develops then this indicates acute cardiac ischaemia.

When to worry about arrhythmias

*In all cases of **wide** QRS complexes **worry**,
give oxygen, get the defibrillator, call for help.*

You may need to intervene if:
- The heart rate is greater than (200 - the patients age). For example a 70 year old has a pulse rate of greater than 130 beats per minute;
- The pulse rate is less than 50 beats per minute;
- The QRS complexes become wide;
- A regular heart rhythm suddenly becomes irregular;
- The ST segments rise above, or fall below, the iso-electric line;
- The patient complains of chest discomfort, angina of finds it "difficult to get his breath";
- The patient complains of nausea or visual disturbances; or his conscious state deteriorates;
- The patient's perfusion status deteriorates or his oxygen saturation falls below 93 per cent.

If the patient's oxygen saturation and his blood pressure are dropping call for help, and fetch the cardiac resuscitation trolley no matter what the rhythm on the ECG.

Treat the patient, not the monitor.

More about arrhythmias in Appendix V

Principles of treating cardiac arrhythmias
INITIALLY:
1. Keep your patient alive. First check the pulse by feeling the carotid artery in the neck. If it is absent or the patient is losing consciousness start your protocol for cardiac arrest.
2. Administer high flow oxygen. Position the patient in a comfortable position. Call for assistance. Take a hard copy of the rhythm. This is called a rhythm strip.

DIAGNOSE THE PROBLEM:
1. Look at the rhythm strip. The interval between the complexes will either be regular, or irregular. If you are unsure, mark the position of a series of three R-wave peaks on the edge of a strip of paper, or better still use

geometry dividers. Slide the paper along to another series of three peaks. Do the peaks coincide? If so, the rhythm is regular.

2. Measure the width of the QRS complexes.
   - Supraventricular tachycardias are usually narrow complex tachycardias (QRS complex less than 120 msecs in width).
   - ventricular tachycardias are usually wide complex tachycardias (QRS complex greater than 120 msecs width);

3. Look for causes of the arrhythmia:
   - hypoxia, hypercarbia, and hypotension;
   - electrolyte imbalance, particularly potassium and magnesium;
   - arrhythmogenic drugs, such as catecholamines and aminophylline.

First keep your patient alive,
only then find out what is wrong.

DESCRIBING ECGS

Learn to recognize and describe ECG traces. Sooner or later you will have to tell someone what is happening over the telephone. This takes practice!

Ask yourself these five important questions:

1   What is the heart rate?
   - a bradycardia is less than 60 beats per minute,
   - a tachycardia is greater than 100 beats per minute,
2. Is the rhythm regular?
3   Is the QRS complex wide or narrow?
4   Is there a P wave in lead II?
5. Are there signs of ischaemia?
   - is the ST segment raised above, or depressed below the isoelectric line?
   - is the ST segment sloping?
6. Is the pulse oximeter showing a decreasing saturation?

THEN:

1. Control the cardiac rate. Usually this will restore tissue perfusion. Then, if possible convert the patients heart to sinus rhythm. This may involve one or more of the following:
   - anti-arrhythmic drugs;
   - cardioversion;
   - overdrive pacing.

Management of arrhythmias

MONITOR: Blood pressure, pulse, respiratory rate, ECG, pulse oximetery, perfusion status. As soon as possible take a 12 lead ECG with long strip from lead II and V$_5$.

MANAGEMENT OF TACHYARRHYTHMIAS

The following table outlines how to manage the various tachyarrhythmias.

SUMMARY OF THE TREATMENT OF TACHYCARDIAS		
ECG rhythm	Broad complex QRS > 120 msec	Narrow complex QRS < 120 msec
Irregular ECG rhythm	Usually a ventricular tachycardia with fusion beats.	Usually: • Atrial fibrillation; • Atrial flutter.
Management	If the blood pressure and perfusion is good then try one of: • esmolol; • sotalol; • propanolol; • metoprolol. And then • amiodarone. If the blood pressure is low, then use cardioversion. Avoid adenosine. Avoid verapamil. Avoid digoxin.	Try, in order: • adenosine; • verapamil; • digoxin. Treat new onset arrhythmias associated with poor peripheral perfusion with cardioversion.
Regular ECG rhythm	Usually a ventricular tachycardia	Usually a supraventricular tachycardia.
Management	Try lignocaine 1.5 mg/kg IV push. Wait 5 – 10 minutes before repeating. Then use adenosine 6 mg stat IV over 1 – 3 seconds. Wait 1 – 2 minutes Then try procainamide IV 20 – 30 mg/minute. If that fails use synchronized cardioversion. Avoid verapamil.	If on a β-blocker, or has a poor cardiac output, then use cardioversion. If the patient's perfusion and blood pressure is good, and he is not on β-blockers, try adenosine, and if that fails then verapamil. May need to stabilize later on digoxin, with or without a β-blocker.

Cardioversion

The acute onset of an narrow complex supraventricular tachycardias (SVT) may cause life threatening hypotension, in which case you will need to immediately *cardiovert* the patient. Give a small dose of a ß-blocker, this will greatly increase your chance of success. The patient will need a brief anaesthetic during this procedure.

MAGNESIUM

Magnesium is a physiological calcium antagonist and its deficiency is associated with cardiac arrythmias. A lack of magnesium can precipitate refractory ventricular fibrillation.

Many elderly patients, those with diabetes, alcoholics, or those treated with diuretics are probably magnesium deplete. Also suspect those who have had large intestinal fluid losses or who are hypokalaemic.

Following any arrhythmia the patient has in the recovery room, and as soon as the arrhythmias is stabilized, give 2 gm magnesium sulphate 20% solution IV slowly over 30 minutes to help prevent recurrence. (Magnesium spreads evenly throughout the extracellular fluid so a large loading dose is required).

Follow-up persistent, or dangerous arrhythmias. Transfer the patient to a high dependency unit where he can have continuing monitoring and support for three or four days.

Cardioversion does not jump start the heart. It produces momentary asystole, and by depolarising all the myocardium simultaneously it gives an opportunity for the natural pacemakers to resume normal activity.

Try the following settings to start with:

Any patient on digoxin	0.1 joule/kg
Atrial flutter	0.1 joule/kg
Ventricular tachycardias	0.5 joule/kg
Atrial fibrillation	1.0 joule/kg

For instructions on cardioversion, defibrillation and a diagram for placing the paddles see page 289.

ADENOSINE OR VERAPAMIL
FOR TREATMENT OF SUPRAVENTRICULAR ARRHYTHMIAS?

ADENOSINE [2]

Adenosine is a naturally occurring purine nucleoside. It is both a precursor and a metabolite of ATP and AMP. It is an important natural occurring vasodilator in the microcirculation allowing more oxygen to reach the tissues. Adenosine also has a chronotropic effect on the heart, slowing the passage of impulses through the sinus and AV nodes, as well as an inotropic effect on the atria, decreasing myocardial work. It also acts on the carotid body to stimulate respiration and decrease blood pressure, and may reduce the pain of myocardial ischaemia.

Adenosine has a plasma half-life of less than 6 seconds. This is very short, so it must be given into a large vein, and then flushed through quickly, otherwise none will reach the target. Initially give a 3 mg bolus. If this is unsuccessful give a 6 mg bolus. If this is not effective follow it with 12 mg bolus, and repeat this 12 mg dose again if necessary. If you have a central venous line then halve the doses. Side effects of the drug include bradycardia and even asystole, but this is usually brief. Awake patients feel flushed due to the vasodilation. Be cautious if patients are on dipyridamole the patient may develop heart block. Adenosine is contraindicated in patients with asthma because if can cause bronchospasm. Other side effects include hypotension, chest pain, dyspnoea and nausea.

Adenosine only slows transmission of impulses through the atrioventricular node, but works equally well with WPW syndrome and supraventricular tachycardias.

VERAPAMIL

Verapamil is a calcium antagonist. Give 0.1 - 0.2 mg/kg slowly over 10 minutes. Verapamil can be dangerous in certain forms of tachycardia. Its inotropic and hypotensive effects cause ventricular depression, and cause complete heart block in patients already receiving beta blockers, or those with wide QRS complex tachycardias. Verapamil is safe in asthmatic patients. It is less effective than adenosine in the patients with WPW syndrome.

HINTS

- If the SVT has been correctly diagnosed both drugs are effective with over 80% of patients converting to sinus rhythm. Adenosine works more rapidly. Using adenosine after verapamil is usually ineffective. The main merit for trying verapamil first is cost. Verapamil is cheap and adenosine is expensive.
- For fast and wide arrhythmia and any arrhythmia which is causing the patient to become hypotensive you must cardiovert him. You must know how to use the defibrillator to do this, so must every technician, nurse and doctor in the operating suite.

MYOCARDIAL ISCHAEMIA AND INFARCTION

In developed countries about 12 - 20 per cent of patients have preoperative evidence of ischaemic heart disease. Perioperative myocardial infarction is the most common cause of death in non-cardiac surgical patients. Be alert for the possibility of myocardial ischaemia, or infarction in any patient known to have coronary artery disease. Myocardial ischaemia during the operation, or in the first few hours after operation put the patient at risk of arrhythmias, ischaemic episodes, or cardiac failure in the first postoperative week.[3] Most postoperative infarcts occur on the second or third postoperative day.[4]

Causes

Myocardial ischaemia occurs for two reasons: either the heart muscle is not receiving enough oxygen (*supply induced ischaemia*), or the heart is working too hard and outstripping its oxygen supply (*demand induced ischaemia*).

COMMON CAUSES OF **SUPPLY** INDUCED ISCHAEMIA INCLUDE:

- hypoxia - anaemia - lung disease;
- tachycardia;
- bradycardia;
- hypotension.

COMMON CAUSES OF **DEMAND** INDUCED ISCHAEMIA INCLUDE:

- hypertension;
- sympathetic drive - pain - hypoxia - hypercarbia - emotional stress;
- shivering and hypothermia.

RISK FACTORS ARE:

- coronary artery disease;
- congestive cardiac failure;
- emergency surgery;
- current, or ex-smoker;
- vascular disease;
- hypertension;
- diabetes;
- painful surgery over age 45 years;
- prolonged surgery over 3 hrs;
- vascular surgery;
- BP unstable during anaesthetic;
- lung disease;
- polycythaemia;
- hyperlipidaemia.

Attempts to quantify risk factors have been made. The index most widely quoted is the Goldman Risk Index.[5] Unfortunately this does not specifically address the risks, or predict the complications that occur in the recovery room.

The surgical patients who are likely to infarct postoperatively are:

- those who have had a myocardial infarct in the past six months, and especially in the past 3 months;
- those with unstable preoperative angina;
- congestive cardiac failure at the time of surgery;[6]
- prolonged, or emergency surgery in a patient with other risk factors;
- intraoperative tachycardia, hypotension or hypertension in patients with other risk factors.

Diagnosis of cardiac ischaemia

Emerging from a general anaesthetic is sometimes extremely stressful, and it is not unusual for a patient to develop signs of myocardial ischaemia for the first time in the recovery room. If the recovery room staff fail to recognize it, the patient will return to the ward at risk of suffering a myocardial infarct in the next few days. About half postoperative myocardial infarcts are clinically silent, and frequently the patients will die from this infarct. Postoperative infarcts are avoidable if the signs of cardiac ischaemia are detected early enough. Ischaemic changes are often present on the ECG for at least 12 hours before the patient suffers his heart attack.

Myocardial ischaemia will not
always proceed to infarction.

The diagnosis of ischaemia and infarction depends on two features:
1. Chest pain.
2. ECG changes.

It is almost impossible clinically to distinguish between myocardial ischaemia and myocardial infarction.

ATYPICAL CHEST PAIN

Reassuring signs that the pain is not angina include:
• Sharp knife-like pain which is aggravated by breathing or coughing;
• Pain localized with one finger;
• Pain reproduced by movement of the arms;
• Pain in the lower abdomen, below the umbilicus;
• Pain radiating to the legs.

If you suspect myocardial ischemia,
give sublingual GTN.

1. CHEST PAIN
ANGINA. Ischaemic chest pain is called *angina*. It feels like a crushing pain behind the sternum, usually described by the patient "as though someone is sitting on my chest," or "a tight band around my chest." It may be accompanied by a pain down the arm or in the jaw. In the recovery room angina is a grave warning sign of impending acute myocardial infarction. In the immediate postoperative phase it is often symptomless;[7] this is so-called silent angina. Sometimes it is known as para-anginal phenomena. The patient does not complain of pain, but looks and feels unwell. He may sweat, appear grey, have a poor perfusion status, feel nauseated, become hypotensive, feel anxious, shake, become short of breath, complain of dizziness, or have an arrhythmia.

MYOCARDIAL INFARCTION. If myocardial ischaemia is not relieved the patient will progress to myocardial infarction with the death of heart muscle. There is clear evidence that repeated episodes of ischaemia cause myocardial infarction.[8] Crushing central chest pain may radiate to the neck, jaw or arms accompanied by sweating, breathlessness, hypotension, hypertension, nausea or arrhythmias. If the patient is able to speak he says that he feels "alarmed" or "terrible", and the pain is the worst he has ever experienced. The pain is diagnostically *not relieved* by glyceryl trinitrate. Insidiously these signs may be absent in the immediate postoperative period, and the infarct may be clinically silent with no pain, only the ECG signs of ST elevation or depression. Suspect silent infarction if a patient becomes hypotensive, has an irregular pulse, starts to sweat or develops pulmonary oedema with wheezing, and basal crepitations in the lung.

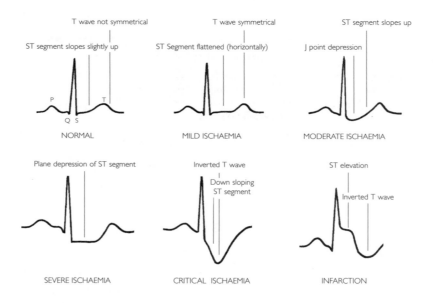

fig 15.4 Progress of ST segment and T-wave in ischaemia

2. ECG CHANGES

Monitoring may reveal arrhythmias and ST and T wave changes.[9] As ischaemia progresses the ST segments first become prolonged (greater than 0.12 seconds), and then depressed by more than 0.5 mm. Postoperative myocardial infarction is usually preceded by prolonged periods of ST depression greater than 0.5 mm.[10]

Management of acute myocardial ischaemia

In the early stages it is impossible to distinguish between reversible ischaemia, and irreversible myocardial infarction, because ST segment changes occurs in both. Myocardial ischaemia with acute ST elevation is potentially reversible, but if it is greater than 2 mm and does not resolve within 5 - 10 minutes then an infarct has probably occurred.

DRUGS USED IN TREATMENT OF ISCHAEMIA

The aim of therapy is to increase the oxygen supply to the heart or reduce the hearts requirements for oxygen. Use glyceryl trinitrate to dilate the coronary arteries and improve the oxygen supply to the heart, or ß-blockers to decrease myocardial contractility and reduce the myocardial oxygen demands.

NITROGLYCERINE can be given as a skin patch, but it is better to give it sublingually, or intravenously. It relaxes all vascular smooth muscle, vasodilating the whole circulation, but it works best on the coronary and pulmonary arterioles.[11] Take care because it will cause profound hypotension in a hypovolaemic patient. It can divert blood to under-aerated parts of the lung causing shunts and hypoxaemia. It works for about 20 - 30 minutes when given sublingually. If you dilute it to 100 microgram per ml, and give it in O.5 ml increments intravenously it will work for about 6 - 8 minutes. Side effects include headaches, flushing, dizziness, and postural hypotension.

Be careful because the vasodilation glyceryl trinitrate causes will produce severe hypotension in patients with severe aortic stenosis, obstructive cardiomyopathies, or mitral stenosis.

BETA BLOCKERS reduce myocardial work, and limit myocardial infarction size[12].

PRINCIPLES OF THERAPY

With the hope of limiting the extent of the ischaemia, or infarct, the aims of treatment in the recovery room are:

- Correct demand induced ischaemia:
  - control the pain;
  - treat hypertension;
  - and reduce myocardial oxygen consumption.

- Correct supply induced ischaemia
  - prevent hypoxia;
  - correct hypotension;
  - correct arrhythmias.

MONITOR:

1. Blood pressure, pulse, respiratory rate, ECG, pulse oximetery, perfusion status. As soon as possible take a 12 lead ECG with long strip from lead II and V5.

2. Computerized ST segment monitoring is good for detecting myocardial ischaemia. If you do not have this option available, use the modified CM5 lead for detecting ST and T wave segment changes. Place the left arm electrode over the fifth left intercostal space in the mid axillary line, and turn the lead select switch to Lead I.

3. Take blood for: baseline troponin-I levels, which is highly specific for myocardial infarction, haemoglobin, haematocrit, serum electrolytes, and blood gases.

INITIALLY:

• Give high flow oxygen by mask;
• reassure the patient;
• place him in the most comfortable position;
• give the patient a glyceryl trinitrate tablet 600 microgram under his tongue. Repeat this every 5 minutes to a maximum of three tablets, or the onset of side effects, such as hypotension or intolerable headache;
• give morphine 0.1 mg/kg intravenously slowly to relieve pain. Repeat in 5 minutes if necessary.

THEN:

1. Control pain, hypoxia, hypertension, hypotension, tachycardia, bradycardia, anaemia, and emotional stress. These insults increase cardiac work, or decrease cardiac oxygen supply.

2. Consider a nitroglycerine infusion if the pain remains uncontrolled. Start with a low dose of 0.5 - 1.5 microgram/kg/min, and increase the dose by 1 microgram/kg/min until the mean blood pressure is 95 - 100 mmHg.

3. Do not use prophylactic lignocaine in patients with ischaemia or infarction unless there are multiple ventricular premature contractions. Even then it is probably better to use a ß-blocker instead of lignocaine.

4. If the pulse rate is greater than 60 bpm consider giving a ß-blocker. Intravenous ß-blockers decrease mortality by about 15 per cent.

5. If the blood pressure greater than 180/100 mmHg consider an infusion of glyceryl trinitrate; start at 5 microgram/kg/min.

6. If pain remains uncontrolled, or the patient has arrhythmias or hypotension, then consider the diagnosis of myocardial infarction. Treat pain with morphine to a maximum of 20 mg intravenously. Monitor the

patient with a pulse oximeter to ensure oxygen saturation does not fall unnoticed. Use dobutamine for blood pressure support (see page 240). Transfer the patient to the intensive care unit for further monitoring.

7. If pain resolves, and there are no arrhythmias, the blood pressure remains stable, and the ECG signs of ischaemia resolve; the patient may return to the ward after being pain free for one hour. Ideally monitor him for three to four days in an intensive care unit where arrhythmias, ischaemia, and cardiac failure can be detected early.

Hints

1. More than half of the patients undergoing vascular surgery have coronary artery disease. They often develop ischaemia in the recovery room.

2. Cardiac ischaemia is most often caused by the combination of tachycardia and hypertension.

3. If the patient is hypertensive you may see ventricular extrasystoles appearing on the ECG. If you reduce the blood pressure or the heart rate, the extrasystoles will usually go away.

4. Hypotension associated with cardiac ischaemia is an ominous sign.

5. Excellent pain relief reduces the risk of demand induced ischaemia.

HEART FAILURE

The heart is composed of two pumps that feed each other. Usually they work in harmony so that the amount of blood they eject is virtually the same. Cardiac failure occurs when the left or right heart fails to maintain its output. (Refresh your memory of Starlings Law of the Heart on page 520). It is unusual for heart failure to occur as a result of coronary artery disease, unless there has been a prior myocardial infarction.

Cardiac failure can be functionally classified into two groups, systolic dysfunction and diastolic dysfunction.[13]

SYSTOLIC DYSFUNCTION is characterized by poor left ventricular contractility, with a left ventricular ejection fraction of less than 40 per cent and a dilated large heart displacing the apex beat. The ventricular dysfunction is usually due to a previous myocardial infarction, and associated coronary artery disease; but it also may be due to alcoholic cardiomyopathy or hypertension. Recovery room management includes ionotropes, diuretics and vasodilators.

DIASTOLIC DYSFUNCTION is characterized by normal left ventricular contractility, with a left ventricular ejection fraction greater than 40 per cent and a normal sized heart. The ventricular dysfunction can be due to intermittent ischaemia; from hypertensive, or hypertrophic cardiomyopathy. Other causes include thyrotoxicosis, myxoedema and Paget's disease. Since the myocardium is contracting adequately, ionotropes are of no use. The management of diastolic dysfunction is to control the cause: reduce the blood pressure if necessary, control cardiac rate, and treat arrhythmias.

There is some overlap between the signs and symptoms of systolic and diastolic dysfunction. A history of myocardial infarction, Q-waves on the ECG and a third heart sound (S₃ gallop) favour systolic dysfunction. Hypertension, a fourth heart sound (S₄ gallop) and normal cardiac size favour diastolic dysfunction.

Pulmonary oedema can occur in either group.

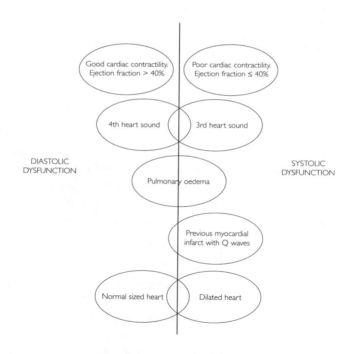

fig 15.5 Relationship Between Signs of Heart Failure

Acute Systolic Dysfunction

Common causes of acute systolic dysfunction
Include:
- myocardial ischaemia;
- myocardial infarction, which may be painless;
- arrhythmias;
- drugs.

With a failing left ventricle, the patient experiences breathlessness and wheeze, these become dramatically worse if the patient lies flat. The patient will be restless, agitated, pale, cyanosed and sweaty. He will be wheezy and have moist sounds in his lungs. His blood pressure may fall, and there may be a tachycardia. Urine output will be low and his perfusion status poor. If the failure is unrelieved he will go on to become severely agitated and distressed, coughing up frothy pink sputum.

Blood gases reveal a metabolic acidosis caused by the poor tissue perfusion; hypoxaemia, and hyperventilation.

A chest X-ray will show pulmonary oedema, pulmonary vascular congestion and possibly cardiac enlargement.

Painless myocardial infarction
may present with pulmonary oedema.

Management of acute systolic dysfunction
MONITOR: ECG, pulse oximeter, non-invasive blood pressure, urine output, blood gases, serum electrolytes and urea, troponin-I levels, and chest X-ray.

INITIALLY:
- Reassure the patient. Sit him up as much as possible. Give high flow oxygen by mask. Inform the anaesthetist.
- Give frusemide 0.5 mg/kg, and repeat it in 20 minutes if the urine output is less than 100 ml/hr.
- Give morphine 0.1 mg/kg intravenously slowly, to relieve distress and slow his rapid breathing. Repeat in 5 minutes if necessary.

THEN:
- A glyceryl trinitrate infusion will help reduce pulmonary vascular pressures (see page 520);

- control arrhythmias if they are present;
- consider cardiac support with ionotropes, such as dopamine or dobutamine (see page 520). You will need a direct intra-arterial blood pressure monitoring if you use ionotropes;
- consider positive pressure ventilation;
- arrange for eventual transfer to the intensive care unit.

CARDIAC FAILURE OR ASTHMA?

Acute left ventricular failure is often confused with an acute asthmatic attack. It is extremely unlikely, that an elderly patient will have his first acute asthma attack in recovery room. To help with the diagnosis, eliminate the possibility of fluid overload; or the possibility of an acute allergic reaction to a drug, blood or plasma expander.

All wheezes are not asthma.

ACUTE DIASTOLIC DYSFUNCTION

Common causes of acute diastolic dysfunction
Include:
- fluid overload;
- myocardial ischaemia;
- gas embolism;
- pulmonary embolism, look for this if the patient is old and bedridden and has come to theatre without ever having been on anticoagulants, especially if he also has deep vein thrombosis;
- arrhythmias.

Features of acute diastolic dysfunction are low blood pressure, nausea, vomiting, and dizziness. The jugular veins are distended and there is a progressive rise in central venous pressure. Peripheral perfusion is impaired, and the urine output low.

Management of acute diastolic dysfunction
MONITOR: ECG, pulse oximeter, non-invasive blood pressure, urine output, blood gases, serum electrolytes and urea, and chest X-ray.
1. Reassure the patient. Lie him flat with his head on a low pillow. Do not tip him head down. Give high flow oxygen by mask. Inform the anaesthetist.

2. Exclude pneumothorax (see page 333), air emboli (see page 335), or pulmonary emboli (see page 336). These conditions occur abruptly and present with acute dyspnoea, tachycardia, hypotension and cyanosis.

3. Give morphine 0.1 mg/kg intravenously slowly to relieve respiratory distress. Repeat 5 minutes later if necessary.

4. Control arrhythmias if present.

VALVULAR HEART DISEASE

An arterial line allows you to see acute changes in the pulse wave form.

Valvular heart disease, such as aortic and mitral stenosis or incompetence have fixed cardiac outputs. Mitral disease is more commonly seen in younger people secondary to rheumatic heart disease. Aortic disease occurs in both young and old and can be caused by other processes such as atherosclerosis.

The blood pressure falls precipitously in patients with valvular heart disease, if either the cardiac output drops, or the patient vasodilates. If a valve is incompetent a bradycardia allows blood time to flow backwards into the ventricle. Tachycardias are particularly hazardous, because there is not enough time for the ventricular contraction to squeeze blood through a narrow valve.

In children, valvular defects are also associated with septal defects and blood will shunt between the left, and right side of the heart. If the child has severe pain, systemic vasoconstriction forces oxygenated blood across the defect into the pulmonary circulation. You need excellent pain control to help prevent this disaster.

The normal area of the mitral valve is 4 cm^2. Symptoms occur when this is reduced to 2.5 cm^2 and are severe at 1 cm^2. The area of the aortic valve is normally 3 cm^2 and problems begin when it is reduced to 1 cm^2.

Patients with aortic or mitral reflux are susceptible to bacterial endocarditis. Make sure they have had antibiotics in theatre, or give them now. Those suffering from mitral valve disease are sometimes in atrial fibrillation, and on digitalis, anticoagulants and ß-blockers.

Patients with aortic valve disease often have cardiac ischaemia. Hypovolaemia or drugs depressing myocardial contraction may lead to myocardial infarction or impaired cerebral perfusion.

The anaesthetist should leave detailed and reasoned limits for acceptable heart rate, blood pressure, and oxygen saturation. Any breathlessness, anxiety, or deterioration in the conscious state is a sign that the circulation may be decompensating. Keep the patient out of pain, because any autonomic stress will cause a tachycardia, or increase cardiac work and destabilize the circulation. Do not discharge the patient to the ward until he is pain free, and has a stable circulation, a good urine output and warm dry hands.

CARDIAC TAMPONADE

Cardiac tamponade occurs when blood, or fluid collects in the pericardial sac compressing the heart. The partly squashed heart cannot produce an adequate cardiac output. This is a complication of thoracic surgery, or following traumatic chest injury. A sudden bleed of 150 - 250 ml into the pericardial sac causes a major fall in blood pressure. Clinically hypotension, tachycardia, dyspnoea, and distended neck veins give a clue. When the patient breathes in, the peripheral pulses may fall by more than 10 mmHg (*pulsus paradoxus*) and may even disappear altogether. The ECG may show electrical alternans with alternating large and small QRS complexes.

Tamponade may accumulate more slowly, such as in renal failure, or with various infections, in which case the pericardial sac can distend to hold more than 1000 mls of fluid, before symptoms become severe.

CARDIOGENIC SHOCK

Cardiogenic shock usually occurs after massive myocardial infarction or in a patient with pre-existing cardiac failure. The patient will feel cold to touch, be pale and sweating, hypotensive, and cyanosed. His blood gases show metabolic acidosis. With cardiogenic shock the myocardial damage is so severe that it overwhelms compensatory mechanisms that would normally maintain cardiac output. Perfusion of kidney, gut, liver and pancreas fails. Skin and muscle circulation may almost cease. Once the left ventricular function falls by about 30 - 40 per cent the vasoconstriction becomes so intense that progressive tissue hypoperfusion occurs. Unless intervention is successful, the patient's condition inevitably spirals down to death.

Management of cardiogenic shock

MONITOR: ECG, pulse oximeter, direct intra-arterial blood pressure, urine output, pulmonary artery wedge blood gases, serum electrolytes and urea, troponin-I levels, and chest X-ray.

IMMEDIATELY:
- Give high flows oxygen of oxygen by mask;
- adjust the patient's posture so he is comfortable;
- call for assistance.

THEN:
- Start a dopamine or dobutamine infusion (see appendix I for instructions on making up these infusions);
- if the patient has ischaemic heart disease start with dobutamine;
- adrenaline, or even noradrenaline, can be added as desperate measure if the blood pressure remains too low;
- transfer the patient to an intensive care unit.

CARDIAC ARREST

Conduct practice drills for cardiopulmonary resuscitation (CPR) at regular intervals. All staff need to be proficient at the management of cardiac arrest. Continual education and practice are the secrets of successful resuscitation. There is no excuse for a disorganized or frenetic resuscitation. Have your trolleys and equipment prepared and check them every day. Put your CPR flow chart on the wall where everyone can see it. Maintaining a clear airway, ensuring adequate ventilation and oxygenation, and giving immediate defibrillation are more important than administering drugs, or inserting intravenous lines.

A heart without oxygen,
will not respond to any form of therapy.

Sources of Cardiac Arrest Protocols
There have been a number of changes to the algorithms (flow charts) for the management of cardiac arrest over the past few years. In the USA, the American Heart Association[14] has issued clear and comprehensive recommendations. These are the definitive word on cardiac arrest, but their length makes them difficult to consult if you are in a hurry. In the UK and Europe, the European Resuscitation Council[15] has issued clear, brief and effective guidelines; these are highly recommended. You may be able to get a copy of their wall chart from Laerdal Medical Ltd. In Australia, the Australian Resuscitation Council[16] have published independent and slightly different guidelines. Obtain a copy of the guidelines applicable to your area.

Paediatric cardiac arrest (see paediatric chapter)

A = AIRWAY
- Airway maintenance is well described with diagrams on page 325. You must be competent at this;
- endotracheal intubation is the best way of maintaining the airway;
- exclude cardiac tamponade, air embolism, and tension pneumothorax.

B = BREATHING
1. Mouth-to-mouth ventilation in a non-intubated patient is easily taught and remembered, but understandably many staff are reluctant to use this. It achieves an inspired oxygen concentration of 16 per cent;
2. It requires considerable skill, and constant practice to use the self inflating bag and mask confidently. Many staff are unable to use these devices effectively to deliver the necessary tidal volumes of 15 ml/kg/min.
3. Try to achieve tidal volumes of at least 15 mls/kg, or as big breaths as you can achieve with the 1600 ml self-inflating bag.
4. If you are alone start the cycle of 2 breaths with mouth-to-mouth breathing followed by 15 sternal compressions.
5. Once the patient is intubated give 5 sternal compressions for every breath.
6. Give 5 initial breaths, preferably of 100 % oxygen, before starting cardiac massage to ensure good oxygenation.

C = CIRCULATION
1. If you have no access to an ECG, remember that 90 per cent of cardiac arrest in adults is VF or VT; and early defibrillation is the key to survival. Use 200 joules, then another 200 joules, and from then on 360 joules. Do not perform chest compressions while you recharge the defibrillator, reassess the ECG trace, and feeling the carotid artery for a pulse, but do keep oxygenating the patient.
2. Adrenaline 1 mg (1 ml of 1:1000 solution) is the first agent to use in cardiac arrest. Only use adrenaline after establishing oxygenation, commencing cardiac compression, and defibrillating the patient. Give subsequent doses at 3 - 5 minute intervals.
3. To stabilize VT, or VF after defibrillation and adrenaline give lignocaine 1.5 mg/kg intravenously and a further 1 mg/kg over the next half an hour. If lignocaine does not work, try bretylium 5 mg/kg intravenously.
4. With asystole, if after 3 doses of adrenaline there is no electrical activity, try a supramaximal dose of adrenaline 5 mg intravenously.

D = DRUGS

1. For intravenous access always try to use veins above the waistline. Follow peripheral drugs with a flush of 30 mls of fluid. The best vein is the external jugular;

2. 10% Calcium chloride, 5-10 mls intravenously, is only useful in hypocalcaemia, hyperkalaemia, or overdose of calcium channel blockers; otherwise do not use it. These problems are more common in renal patients;

3. Sodium bicarbonate is only indicated for hyperkalaemia, or acidosis after prolonged (10 minutes) arrest. It is a drug to use cautiously. If the pH is below 7.1 sodium bicarbonate may be useful. Start with 0.1 mmol/kg intravenously, repeat at 2 minute intervals to a maximum of 0.3 mmol/kg,

4. Adrenaline, lignocaine and atropine can be given down an endotracheal tube. Absorption is unreliable and about 2 - 3 times the intravenously dose is needed. Dilute the drug in 10 mls of normal saline.

5. Many other antiarrhythmics (such as magnesium, bretylium, amiodarone, and sotalol) have been proposed for use in refractory VF; to date, there have been no trials to prove their usefulness.

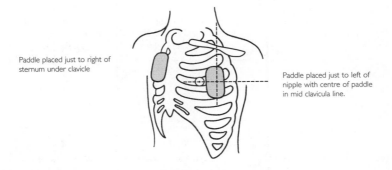

Paddle placed just to right of sternum under clavicle

Paddle placed just to left of nipple with centre of paddle in mid clavicula line.

fig 15.6 Where to place the defibrillator paddles

CARDIOVERSION (DEFIBRILLATION)

1. Apply moist gel pads to the upper chest. One just to the right of the sternum and under the clavicle. The other to the left of the nipple, with the centre of the paddle in the mid clavicular line (over the apex of the heart).

2. Press the paddles over the gel pads firmly taking care not to spread the gel over the skin.

PROTOCOL FOR AN ADULT CARDIAC ARREST

Treatment of Ventricular Fibrillation (VF)	Treatment of Asystole	Treatment of Electromechanical Dissociation
Precordial thump	Exclude 4 Hs; hypothermia, hypoxia, hyperkalaemia, hypokalaemia.	
↓ 5 breaths of 100% oxygen	↓ 5 breaths of 100% oxygen	↓ 5 breaths of 100% oxygen
↓ Defibrillate x 3 160 J 160 J 320 J	↓ Adrenaline 1 mg IV bolus and repeat every 3 minutes	↓ Adrenaline 1 mg IV bolus and repeat every 3 minutes
↓ Adrenaline 1 mg IV	↓ Atropine 1.2 mg IV bolus	↓ Adrenaline 1 mg IV bolus and repeat every 3 minutes
↓ Defibrillate 360 J within 30–60 sec	↓ Adrenaline 1 mg IV bolus and repeat every 3 minutes	↓ Adrenaline 1 mg IV bolus and repeat every 3 minutes
↓ Lignocaine 1.5 mg/kg at 3–5 minutes	↓	↓
↓ Consider bicarbonate 0.25 mmol/kg IV over 5 minutes	↓ Consider bicarbonate 0.25 mmol/kg IV over 5 minutes	↓ Consider bicarbonate 0.25 mmol/kg IV over 5 minutes

3. Check the ECG and confirm there is no carotid pulse.
4. Select the non-synchronized (VF) setting.
5. Charge to the required energy level. Use 200 joules initially. Say "Charging!"

6. Announce that the shock is to be given and make sure everyone is standing clear of the trolley. Say "Stand clear!"
7. Press the paddle buttons simultaneously. Say "Shocking now!"
8. Check the ECG, and carotid pulse after each shock. Say "Check the pulse!"
9. Repeat if unsuccessful. and use 360 joules then a maximum of 400 joules during cardiac arrests.

If the heart has been stopped for some time it will be more difficult to start again and success will depend on oxygenating the heart muscle.

When to stop?
In adults, survival is unlikely if the patient has failed to demonstrate a return to spontaneous circulation within 20 minutes, and is over the age of 45 years, and there is no evidence of drowning, drug overdose, local anaesthetic cardiotoxicity, or hypothermia.

TERMINOLOGY

Asystole means the heart has stopped (cardiac arrest). The ECG shows a straight or gently undulating line with no electrical activity.

Atrial ectopics occur when the impulse arises in odd places within the atria and not in the SA node.

Atrial fibrillation (AF) occurs where the atrial excitation wave is unco-ordinated and atria ceases to contract. No P-waves can be seen on the ECG and the ventricles contract irregularly. If the chest is opened the atria looks as though they are shivering.

Atrial flutter occurs where the atria are contracting ineffectively fast. It is seen as a saw-toothed picture between the QRS complexes.

Bradycardia is a heart rate less than 50 beats per minute.

Complete heart block is where no P-waves can be seen and the ventricles beat at their intrinsic rate of about 25 - 35/minute.

Ectopic beats arise where they should not. They are "out-of-place" beats.

Electromechanical dissociation (EMD) occurs where a formed wave can be seen on the ECG, but there is no detectable peripheral pulse. This is usually fatal.

Heart block is where the P-waves are further away from the QRS complex than normal. They might be a constant distance from the QRS complex (serious) or they may vary (dangerous).

Idioventricular rhythm occurs when all the higher pacemakers are suppressed, and the ventricle contracts at its intrinsic rate of 25 - 35/minute.

Multifocal premature beats (MPBS) are signs of a very irritable myocardium. Premature excitations are ectopic beats arising from many different sites in the ventricles. It needs urgent treatment.

Nodal rhythms occur where the AV node triggers the beat instead of the SA node. The P-waves are either absent (hidden in the QRS) or upside down.

Premature atrial contraction occurs when the atrial beat does not arise in the SA node, but somewhere else in the atria. Sometimes it is the result of a wave in the AV node taking a U-turn.

Pro-arrhythmias are drug induced arrhythmias. They occur in about 10 per cent of patients on antiarrhythmic agents.

R-on-T phenomenon with the R wave snuggles right up next to, or even inside the T-wave. This is a dangerous sign as the patient may flip into ventricular fibrillation, or a ventricular tachycardia. Treat this urgently.

Sick sinus syndrome is a condition of sinus bradycardia or even sinus arrest, following a supraventricular tachycardia. Sometimes this is known as the *tachycardia-bradycardia syndrome*.

Sinus rhythm occurs when the sino-atrial node dictates the heart rate at a regular rhythm between 50 -100/minute.

Sinus bradycardia is a bradycardia where the P-waves are a normal distance from the QRS complex.

Sinus tachycardia is where the heart rate is greater than 100/minute. The P-waves and QRS waves are normal.

Supraventricular arrhythmias arise in the atria.

Supraventricular tachycardia (SVT) is a heart rate of 150 - 250/minute. The P-waves are usually, but not always, still visible. There are a number of causes.

Tachycardia is a heart rate greater than 100/minute.

Tachycardia bradycardia syndrome - see sick sinus syndrome

Torsades de pointes (twisting of the points) is a very fine ventricular tachycardia with rapidly changing QRS shapes. It looks as though they are rotating about a baseline.

Ventricular fibrillation (VF). If the chest is open the heart muscle is seen to be writhing like a bag full of earthworms, and there is no cardiac output.

Ventricular premature beats (VPBs) are wide, bizarre QRS complexes with a down sloping ST segment, and not preceded by a P wave. They indicate an irritable myocardium, where the ventricle has contracted without a normal triggering sequence. Sometimes these are known as ventricular ectopics, or ventricular extrasystoles (VEs), or even premature ventricular contractions (PVCs). Suspect myocardial ischaemia.

Ventricular tachycardia (VT) occurs when there are runs of more than three VPBs together.

Wolff-Parkinson-White (WPW) syndrome is one of the pre-excitation syndromes heart, where the ventricle is prematurely activated because the impulse has taken a shortcut through an accessory pathway. Usually the PR interval is short (0.1 - 0.2 seconds), and there is a wider QRS complex.

1. Griffith MJ, Carrat CJ, (1994) *Lancet* 343:386.
2. Lang R, (1998) *Australian Anaesthesia* 139-50.
3. Roy WL, Edelist G. (1979) *Anesthesiology*, 51: 393-7.
4. Ashton CM, Petersen NJ, *et al.* (1993). *Annals of Internal Medicine*, 118:504-10.
5. Goldman L, Caldera DL, *et al.* (1977). *New England Journal of Medicine*, 297:845-50.
6. Mangano DT, Browner WS, *et al.* (1990). *New England Journal of Medicine* 118:504-10.
7. Ashton CM, Petersen NJ, *et al.* (1993). *Annals of Internal Medicine*, 118:504-10.
8. Braunwauld E, Kloner RA. (1982). *Circulation*, 66:1146-9.
9. Hales P. (1992). *Australian Anaesthesia* 1992, pp 210-15, published by the Australian and New Zealand College of Anaesthetists, Melbourne, Australia.
10. Landsberg G, Luria MH, *et al.* (1993). *Lancet*, 20:715-9.
11. Pearl RG, Rosenthal M. (1982). *Annals of Internal Medicine*, 99:9-13.
12. Frishman WH. (1988). *Medical Clinics of North America*, 72:37-75.
13. Goldsmith SR, Candace D. (1993). *American Journal of Medicine*, 95:645-55.
14. Guidelines for Cardiopulmonary Resusctitation. (1992). *Journal of the American Medical Association*, 268: 2171-298.
15. Guidelines for Basic and Advance Life Support. *European Resuscitation Council (1992). Resuscitation*, 24: 103-22.
16. The Australian Resuscitation Council Guidelines. (1993). *Medical Journal of Australia*, 159: 616-21.

16. RESPIRATORY PHYSIOLOGY

HYPOXIA AND HYPOXAEMIA

Above all else you must make sure that patients under your care do not become hypoxic. The onset of hypoxia is subtle. It is frequently neither obvious nor predictable, but it quickly maims or kills. It occurs more commonly in the recovery room than any where else in the hospital. If you thoroughly understand how and why hypoxia occurs, and how to recognize it you will be better equipped to prevent it.*

The prime responsibility of the recovery room
is to prevent hypoxia.

THE PHYSIOLOGY OF HYPOXIA AND HYPOXAEMIA

Oxygen is transported to the tissues bound to haemoglobin inside red blood cells (*erythrocytes*). When haemoglobin is filled to its capacity with oxygen it is said to be *fully saturated*. We measure the per cent oxygen saturation of haemoglobin with a pulse oximeter. Normal values exceed 98 per cent. *Hypoxaemia* occurs in a normal patient when the haemoglobin's oxygen saturation is 90 per cent, or less.

Two terms are often used, hypoxia and hypoxaemia. They do not mean the same thing.

Hypoxia occurs when tissues do not receive enough oxygen to meet their metabolic needs. Tissues such as brain, kidney and heart with a high metabolic rates are easily damaged by hypoxia; while others such as skin, and fat are more tolerant.

In contrast, *hypoxaemia* is something we measure. It occurs when the partial pressure of oxygen in the arterial blood (PaO_2) falls below 60 mmHg (7.89 kPa).[1]

Hypoxaemia does not necessarily mean the tissues are hypoxic, and tissues can be hypoxic in the absence of hypoxaemia; for example in an anaemic patient the PaO_2 and oxygen saturation may be normal, but because there are fewer red blood cells to carry oxygen, the tissues may become hypoxic.

Each minute a resting adult uses about 250 mls of oxygen and produces about 200 mls of carbon dioxide. Every 100 mls of blood, fully loaded with oxygen, carries about 20 mls of oxygen bound loosely to haemoglobin inside the red cells. Without haemoglobin the same 100 mls of blood could only carry 0.03 ml of oxygen dissolved in the plasma.

---

* You may wish to refresh your memory of terms, symbols and normal values which are summarized at the end of the chapter.

Oxygen Transport

The most important task of the recovery room is to ensure enough oxygen from the outside air reaches the mitochondria in the cells. There are four steps to this task.

1. Breathing
2. Gas transfer between the lungs and blood.
3. Carriage of oxygen to the tissues.
4. Mitochondria in the cells using oxygen as an energy source.

1. Breathing

Breathing is the process by which oxygen rich air is *inspired*, and carbon dioxide laden air is *expired*. The principle respiratory muscles are the diaphragm, and intercostal muscles. As these contract, the intrathoracic volume increases, and air is sucked into the upper airways where it is humidified. The air passes on through the larynx down through the lower airways to the alveoli where gas exchange occurs. The total surface area of the alveoli available for gas to *diffuse* into, or out of the capillaries is huge, traditionally quoted as about 90 square metres (the size of a tennis court). The lungs needs such a large surface area because oxygen (in contrast to carbon dioxide) is not a very soluble gas. Oxygen diffuses slowly and carbon dioxide diffuses fast.

If the patient is working hard to breathe (for instance after exercise, or with asthma) then *accessory muscles*, the strap muscles in the neck and the abdominal muscles, can be *recruited* to assist. If you see these muscles contract it means the patient is in severe respiratory difficulty.

The normal respiratory rate is about 12 - 15 breaths per minute. Each breath contains about 400 mls of air (called the *tidal volume*). Half this volume of air reaches the alveoli to give up part of its oxygen to the blood. At the same time, carbon dioxide leaves the blood, and is excreted in the expired air. The air remaining in the airways, and not involved in exchange, is called *dead space air*. If the tidal volume is less than the dead space, no fresh air will reach the alveoli, and no waste carbon dioxide can escape. If the tidal volume falls, and carbon dioxide concentration in the alveolus rises, the patient is said to be *hypoventilating*.

At the end of a quiet expiration, about 3 litres of air remain in the lungs. This volume is called the *functional residual capacity* (FRC). The residual air continues to take part in the gas exchange, and acts as a small oxygen store when we breathe out. If it were not for the FRC acting as a residual store of oxygen, we would turn blue every time we breathed out, and pink when we breathed in again. As we age and our lungs lose their elasticity more gas remains in the lungs and the FRC gets bigger. Infants have proportionally the same FRC as an adult, but their oxygen consumption is twice an adult's rate, so hypoxia develops much faster in infants, and neonates than in adults.

Air stored in the functional residual capacity is lower:
• during and directly after anaesthesia;
• after abdominal and thoracic surgery many alveoli collapse which reduces the amount of useable lung;
• if the patient is lying down, his abdominal contents push up the diaphragm reducing the amount of functioning lung. This becomes a major problem in the obese.

A patient with a small functional residual capacity, does not tolerate a slow respiratory rate well.

CONTROL OF BREATHING
Respiratory centres in the brain stem regulate breathing. They act like a biological computer which receives (*input*) messages from the lungs and elsewhere, analyses and organises them (*processor*), and then activates nerves (*output*) to instruct airways to constrict or dilate, muscles to contract, and if necessary co-ordinate a cough, a sigh, or recruit the accessory muscles. Furthermore the respiratory centres also communicate with the cortex so that you can voluntarily take a deep breathe and hold it, or let out air gradually so that you do things such as talk, shout, whistle or whisper.

The input to the respiratory centres comes from *chemoreceptors*; *stretch receptors* in the lung and intercostal muscles, and *epithelial receptors*. Chemoreceptors in the brainstem are more sensitive to a rising PCO_2 while chemoreceptors in the carotid sinus are more sensitive to a low PO_2. The respiratory centre takes a lot of notice of the brainstem chemoreceptors and a small rise in arterial PCO_2 will cause a big rise in respiratory rate and depth. In contrast the arterial PO_2 has to fall to at least 55 mmHg (7.24 kPa) before the carotid sinus chemoreceptors become the main drive to respiration. Opioids depress the carbon dioxide receptors in the brainstem, while volatile anaesthetic agents depress the oxygen chemoreceptors in the carotid sinus. These depressive effects can last for some hours after the end of anaesthesia, and may contribute to post-operative respiratory depression. Stretch receptors in the lung (J-receptors) and in the intercostal muscle (muscle spindles) give information about the work and rate of breathing. If the work of breathing rises or the rate falls, you will feel breathless. *Dyspnoea* is the subjective feeling of breathlessness, and is an important sign that the subject is working harder to breathe. Epithelial receptors guard your airway and signal the brainstem to cause sneezing, coughing, breath-holding, and laryngospasm. If the throat has been sprayed with local anaesthetic such as lignocaine the epithelial receptors will not function and the patient is at higher risk of aspiration.

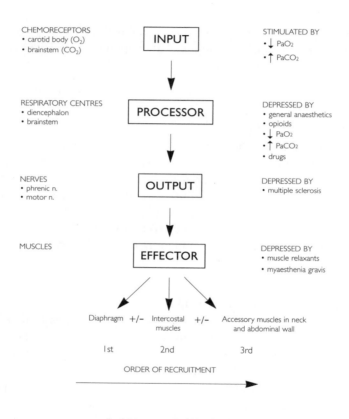

fig 16.1 Control of breathing

If you are having difficulty in diagnosing the cause of respiratory depression, work through the pathways involved: input, processor, and output as well as problems in the lungs themselves. Diseases affecting nerves (such as multiple sclerosis) or muscle (such as myasthenia gravis) or the residual effects of muscle relaxants, will weaken respiratory effort.

2. Gas transfer between the lung and the blood

Three terms: *concentration*, *tension* and *partial pressure* all mean roughly the same thing. They are used to express how much gas is present in every litre of a mixture of gases.

DALTON'S LAW OF PARTIAL PRESSURE

The concentration of a gas in either air or a solution is measured by its *partial pressure*. This pressure is stated in millimetres of mercury (mmHg) or kilopascals (kPa). In a mixture of gases the partial pressure of a particular gas is the pressure that the gas would exert if it alone occupied the space available to it. Nearly 200 years ago John Dalton, in his *Law of Partial Pressures*, said "if you add up the partial pressures of all the gases in a mixture of gases you will get the total pressure they exert." At sea level the total pressure exerted by all the gases in the atmosphere is 760 mmHg (100 kPa), but oxygen only exerts a pressure twenty one percent of this: $\frac{21}{100} \times 760 = 160$ mmHg. By the time oxygen gets to the alveoli, carbon dioxide and water vapour have diluted its concentration and partial pressure of oxygen will be only 110 mmHg (13.29 kPa).

Although we can measure partial pressures of oxygen (PO_2) we customarily use the inspired fractional concentration of oxygen (FIO_2) to state its concentration in the inspired air. Since air is 21% oxygen, the $FIO_2 = 0.21$. An ordinary face mask used in recovery room delivers an FIO_2 of about 0.36 at a flow rate of 6 l/min.

For a healthy person breathing air ($FIO_2 = 0.21$), the normal arterial partial pressure of oxygen (PaO_2) is about 100 mmHg. (13.1 kPa). This declines with age, and at 80 years will be about 80 mmHg (10.5 kPa). The following formula gives the normal arterial PaO_2 at any age

$$PO_2 \text{ at given age} = 104 - \frac{\text{Age in years}}{4}$$

Giving patients supplemental oxygen raises their FIO_2. In a normal person if the FIO_2 increase, the partial pressure of oxygen in the arterial blood rises proportionally. This is not so in a patient with sick lungs. The reason for this is a process called *shunting*.

SHUNTING AS A CAUSE OF HYPOXIA

In the normal lung less than five percent of the blood bypasses oxygenated alveoli, however in pulmonary disease a much larger proportion of blood may miss out being oxygenated as it *shunted* through the un-aerated alveoli. This means that blue oxygenated blood enters some of the pulmonary capillaries, and emerges still blue at the venous end to mix with red oxygenated blood from properly aerated alveoli in the pulmonary venous blood. This *venous admixture* causes the arterial PO$_2$ fall. Unfortunately the more severe the lung disease or cardiac failure, the greater is the effect of *shunting*, and the less effective is supplemental oxygen.

CAUSES OF FAILURE TO OXYGENATE BLOOD

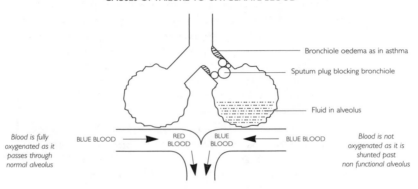

fig 16.2 Shunting

Partial collapse, *micro-atelectasis*,* is the collapse of random tiny segments of lung.

This occurs because surfactant secretion falls during general anaesthesia making the lungs stiffer and less compliant. Blood passing through the collapsed alveoli them cannot take part in gas exchange. When the patient deep breathes and coughs after their anaesthetic the alveoli are stimulated to secrete surfactant.

---

* Just like small bubbles, alveoli tend to collapse as their walls get stuck together by *surface tension*. To overcome this the lung secretes a detergent like substance, a mixture of phospholipids, called surfactant that decreases surface tension. If it weren't for *surfactant* it would be impossible to generate enough muscular effort to breath in.

Following abdominal and thoracic operations the diaphragm does not work properly. Deep breathing and coughing temporarily improve oxygen saturation by blasting open collapsed airways and alveoli.

Encourage the patient to
deep breath and cough.

HYPOVENTILATION AS A CAUSE OF HYPOXIA

Carbon dioxide (CO_2) is produced in the tissues, and carried in the blood to the lungs to be excreted. As the carbon dioxide diffuses from the blood into the alveoli, it displaces the other gases there; and the oxygen tension decreases. *Hypoventilation* is a very precise term. By definition, if the arterial partial pressure of carbon dioxide ($PaCO_2$) is raised the patient is said to be *hypoventilating*.

Although best considered as separate entities, hypoventilation and hypoxia are inter-related. As the alveolar PCO_2 rises, so the alveolar PO_2 falls. They conform exactly to Dalton's Law of Partial Pressures.

HYPOVENTILATION AS A CAUSE OF HYPOXIA

How can we work out if hypoxia is due to hypoventilation alone, or if the lungs are damaged and unable to transfer oxygen properly? The easy way is to see if the value of the partial pressure of oxygen in the blood (PaO_2) is reasonably close to the partial pressure of oxygen in the alveoli (PAO_2). If they are not close together, then some blood is bypassing aerated alveoli and is not being oxygenated. With a little practice you will be able to do the following calculations in your head.

1. Work out the inspired PIO_2. If the patient is not on supplemental oxygen and is breathing air the PIO_2 at sea level (atmospheric pressure =760 mmHg) will be 160 mmHg. This is a figure worth remembering.
2. Take a set of blood gases.
3. Estimate the partial pressure of carbon dioxide in the alveolus (PAO_2) To do this subtract the partial pressure of carbon dioxide measured in the blood ($PaCO_2$) from partial pressure of the inspired oxygen (PIO_2).
4. Calculate the percentage difference between the estimated PAO_2 and the measured PIO_2. If the PaO_2 is greater than 80% of the estimated alveolar PAO_2, there is probably little shunting in the lungs and they are essentially normal. If the PaO_2 is less than 80% of the estimated alveolar PAO_2 then there is something wrong with the lungs.

CASE 1

Mary has had her varicose veins tied and is breathing air:
(Atmospheric pressure is 760 mmHg)

1. Calculate the $\qquad$ $PIO_2 = \dfrac{21}{100} \times 760$ $\qquad$ = 160 mmHg

2. Measure blood gases: $PaO_2 = 100$ mmHg
$\qquad\qquad\qquad\quad$ $PaCO_2 = 40$ mmHg

3. Estimate the $\qquad$ $PAO_2 = 160 - 40$ $\qquad$ = 120 mmHg

4. Calculate the PAO_2 as a percentage of the PaO_2
$\qquad$ $PAO_2\%$ of the $PaO_2 = \dfrac{100}{120} \times 100$ $\qquad$ = 83%

ANALYSIS OF MARY'S BLOOD GASES

The $PaCO_2$ is 40 mmHg so Mary's ventilation is normal.

Her PaO_2 is 100 mmHg on air so she is not hypoxaemic.

This PaO_2 is greater 80% of the measured estimated alveolar PAO_2, so the lungs are functioning satisfactorily.

CASE 2

Peter is 66 year old smoker who just returned from theatre following an inguinal hernia repair. He is breathing 35% oxygen and has just received some IV morphine.
(Atmospheric pressure is 760 mmHg)

1. Calculate the $\qquad$ $PIO_2 = \dfrac{35}{100} \times 760$ $\qquad$ = 266 mmHg

2. Measure blood gases: $PaO_2 = 80$ mmHg
$\qquad\qquad\qquad\quad$ $PaCO_2 = 50$ mmHg

3. Estimate the $\qquad$ $PAO_2 = 266 - 50$ $\qquad$ = 216 mmHg

4. Calculate the PAO_2 as a percentage of the PaO_2
$\qquad$ $PAO_2\%$ of the $PaO_2 = \dfrac{80}{216} \times 100$ $\qquad$ = 37%

ANALYSIS OF PETER'S BLOOD GASES

The $PaCO_2$ is 50 mmHg, therefore Peter is hypoventilating.

The PaO_2 is 80 mmHg on 35% oxygen, therefore he is not hypoxaemic.

PaO_2 is 37% of his estimated alveolar PAO_2. This is a lot less than 80% so not only is Peter hypoventilating, but he also has something structurally wrong with his lungs. We should be thinking about aspiration, pneumonia, pre-existing lung disease and all the other pathology that could be involved. He will certainly need supplemental oxygen in the ward.

DIFFUSION HYPOXIA

Diffusion hypoxia is a particular hazard in the very young and the very old. For about 5 - 10 minutes after the end of a general anaesthetic, nitrous oxide diffuses back from the circulation into the lungs, diluting the inspired air and reducing the oxygen concentration in the lung. This is one good reason to give high concentrations of oxygen for the first 10 minutes after discontinuing an anaesthetic.

ALVEOLAR AIR EQUATION

A more accurate, but more difficult, way to determine alveolar PO_2 is to calculate is to use the Alveolar air equation.

$$PAO_2 = PIO_2 - \frac{(PaCO_2)}{R}$$

PAO_2 = the alveolar partial pressure of oxygen

PIO_2 = the partial pressure of inspired oxygen

$PaCO_2$ = the partial pressure of carbon dioxide in arterial blood

R = the respiratory quotient, normally about 0.8

---

3. Oxygen supply to the tissues.

Oxygen diffuses across the epithelial lining cells of the lung, then into the red cell where, loosely bound to haemoglobin, the blood flow carries it to the tissues.

There are four factors involved in the supply oxygen to the tissues: healthy lungs, good cardiac function to pump the blood to the tissues, enough haemoglobin to carry the oxygen; and a variety of metabolic factors.

LUNG FUNCTION

Good lung function allows the haemoglobin to be fully saturated with oxygen. The haemoglobin's oxygen saturation can be measured with a pulse oximeter. Respiratory failure or low inspired oxygen tensions causes *hypoxic hypoxia*.

CARDIAC FUNCTION

Cardiac output determines the speed at which the oxygen carrying haemoglobin reaches the tissues. In cardiac failure, blood is pumped more slowly through the tissues, and the oxygen supply falls. This type of hypoxia is called *stagnant hypoxia*.

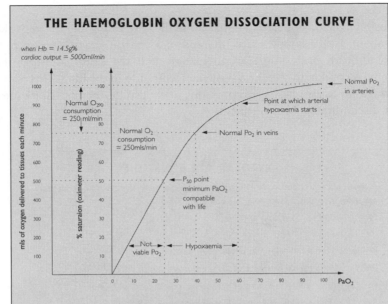

THE HAEMOGLOBIN OXYGEN DISSOCIATION CURVE

when Hb = 14.5g%
cardiac output = 5000ml/min

fig 16.3 Haemoglobin oxygen dissociation curve.

You will need to understand this graph if you are to make sense of how oxygen gets into the tissues. The graph matches the haemoglobin's saturation with oxygen (on the vertical axis) to the pressure it exerts as it attempts to leave the haemoglobin (on the horizontal axis). For example if haemoglobin is 90 per cent full of haemoglobin, the push oxygen will exert as it leave the haemoglobin is about 60 mmHg. For oxygen to get into, and be used by the cells, it has to be delivered both, in sufficient quantity, and with enough pressure. It is the partial pressure of oxygen in the capillary that provides the force to drive oxygen from the red cell into the tissues, through the cell membrane, through the cytoplasm and on to the mitochondria.

The shape of the curve changes with the pH of the blood, and the patient's temperature. Patients in recovery room are often moderately acidotic and hypothermic. Acidosis causes the arterial PaO_2 to be higher than normal at a given saturation. This is a good thing, since the extra pressure increases tissue oxygenation. On the other hand hypothermia decreases tissue oxygenation, but also reduces the tissue's oxygen consumption.

HAEMOGLOBIN

Normally there is about 120 - 160 grams of haemoglobin in a litre of blood. Lack of haemoglobin mass causes *anaemic hypoxia*.

METABOLIC FACTORS

Each gram of haemoglobin carries about 1.34 mls of oxygen. Some metabolic disturbances such as alkalaemia, and hypothermia, decrease the amount of oxygen carried by haemoglobin. These factors predipose to metabolic hypoxia.

OXYGEN FLUX

Mathematically these four factors can be combined as the oxygen flux equation. The equation will help you to work out why patients suddenly deteriorate in the recovery room.

Oxygen supply to tissues	=	Cardiac output	×	Haemoglobin concentration	×	Haemoglobin saturation %	×	Oxygen carrying capacity of haemoglobin
1000 ml/min	=	5000 ml/min	×	145 gm/1000 ml	×	98.5/100	×	1.34 ml/gm

Only about 250 ml of the 1000 ml of oxygen normally carried to the tissues each minute is used. Haemoglobin enters the tissues almost 100 per cent saturated and leaves about 75 per cent saturated, that is about three quarters full.

Notice the multiplication signs. These show how the four components *multiply* together to cause tissue hypoxia. A failure of more than one component makes the oxygen supply *many times* worse. If the oxygen supply falls below about 400 ml per minute, the patient will probably die. This corresponds to an arterial PaO_2 of 25 mmHg (3.29 kPa) which is too low for survival. Such a low PaO_2 can occur insidiously in a sick patient.

AN EXAMPLE OF INSIDIOUS HYPOXIA.

Consider Claude, aged 72 years, who has heart disease. He comes to the recovery room following emergency vascular surgery. He has a cardiac output of 4000 ml/min, a haemoglobin of 88 gm/l, and an arterial blood gas saturation of 90 per cent. Claude will have a tissue oxygen supply of 410 ml/min and will be near death.

Oxygen supply to tissues	=	Cardiac output	×	Haemoglobin concentration	×	Haemoglobin saturation %	×	Oxygen carrying capacity of haemoglobin
410 ml/min	=	4000 ml/min	×	88 gm/1000 ml	×	90/100	×	1.34 ml/gm

Yet any one of those factors alone would not be an overwhelming threat to life.

NORMAL

Many red cells, all fully oxygenated.
Haemoglobin 14gm/decilitre.
Pulse oximeter reads 99%
PaO_2 100 mmHg
Oxygen content of blood 20ml/100ml

No Hypoxia
No Hypoxaemia

Haemoglobin has 4 oxygen
molecules bound.

ANAEMIA

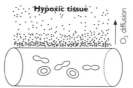

Few red cells, all fully oxygenated.
Haemoglobin 7gm/decilitre.
Pulse oximeter reads 99%
$PaO_2 = 100$ mmHg
Oxygen content of blood 10ml/100ml

Hypoxia
No Hypoxaemia

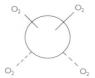

Haemoglobin has 4 oxygen molecules
bound, but there are fewer
haemoglobin molecules.

HYPOXAEMIA

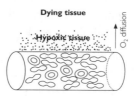

Many red cells, partially oxygenated.
Haemoglobin 14gm/decilitre.
Pulse oximeter reads 55%
$PaO_2 = 33$ mmHg
Oxygen content of blood 11ml/100ml

Hypoxia
Hypoxaemia

Haemoglobin has only 2 molecules of
oxygen bound, and these it is
reluctant to release.

fig 16.4   Tissue oxygen supply in normal, anaemic and hypoxaemic tissue

TISSUE OXYGEN SUPPLY AND PO_2 OF BLOOD ENTERING CAPILLARY BEDS

Tissue oxygen supply	Haemoglobin saturation	PO_2 of blood entering capillary beds
1000 ml/min	100%	100 mmHg (13.3 kPa)
750 ml/min	75%	40 mmHg (5.3 kPa)
400 ml/min	40%	about 25 mmHg (3.3 kPa)*

* allowing for the Bohr effect induced by hypoxic tissue acidosis enables haemoglobin to give up its oxygen more easily. Acidosis actually helps haemoglobin release oxygen to hypoxic tissue. The Bohr effect occurs because the globule shape of the haemoglobin molecule is distorted by acidosis or alkalosis and this alters the way it picks up, holds on to, and releases oxygen.

In summary the combination of two or more of the following may be lethal.
- anaemia;
- heart failure;
- poor lung function;
- hypothermia, alkalosis.

EXTRACTION FAILURE

Massive blood transfusion can lead to hypoxia. The transfused red cells will pick up oxygen, but only release it reluctantly in the tissues. In patients dying from septicaemia, or severe shock, the cells are so sick that they cannot use oxygen even if it is delivered to them. The cells cannot extract oxygen from the haemoglobin. Comparing the oxygen content of arterial blood and mixed venous blood gives the *extraction fraction* (Tx). This is an indication how much oxygen is being used by the tissues.

4. How the cell obtains and uses oxygen

Once in the tissues oxygen diffuses into the cell's mitochondria, where it is used for biochemical reactions involving *oxidative metabolism*. In effect 80 per cent of the oxygen 'burns' with carbon in sugars, fats and proteins to form carbon dioxide, while the remainder of the oxygen mops up hydrogen ions, and is converted into water. The oxidation takes place in carefully graded steps so that not too much heat is released at once. These processes release a lot of energy, most of which is stored in high energy phosphate compounds. These act like re-chargeable batteries, and are used all through the cell for starting and maintaining chemical reactions.

At the arterial end of a capillary the PaO_2 is about 100 mmHg. As the red cell moves along the capillary it unloads oxygen, and picks up carbon dioxide. The PO_2 progressively falls so that by the time it has reached the venous end of the capillary the P_vO_2 is only about 40 mmHg. In technical terms the partial pressure of oxygen establishes a *concentration gradient* down which oxygen diffuses to reach the mitochondria inside the cells.

Put more simply, the partial pressure pushes oxygen from the haemoglobin on its microscopically long journey through membranes, and across fluid spaces to reach the mitochondria. The higher the pressure, the bigger the push, and the further the oxygen will diffuse. Cells close to the capillary receive a good oxygen supply, and those further away receive less.

Around the capillary it is possible to describe a cylinder, known as a *Krogh cylinder*, of oxygen tension in the tissue. Cells inside the cylinder are well oxygenated; but at the periphery of the cylinder the oxygen tension falls, and the cell's oxygen supply becomes more tenuous. To compensate for this the cylinders overlap one another so that the more peripheral cells get their oxygen supply from a number of adjacent cylinders.

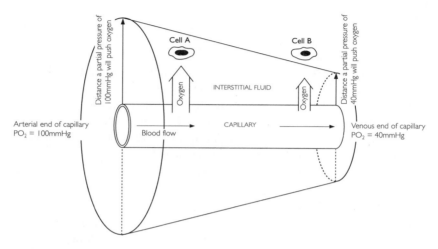

Cell A and Cell B are both the same distance from the capillary but the oxygenation of Cell A is much better than Cell B.

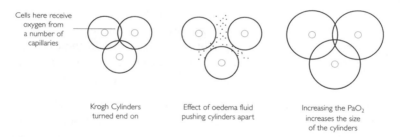

Cells here receive oxygen from a number of capillaries

Krogh Cylinders turned end on

Effect of oedema fluid pushing cylinders apart

Increasing the PaO₂ increases the size of the cylinders

fig 16.5 Krogh cylinders

Two things can jeopardize the oxygen supply to the cells. Firstly the cylinders may be pushed apart by oedema fluid, as happens in cerebral oedema. The cells become hypoxic, and are unable to maintain their function. Secondly, as the patient becomes hypoxaemic, the PaO_2 falls, and as the diameter of the Krogh cylinders contracts, the cells become hypoxic.

By administering a higher concentration of inspired oxygen, we can increase the size of the Krogh cylinders, and improve tissue oxygenation. This is important after surgery where tissue trauma causes oedema. It is of crucial importance after head injury, where cerebral oedema jeopardizes cells on the margins of the Krogh cylinders.

Once the oxygen supply falls the hypoxic cells, will for a short time, shift to anaerobic metabolism to provide the power to run their processes. However if there is no oxygen to mop up the hydrogen ion produced by the cells, the hydrogen ion overflows into the tissue fluids and eventually causes acidaemia. As the hydrogen ion accumulates in the tissues its strong positive charge starts to bend proteins out of shape. Enzymes no longer function properly and this further upsets cellular function.

PROBLEMS WITH OXYGEN

Flammable material will burn briskly in oxygen, but oxygen itself will not burn. Keep naked flames and sources of electrical sparks at least 2 metres away from a source of oxygen.

Oxygen toxicity of the newborn

If exposed to high oxygen concentrations, premature babies and neonates (less than 1500 gm) are at particular risk from retrolental fibroplasia (also called *retinopathy of prematurity* or ROP), and will go permanently blind.

OPTIMAL PAO$_2$ FOR THE NEWBORN			
Baby's age	PaO$_2$(mmHg)	PaO$_2$ (kPa)	Hb saturation %
Pre term	40-60	5.3-8.0	70-90
Full term	50-70	6.6-9.2	84-92

Adult oxygen toxicity

Older patients receiving 100% oxygen for longer than 4 - 6 hours run the risk of progressive lung damage.

Carbon-dioxide resistant patients

In a normal person, a small rise in PaCO$_2$ will stimulate the respiratory centres to increase the rate and depth of breathing. Patients with chronic obstructive airway disease have chronically raised PaCO$_2$, (*blue-bloaters*), may stop breathing if given more than 28% inspired oxygen These patients have adapted to a high PaCO$_2$, and will no longer increase their respiratory effort if it rises. Instead, they depend on a low PaO$_2$ for their respiratory drive. Blue bloaters are easily recognized, because they almost invariably have pulmonary hypertension, with right heart failure (so called *cor pulmonale*). They are cyanosed, plethoric, can only say a few words between gasps, and frequently have oedematous ankles. It is a common error to deprive them of supplemental oxygen, 'just in case they stop breathing'. Watch them closely, and if their respiratory effort starts to fail, their oximeter reading falls, or they become drowsy (a sign of rising $PaCO_2$); then assist their breathing with a bag and mask. This is a difficult problem, because once intubated and stabilized on a ventilator, these patients can be almost impossible to wean. Many physicians try to get by with other measures, for example an intravenous respiratory stimulant such as doxapram.

RESPIRATORY SYMBOLS AND DEFINITIONS

SYMBOLS

O_2	=	oxygen
CO_2	=	carbon dioxide
H_2O	=	water

Upper-case letters are used to describe substances in the gaseous phase.

P	=	partial pressure (tension) of a gas
A	=	alveolar
I	=	inspired gas
E	=	expired gas
V	=	volume in litres
T	=	tidal

Lower-case letters are used to describe substances in the liquid phase.

a	=	arterial
v	=	venous
c	=	capillary

In a mixture of gases the *partial pressure* of a particular gas, is the pressure that gas would exert if it alone occupied the space available to it.

PO_2	=	partial pressure of oxygen.
PaO_2	=	partial pressure of oxygen in arterial blood.
$PaCO_2$	=	partial pressure of carbon dioxide in arterial blood.
FIO_2	=	fractional inspired content of oxygen. Air is about 21% oxygen, so breathing air the FIO_2 = 0.21
H^+	=	hydrogen ion.
$[H^+]$	=	hydrogen ion concentration.
pH	=	a non-linear scale for measuring hydrogen ion concentration.
FRC	=	functional residual capacity

UNITS

$cm\ H_2O$	=	centimetres of water pressure.
mmHg	=	millimetres of mercury pressure.
kPa	=	kilopascals of pressure. 7.60 mmHg = 1 kPa 1.32 mmHg = 10 cm H_2O

In the UK the kilopascal (kPa) is the preferred unit for measuring pressure.

DEFINITIONS

Apnoea is the complete absence of breathing.

Breathing is the mechanical act of moving air in and out of lungs.

Hypercarbia is an excess of carbon dioxide in the body.

Hypoxaemia occurs when the PaO_2 falls below 60 mmHg (7.89 kPa)

Hypoxia occurs when there is not enough oxygen to allow the cells carry out their normal function.

Hypoventilation is failure of lungs to eliminate carbon dioxide. It is measured by a rise in the partial pressure of carbon dioxide in the arterial blood.

Respiratory rate (RR) is the number of breaths taken each minute.

Tidal volume (TV) is the amount of air moved into or out of the lungs with each breath.

Minute volume (MV) is the volume of air moved into or out of the lungs in one minute. MV = RR x TV

Dyspnoea occurs when the patient feels he cannot get his breath.

1 McKenzie AJ. (1987). *Anaesthesia and Intensive Care*, 17:412-17.

17. RESPIRATORY PROBLEMS

More than one-third of patients presenting for surgery have respiratory disease that either limits their day-to-day activity, or requires on-going treatment. The effects of chronic cigarette smoking, and asthma are common problems, which should be identified in the preadmission clinic and optimized before surgery.

Airway management is the most important skill required by recovery room. No staff should be left alone with unconscious patients until they are confident that they can maintain an airway, and cope with airway emergencies. Not only should you watch your patients carefully, but you should also listen carefully to detect airway obstruction, or sputum retention the moment it occurs.

Keep special trolleys set-up for intravenous access, reintubation, bronchoscopy, and insertion of chest drains. See appendix VII for examples of these trolleys. Instructions for inserting a thoracic drain are on page 96.

A high capacity sucker must be instantly available to remove foreign material from the patient's airway. Place the sucker under the right hand side of the patient's pillow where it can be quickly found. Patients have died because the sucker was out of reach, or not turned on.

Wherever possible nurse comatose patients on their side in the *recovery position*. Even conscious patients are safer like this. Patients lying on their backs are always at risk of airway obstruction and aspiration pneumonitis. They are also more likely to develop postoperative chest infections.

Problems encountered in the recovery room include:
• cyanosis;
• dyspnoea;
• coughing;
• sputum retention;
• wheezing;
• obstructed airway, stridor and laryngospasm;
• laryngeal and pharyngeal oedema;
• vocal chord paralysis;
• foreign body aspiration and the coronor's clot;
• aspiration pneumonitis;
• pneumothorax;

- embolism;
- hypoxia, hypoxaemia and hypoventilation;
- respiratory failure.

Sometimes these problems are self-limiting, and easy to assess and manage. Sometimes they are the signs of serious problems. Initially, treat the symptoms, and use your monitors, to help you to work out what is happening.

First save the patient's life,
then find out what is wrong.

- Keep the patient on his side;
- clear his airway with the sucker;
- give high flow of oxygen by mask;
- check his blood presure, pulse and oxygen saturation;
- check that the intravenous line is running well;
- monitor his ECG, look for signs of ischaemia or arrhythmias;
- if at all worried call for help.

A ROUGH ESTIMATION OF POSTOPERATIVE REDUCTION IN RESPIRATORY FUNCTION		
Site of incision	Preoperative FEV$_1$	Estimated postoperative FEV$_1$ as percentage of preoperative level.
Upper abdominal	100%	25 – 35%
Lower abdominal	100%	45 – 55%
Thoracic	100%	55 – 65%
Elsewhere	100%	10%

General anaesthesia causes respiratory depression, drying of secretions and bronchial cilial dysfunction. The alveolar cells stop producing surfactant. Muscle relaxants may cause residual muscle weakness. Pain may inhibit the ability to deep breathe and cough. The net effect of these problems is a patient who may breathe more slowly and less deeply than normal, be reluctant to cough, and have sticky sputum which blocks small airways causing segments of the lungs to collapse. The problems are worse the closer the surgical incision is to the diaphragm, and are especially severe with subcostal incisions such as open cholecystectomy.

ESTIMATION OF POSTOPERATIVE
RESPIRATORY FUNCTION

A useful, but rough guide can be obtained preoperatively by measuring the patient's forced expiratory volume over one second (FEV_1) with a spirometer. This is a dynamic test which is influenced by the amount of airway obstruction. Normally the FEV_1 should be at least 70 – 80% of the forced vital capacity (FVC). Using table (page 000), estimate the patient's postoperative FEV_1.

If predicted FEV_1 < 10 ml per kg ventilatory support likely to be needed.

If predicted FEV_1 10 – 15 ml per kg, then reassess in the recovery room.

If predicted FEV_1 > 15 ml per kg, then respiratory failure is unlikely.

Example case:

Consider Alice, a 60-year-old woman who smokes, weighs 60 kg, and is to have an open cholecystectomy.

Data:

$$\text{Weight} = 60 \text{ kg}$$

Smoker 25% function

(a non-smoker would have 35% function)

$$\text{Her preoperative } FEV_1 = 3200 \text{ ml}$$

$$\text{Estimated postoperative } FEV_1 = 3200 \times 25/100$$

$$= 800 \text{ ml}$$

$$FEV_1 \text{ per kg} = 80/60$$

$$= 13 \text{ ml/kg}$$

At a predicted postoperative FEV_1 of 13 ml/kg this woman will need reassessment in the recovery room. On admission to the recovery room she was stable, but within 30 minutes her respiratory rate rose to 28 breaths per minute and her oxygen saturation fell to 90%. Her pain was then managed with intercostal blocks, and she was encouraged to deep breath and cough. She improved rapidly, but was sent to a high dependency nursing ward for close observation for the next 36 hours.

Factors that suggest the need for respiratory support are:
- a respiratory rate > 25 breaths per minute;
- an oxygen saturation < 92%;
- inability to take a deep breath and cough effectively;
- an alveolar–arterial oxygen gradient of greater than 250 mmHg when the patient is receiving 100% inspired oxygen.

If the predicted FEV_1 were to be much less than 10 ml/kg then consider keeping the patient intubated and ventilated, and reassessing them in the intensive care unit.

Cyanosis

Cyanosis is a bluish colouration of the skin or mucous membranes. If in doubt, compare the colour of the patient's tongue with that of a staff member. Treat the cyanosis as a life threatening hypoxia until you are sure of the cause.

Immediately: call for help, check carotid pulse,
clear and maintain an airway,
support breathing, and give high flow oxygen.

MONITOR: pulse rate and rhythm, respiration, blood pressure, ECG, pulse oximeter, blood gases.

PHYSIOLOGY OF CYANOSIS

Cyanosis is not seen until the patient has at least 3 grams of deoxyhaemoglobin in their blood. This corresponds approximately to a PaO_2 less than 50 mmHg (6.6 kPa) and a pulse oximetry reading of less than 85%. Occasionally central cyanosis is caused by drugs, such as methylene blue, or prilocaine, or it can be a result of an incompatible blood transfusion. Anaemic patients may not become cyanosed, even when dangerously hypoxic.

Good lighting is needed to detect cyanosis. Although daylight is preferable, it is usually not possible. As an alternative your recovery room should be lit by special daylight fluorescent tubes which have less blue light in them than normal fluorescent tubes. The yellow light from a normal light bulb also makes cyanosis difficult to see.

Methaemoglobinaemia may present as cyanosis. The drugs prilocaine, benzocaine and nitroglycerine can oxidize haemoglobin from the ferrous (Fe^{++}) to the ferric (Fe^{+++}) form. The methaemoglobin so formed will not release oxygen to the tissues, and causes hypoxia. The arterial blood looks dark, almost brown. The pulse oximeter gives a saturation reading of about 85% irrespective of the true saturation. If you suspect this problem take a blood sample for methaemoglobin levels. Repeat this at 2 hours and 8 hours. A level greater than 15% will cause hypoxia, greater than 60% is dangerous, greater than 70% can be fatal. Treat with methylene blue 1 mg/kg IV over 10 minutes. Methylene blue itself makes the patient appear cyanosed. Excess methylene blue can convert haemoglobin into the ferric form. Measure blood gases, the PaO_2 may well be normal, but if the patient is hypoxic then an acidosis will develop.

Causes include:
- hypoventilation caused by residual anaesthetic drugs, muscle relaxants, opioids, or benzodiazepines;

- airway obstruction, such as laryngospasm, asthma or inhaled vomitus;
- lung disease, such as pneumonia, lung collapse or pulmonary oedema;
- mechanical problems, such as haemo- or pneumothorax;
- cardiac failure, air embolism, or fat emboli;
- abnormal haemoglobin, such as incompatible transfusion with massive haemolysis, methaemoglobin, sulphaemoglobin or carboxyhaemoglobin.

There are two types of cyanosis, *central cyanosis* and *peripheral cyanosis*.

Central cyanosis is seen as blue lips, tongue and mucous membranes. It is a sign of severe hypoxia

Peripheral cyanosis causes blue hands, feet and finger nail beds. If the patient has central cyanosis he will have peripheral cyanosis too. But peripheral cyanosis can occur without central cyanosis and may indicate that the patient is cold, has venous congestion or is shocked. Cyanosis is difficult to detect in a dark skinned person. Check his nail beds, the insides of his mouth, or the inner part of his eyelid; even so you cannot always be sure. A pulse oximeter is not influenced by skin colour, and will give and accurate reading.

DYSPNOEA

Dyspnoea occurs when the patient has to work harder than normal to breath. It is a subjective feeling, not an observation. The patient *feels* short of breath and calls it *air hunger*, medical staff refer to it as *respiratory distress*. The patient's distress ranges from just being uncomfortable through to extreme panic as he struggles for every breath and is unable to talk.

A patient may be dyspnoeic, but not hypoxaemic (eg. an asthmatic on high inspired oxygen concentrations); or hypoxaemic and not dyspnoeic (eg. opioid induced respiratory depression). Read the previous chapter for an explanation of hypoxaemia.

DIAGNOSING THE CAUSE OF DYSNOEA

Is this patient's dyspnoea part of a larger disease process? Work through the possible causes in an anatomical sequence from the brain to the lung.

Causes of dyspnoea include:
1. Certain emotional states. The patient may be stressed or agitated about the outcome of their operation. This causes *hysterical hyperventilation*. Overbreathing makes the patient dysnoeic and aggravates the problem. This is an uncommon problem in recovery room. Hold the patient's hand, reassure him and if necessary settle him with a small dose of opioid.

2. An acutely raised arterial PCO_2. This occurs after laparoscopic investigations where CO_2 has been used to inflate the abdominal cavity. Less predictably a low arterial PO_2 may cause dyspnoea especially if it is associated with metabolic acidosis such as occurs in haemorrhagic shock.

3. Increased muscular effort to breath. Consider airway's obstruction; pneumothorax, and haemothorax.

4. The residual effects of muscle relaxant drugs causing patients to struggle for breath; typically their movement is jerky and floppy like a puppet on a string.

5. Excess fluid in the interstitium or alveoli of the lung making the lungs stiffer (*decreased lung compliance*). This occurs in pulmonary oedema, or pneumonia.

6. Inflammatory mediators such as histamine, prostaglandins and bradykinins stimulate interstitial lung receptors to signal the brain to increase respiratory rate. This occurs in pulmonary, fat or air embolism, and also in anaphylaxis, pulmonary aspiration and asthma.

COUGHING

Coughing is a sign of irritation in the larynx or lower airway.

It is a protective reflex and its function is to eject foreign material. With excessive coughing the patient is unable to get his breath, becomes distressed, and turns purple in the face from vascular engorgement. He may become cyanosed and hypoxic. Coughing can tear stitches especially following plastic facial surgery, middle ear surgery, or disrupt a repair of a retinal detachment. It might also break ribs (*cough fractures*) in the elderly, contribute to cardiac arrhythmias, and disrupt abdominal sutures.

Causes include:
• laryngoscopy, bronchoscopy or abrasion of the airway during intubation;
• oedema or inflammation of the bronchi and bronchioles, as in asthma and pulmonary oedema;
• aspiration of material into the respiratory tree. This occurs because the patients protective laryngeal reflexes are depressed after general anaesthesia or even sedation. Small amounts of material aspirated from the upper airway trigger coughing. If your patient starts coughing abruptly then this is the most likely cause. Aspiration pneumonitis

occurs if large amounts of material are inhaled through the larynx into the lower airway.

Coughing can be a problem after a rigid bronchoscopy. The patient may not have time to catch his breath between paroxysms, and become cyanosed, hypoxic and distressed. Give high concentrations of humidified oxygen. The patient will often attempt to sit up, and may become even more agitated if you try to restrain him. Be careful that he does not fall off the trolley, make sure the trolley sides are up and a strong attendant is there to help. Recall the anaesthetist and give 1% lignocaine 1 mg/kg intravenously. This usually settles these patients. Occasionally the patient may need to be intubated to regain control.

Remember to wear goggles when receiving a bronchoscopy patient. Take very great care that nothing coughed from the patient's airways touches you. As soon as possible wash thoroughly, including your hair, and change your clothes.

PATTERNS OF BREATHING

Expose the patient's chest and watch the way in which the patient breaths carefully. Listen to the air entering and leaving his mouth. Sometimes dyspnoea is confused with a particular pattern of breathing, which if recognized can help you diagnose the underlying cause.

KUSSMAUL'S breathing is a sign of metabolic acidosis. The patient breathes deeply and feels breathless.

CHEYNE-STOKES breathing is easily recognized, because the patient takes a series of breaths, and then stops briefly, only to resume breathing again within a few moments. It is of concern in head injured patients or following neurosurgery.

SEE-SAW breathing is a sign of an obstructed airway. In attempting to breathe the patients chest will fall as his abdomen rises giving an impression of a rocking movement. You will not feel air passing in or out of the mouth. Normally the chest and abdomen rise and fall together.

PLEURITIC PAIN limits breathing to sharp suddenly curtailed inspiratory gasps. This occurs in patients with chest drains, after thoracic surgery or a pneumothorax. A pneumothorax makes it difficult for a patient to breath in.

OBSTRUCTIVE lung disease imposes a pattern of slow deep breaths.

RESTRICTIVE lung disease imposes a pattern of rapid shallow breaths.

MANAGEMENT

If coughing becomes a problem, or is threatening oxygenation:

1. Sit the patient up.

2. Give high flow oxygen by mask.

3. Attach a pulse oximeter and ECG.

4. Ask the anaesthetist to examine the airway with a laryngoscope to check for foreign material.

5. If the coughing is due to simple irritation of the mucosa, give lignocaine 1.5 mg/kg IV over 30 seconds.[9] This will quickly resolve the patient's cough.

6. If the patient becomes hypoxic or develops cardiac arrhythmias, it may be necessary to sedate, and re-intubate him and re-assess the situation.

Morphine is a good cough suppressant, but pethidine is not. If a patient is producing excessive sputum it is unwise to suppress his cough reflex. The accumulating secretions may block airways causing lower lobe collapse, and pneumonia. Coughing can sometimes develop into stridor with laryngeal spasm, a life threatening situation (see page 323).

SPUTUM RETENTION

Sputum retention is common in all patients who smoke and those with chronic bronchitis. Humidified oxygen helps, avoid anticholinergic drugs which make the sputum thick and sticky. Sometimes the patient wants to cough, but he cannot. This is a problem in people with severe emphysema or chronic bronchitis. These patients cannot raise enough of a cough impulse to get thick tenacious sputum through their larynx. They may require a cricothyroidotomy with a Minitrak® to keep their airway clear of mucus.

Some elderly patients with brain stem ischaemia are not distressed, and will lie there oblivious of the gurgle every time they breathe. These patients have such poor laryngeal, and pharyngeal protective reflexes that you will be able to open their mouths, and with the help of a laryngoscope and Magill forceps, pass a sucker through their vocal cords to aspirate the retained mucus. Pre-oxygenate the patient thoroughly first. If the patient coughs, well and good, but take care not to distress him. If this fails a Minitrak® may be necessary to keep the airway clear of mucus.

Patients with chronic obstructive airways disease pose particular problems in the recovery room. One of which is sputum retention. Read more about these patients in the chapter on pre-existing diseases.

CRICOTHYROID PUNCTURE

There are a number of commercially available tracheostomy sets which are designed for quick and easy insertion. However, in an emergency situation, where the patient is becoming cyanosed, or his conscious state is deteriorating, you may not have time to organize this. You may have to perform an acute cricothyroid puncture.

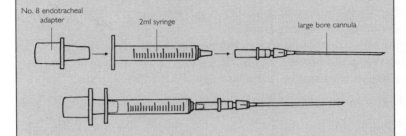

fig 17.1 Improvised cricothyroid puncture set

Take the largest bore intravenous cannula you have, (preferably 10 G or bigger) and insert it through the cricothyroid membrane into the trachea. Attach the barrel of a 2 ml syringe into the needle and then jam a No. 8 endotracheal 15 mm adaptor into the barrel of the syringe. It will now be possible to attach the cannula to a self-inflating bag or T-piece to support the patient's oxygenation until a tracheostomy or other means of establishing an airway can be achieved.

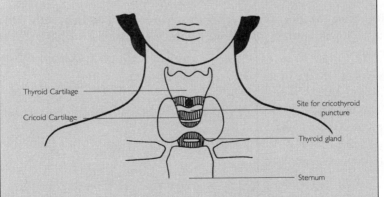

fig 17.2 Location of cricothyroid puncture

WHEEZING

Wheezing is a sign of irritation, inflammation or oedema of the bronchioles. Air passing along these fine tubes causes the walls to vibrate like the reed on a clarinet producing an audible wheeze. If you have ever stretched the neck of a balloon and allowed it to deflate you will understand the how the noise of a wheeze is generated.

Wheeze may be accompanied by:
• dyspnoea and breathlessness;
• use of sternomastoid and accessory muscles of respiration;
• agitation and distress;
• cyanosis is a dangerous and late sign.

The first line treatment of wheezing in the recovery room is to:
IMMEDIATELY:
• check that the central venous line has not become disconnected;
• if the patient is still comatose and lying on his back, roll him into the recovery position;
• give high inspired oxygen concentration;
• consult the anaesthetist.

MONITOR:
Pulse, respiratory rate, blood pressure, perfusion status, ECG, pulse oximeter. If the wheeze is severe or the oxygen saturation is below 90 per cent, then consider blood gases, and a chest X-ray.

Diagnosing the cause of wheeze in the recovery room is frequently difficult, but you will need a diagnosis before you can start effective specific treatment .

Causes of wheeze in the recovery room include:
• aspiration;
• anaphylaxis;
• pulmonary oedema;
• asthma;
• pulmonary embolism.

If a patient is breathing quietly one moment, and wheezing the next then consider aspiration. If the wheeze is localized to one lung, or a segment of one lung, consider aspiration, or pulmonary embolism. If the wheeze is in both lungs consider anaphylaxis or cardiac failure with aspiration always a possibility. Aspiration is by far the commonest cause of wheeze in the recovery room. Think of this first, especially if the patient is not particularly distressed. Unfortunately wheeze is often diagnosed and treated as asthma, even if the patient has never had asthma before in his life. Acute first onset asthma is most unlikely to occur in the recovery room.

In acute left ventricular failure a chest X-ray will show acute pulmonary oedema. In contrast, aspiration pneumonia will not show up on a chest x-ray for several hours, and a pulmonary embolism may never show anything at all.

True asthma is rarely a problem in recovery room.
Before making this diagnosis think again.

Anaphylaxis always follows a moment or two after something is given intravenously such as penicillin, blood, or a plasma expanders like Haemaccel® to which the patient is allergic. Wheezing is accompanied by profound hypotension, and cardiovascular collapse. For more about anaphylaxis (see page 462).

Acute left ventricular failure with pulmonary oedema is usually the result of fluid overload during or after the anaesthetic. Check the patient's blood loss against the fluids given. If more than 2 litres of fluid, consider pulmonary oedema. Listen to the chest, you will hear crepitations. Other causes of acute left ventricular failure are myocardial ischaemia or infarction so do a 12 lead ECG and compare it with the preoperative ECG. Do a chest x-ray. Pulmonary oedema will show as a white and fluffy pattern spreading out from the hilar of the lungs.

Asthma[1] is not usually a problem in the recovery room. Asthmatics emerging from general anaesthesia are probably as wheeze free as they ever will be, because volatile anaesthetics are extremely good bronchodilators. If a severe asthmatic patient becomes dyspnoeic consider the possibility of a pneumothorax. This could have occurred, unsuspected, during the anaesthetic especially if the patient has been ventilated.

Never sedate a wheezing patient.

OBSTRUCTED AIRWAY, STRIDOR AND LARYNGOSPASM[2]

The airway can become obstructed either totally or partially, at any point between the lips or nose, and the alveoli. The commonest points are in the oro-pharynx, and at the airway's narrowest point in the larynx.

As air passes at high velocity through a narrowed airway it becomes more turbulent creating a noise which you can easily hear. Low velocity flow burbles through semifluid mucus plugs causing *rales*, while high flow through narrow tubes cause them to vibrate like reeds in a clarinet causing wheezes. Turbulent flow through obstruction in the region of the larynx cause *stridor*.

Tidal air exchange can be easily felt in the palm of the hand. Complete obstruction of the airway is revealed by the absence of air coming and going from mouth and nose.

See-saw breathing is a sign of life threatening airway obstruction (see page 319).

> *Complete airway obstruction is silent,*
> *and quickly and quietly will kill the patient.*

Causes of airway obstruction include:
- clenched teeth;
- tongue obstructing oropharynx;
- forgotten throat pack after nose or throat surgery;
- laryngospasm;
- laryngeal oedema after airway or neck surgery;
- sleep apnoea;
- tracheomalacia occurring after the relief of long standing tracheal compression;
- foreign body at any point in the airway.

Neonates and infants are obligate nose breathers. They cannot breathe through their mouths, so if their nose becomes obstructed they will struggle for breath. Their whole chest wall may be drawn in by their inspiratory effort.

Patients awakening from anaesthesia frequently clench their jaws tightly. If they are still intubated they can bite hard on their endotracheal tube, or laryngeal mask, obstructing it. Prevent this by inserting a Guedal airway along side the endotracheal tube, or folded gauze pad between their teeth. Leave a piece of gauze outside the mouth to remind you that it is in position, and note this on your observation sheet.

The main cause of airway obstruction in the recovery room is due the tongue falling back into the pharynx to obstruct the airway. This is far more likely to occur if patients are lying on their backs. To relieve this sort of obstruction, first gently extend the neck, place your fingers behind the angle of the mandible and lift it forward. You must be familiar with how to deal with this problem.

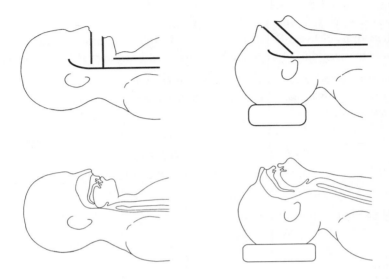

fig.17.3 Effect of extending neck and placing head on low pillow

Anticipate anatomical difficulty in maintaining airways in patients with:
• short or fat bull necks;
• stiff necks;
• previous cervical spinal surgery or injury;
• atlanto-axial instability;
• prominent protuberant upper teeth;
• underslung jaws or with receding chins;
• Down's syndrome;
• Turner's syndrome;
• patients who cannot open their mouths widely.

Initial management of the obstructed airway:
• inspect the patient's airway with a laryngoscope;
• suck out any secretions or foreign bodies;
• give 100% oxygen by mask;
• firmly lift the patient's jaw forward by inserting the fingers behind the angle of the mandible and pulling firmly upwards; in general the ears should be lifted anterior to the clavicles.

- insert an oral Guedal or similar airway;
- sometimes a well lubricated nasopharyngeal airway can be useful in maintaining a difficult airway.

Cyanosis and falling oxygen saturation are late and alarming signs of airway obstruction, and may be accompanied by ECG signs of ischaemia such as sinus tachycardia, which will soon be followed, more ominously, by a nodal bradycardia. ST depression is a sign of severe myocardial ischaemia.

If the airway obstruction is severe a young or muscular patient may do vigorous valsalva manoeuvres against a closed glottis. This can cause pulmonary oedema[3].

Patients with arthritis in their hands
can have unstable cervical spines - be gentle.

How to secure an emergency airway
(see cricothyroid puncture page 321).

Stridor
Stridor is a crowing noise made by turbulent air flowing through a narrowing in the larynx or upper airway. It is caused by partially obstructed airway, and includes *laryngospasm* and snoring. This can become very serious if not relieved quickly. Call for help.

Stridor is a medical emergency.

Laryngospasm
Laryngospasm is one of the causes of stridor. It is a common and dangerous problem, and a sign that something is irritating the upper airway, or some foreign material is present. The intrinsic laryngeal muscles reflexely contract to close the larynx and prevent foreign material passing when he attempts to breathe in. The patient makes a harsh crowing noise and air flow is obstructed. This is called *inspiratory stridor*. The patient is usually agitated, and panicky because he can not breathe.

Irritation induced laryngospasm follows extubation, especially if there has been an earlier difficult or traumatic intubation. It also sometimes follows bronchoscopy, and pharyngeal or laryngeal surgery. It is particularly common in children after upper airway surgery. It occurs in about 20 per cent of children after tonsillectomy.

INITIAL MANAGEMENT:
- Get help; you will need two assistants. The first assistant should attach an ECG, pulse oximeter and measure the pulse rate and blood pressure. Your second assistant should fetch the emergency trolley (cart), and prepare to draw up drugs;
- meanwhile inspect the patient's airway with a laryngoscope;
- suck out any secretions or foreign bodies;
- give 100% oxygen by mask;
- firmly lift the patient's jaw forward by inserting the fingers behind the angle of the mandible and pulling firmly upwards. In general the ears should be anterior to the clavicles;
- once you are sure the airway is clear, use a bag and mask to apply firm positive airway pressure in an attempt to relieve the spasm.

Further management if the above is unsuccessful:
- your assistants should prepare for urgent intubation;
- try lignocaine 1.5 ml/kg IV as a bolus. This will often relieve laryngospasm [4,5];
- should this fail the patient will need to be intubated to establish an airway.

SNORING
Snoring is another cause of stridor caused by partial obstruction of the upper airway. Usually it is caused by a combination of the tongue dropping back to obstruct breathing through the mouth, and the soft palate colluding to partially block breathing through the nose.

Do not allow patients to snore
in the recovery room.

LARYNGEAL OR PHARYNGEAL OEDEMA

Laryngeal oedema is caused by mucosal swelling. The function of the larynx is disturbed for at least four hours after tracheal extubation; even if the patients appear alert[6]. During this time the patient should remain under observation. This is especially important in child day cases who have been intubated.

Oedema in the upper airways occasionally follows extubation in children, and especially neonates and infants. A small amount of reactive oedema will intrude on the narrow lumen rapidly occluding it.

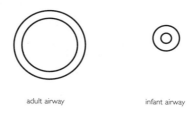

adult airway   infant airway

fig 17.4 The effect of 1 mm oedema in an adult and in an infant. In contrast to the adult, the infant's airway is critically narrowed.

In adults other causes are:
- operations on the neck such as thyroidectomy, or carotid endarterectomy;
- airway burns;
- trauma to the neck;
- subcutaneous surgical emphysema.

MANAGEMENT OF AIRWAY OEDEMA (CROUP) IN CHILDREN

Mild cases will respond to warmed humidified oxygen enriched gas mixtures. However it may be necessary to use nebulised adrenaline. Take two 1 ml ampoules of 1 in 1000 adrenaline and make it up to 5 ml in normal saline. Give this by oxygen driven nebuliser at a 5 l/min flow to a face mask. The effect lasts about 2 hours. Although this sounds a big dose for a small child it has been found to be very effective.[7]

VOCAL CORD PARALYSIS

This is a rare complication following intubation. It is occasionally seen after thyroid surgery if the recurrent laryngeal nerve has been damaged.

Unilateral vocal cord paralysis is usually a benign condition which presents as hoarseness in the recovery room and resolves over several weeks. If the cords have been damaged the patient will be unable to say "Eeeeee" in a high pitched voice.

Bilateral vocal cord paralysis is more serious and presents as upper airway obstruction as soon as the patient is extubated. The methods of maintaining the airway already described above will not be effective, although assisted ventilation with a face mask and self-inflating bag may overcome the obstruction. Laryngoscopy will show motionless vocal cords lying slightly apart (*adducted*), revealing a very narrow v-shaped aperture. The patient will require re-intubation and a tracheostomy.

ASPIRATION OF FOREIGN BODIES

Foreign bodies inhaled into the trachea and lower airways may cause stridor, partial or complete collapse of one or both lungs, or aspiration pneumonitis.

The foreign body can be:
• vomit, gastric contents, blood, secretions;
• pharyngeal or laryngeal oedema;
• a piece of tooth, a forgotten throat pack, a fragment of adenoid tissue, the coroner's clot.
If there is any evidence of aspiration of a foreign body, then the patient should be re-anaesthetized and bronchoscoped to clear the airway. Every recovery room should have a bronchoscope ready for this eventuality.

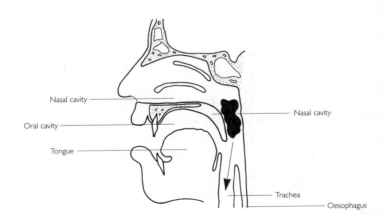

fig 17.5 The coroner's clot.

CORONER'S CLOT

Following bleeding into the upper airway large blood clots can hide in the nasal pharynx. Even if the pharynx is directly examined with a laryngoscope, these may be missed. On returning to the recovery room the coroner's clot can be come dislodged, and without warning aspirated into the trachea totally blocking the airway. Especially after surgery on the upper airway, and before the patient returns to the recovery room, the anaesthetist should gently use a dental sucker to explore the nasopharynx.

ASPIRATION PNEUMONITIS[8]

Aspiration of large amounts of acid gastric contents is a frightening complication of anaesthetia. Acute chemical aspiration pneumonitis can be fatal. Suspect aspiration if the patient has just vomited or regurgitated becomes wheezy, coughs vigorously, develops a tachycardia and becomes cyanosed. These initial symptoms usually improve with humidified oxygen and bronchodilators but several hours later the full syndrome will develop with tachopnoea, the use of accessory strap muscles to help him breath, severe hypoxia and respiratory failure.

The cyanosis of severe aspiration pneumonitis
is not relieved by oxygen therapy.

The incidence of a life threatening aspiration pneumonitis is reported to be between 1 in 1000 to 1 in 10 000 cases. Mortality is quoted to be between 3 and 70 per cent depending on the severity of the lung damage. The minimum amount of fluid aspirated to cause substantial damage to the lungs is thought to be about 0.4 ml/kg (about 25 ml in the average adult). The situation is much worse if the aspirated fluid is acid with a pH less than 2.5. Aspiration of particulate matter like partially digested fluid or blood causes more complications than aspiration of clear fluid.

It is not possible to accurately predict which patient is going to aspirate, but some of the identifiable risks are:
• emergency surgery;
• obesity;
• hiatus hernia;
• pregnancy;
• bowel obstructions;

- trauma surgery;
- a full stomach;
- and diabetes especially when there are automatic or other neuropathies;
- abnormal pharyngeal, laryngeal, or upper airway anatomy (especially in children);
- neuromuscular disease, such as multiple sclerosis or motor neurone disease;
- scleroderma.

Aspiration of acid gastric content in pregnancy or the pueperium causes a devastatingly destructive and often fatal pneumonitis called *Mendelson's syndrome.*

Nurse all patient in the recovery position until they are fully conscious, able to lift their heads, and cough and deep breath on command. Unconscious or obtunded patients, lying on their backs in recovery rooms, are candidates for aspiration pneumonitis. These cases of 'aspiration pneumonitis waiting to happen', are largely avoidable.

> *Patients who look to heaven,*
> *go to heaven.*

Aspiration sometimes occurs without anyone being aware of it before the patient reaches the recovery room. Even small amounts of fluid aspirated into the lower airway can cause postoperative chest infection. It is often assumed that this disaster is due to some lapse by the anaesthetist, but this is not necessarily so.

> *Any sedated patient is at risk of aspiration.*

PROPHYLAXIS AGAINST ASPIRATION

'At risk patients' can be protected by the use of H_2 receptor antagonists such as ranitidine but this must be given 2 - 3 hours before surgery. Ranitidine has a long action and its effect persists into the recovery room.

Preoperative sodium citrate raises the pH of gastric contents and reduces acidity. 30 mls of 0.3 molar sodium citrate given 20 minutes before the induction of anaesthesia is also useful and quicker acting.

INITIAL MANAGEMENT
- This is an emergency get help;
- roll the patient onto his side, and tilt him into a head down position so that fluid drains out the mouth instead of into the trachea;
- clear the airway with a wide bore sucker;
- give high flow oxygen;
- attach an ECG, pulse oximeter, and automated blood pressure machine, prepare to take blood gases and perform a chest X-ray to help with diagnosis.

FURTHER MANAGEMENT
1. Consider bronchoscopy, but do not perform general tracheo-bronchial lavage[9]. Initially it is better to use fibreoptic bronchoscopy to assess the situation, than a rigid bronchoscopy, because the jet injector used to oxygenate the patient during rigid bronchoscopy will force aspirated material deep into the lungs. It may be necessary to selectively unblock a major bronchus. Use 5 to 10 ml of saline followed immediately by suction. Repeat until the aspirate is clear. Take samples of bronchial aspirate for culture and antibiotic sensitivity.

2. Use bronchodilators such as inspired salbutamol. They will help counteract the bronchial oedema and improve oxygenation.

3. Corticosteroids prevent localization of the inevitable infection, and impair lung defence mechanisms. They are contraindicated.

4. Antibiotics are not recommended at this early stage, because they select out resistant bacteria. The patient will almost certainly get a mixed flora bacterial pneumonia, including anaerobes. If possible take specimens of tracheal aspirate for culture. Take blood cultures to reveal the major invasive pathogen. Most physicians delay the use of antibiotics until the patient develops a fever. Rational antibiotic therapy is best based on microbiological evidence. Aerobic gram-negative bacteria are an uncommon cause of aspiration pneumonia despite being frequently found on gram-stains of the sputum. Gram negative pneumonia is more common in alcoholics.

ANTIBIOTICS FOR ASPIRATION PNEUMONITIS

Use benzylpenicillin 1.2 gm IV 4 - 6 hourly plus metronidazole 500 mg IV twelve hourly for 48 hours, then use metronidazole 400 mg orally for 10 - 14 days. For those patients who are allergic to penicillin use clindamycin 600 mg intravenously 8 hourly, followed by clindamycin 300 to 450 mg orally for a total period of 14 days.

5. Transfer all these patients to the high dependency unit (HDU) for observation. If at all possible avoid ventilating the patients because it abolishes the vital ability to deep breathe and cough. If the patient has a PaO_2 less than 70 mmHg (9.2 kPa), transfer the patient to ICU, this patient will need ventilating.

6. A chest X-ray immediately after aspiration will not reveal the extent of the damage, because it takes some hours for radiological signs to develop. The right, middle and lower lobes are most commonly affected. It is, however, very useful to distinguish between aspiration and other disasters such as pulmonary oedema or pneumothorax where you will see changes almost immediately.

PNEUMOTHORAX

When air, which is normally confined to the lung, escapes into the pleural space and is trapped there it causes a *pneumothorax*. Pneumothorax is usually accompanied by pleuritic pain that is so sharp and severe that the patient dare only to breathe in short shallow pants, and stops abruptly with a grunt when he feels pain. Other signs include an unexplained tachycardia, hypotension, wheeze, short sharp inspiratory movements, cyanosis and sometimes *surgical emphysema*.

SURGICAL EMPHYSEMA

Surgical emphysema occurs when air or gas escapes into the tissues. There is a peculiar crackling feeling to the skin and subcutaneous tissues. The most likely cause is a breach in the pleura and a hole in the lung during operations on the neck, rib resection, kidney operations, trauma to the rib cage; and following external cardiac massage where ribs are fractured. It also occurs with distension and rupture of alveoli if the expiratory limb of the anaesthetic circuit or ventilator becomes obstructed. The gas tracks along the sheaths of the blood vessels to the hilum of the lung, from where it spreads to the neck and chest wall. Sometimes the crackling crepitations can be felt in the suprasternal notch. This is diagnostic of air in the mediastinum and may follow a ruptured bronchi, or mid-line trauma such as a stab wound.

A pneumothorax may occur:
- during the insertion of intercostal, cervical, or supraclavicular brachial plexus blocks;
- during the insertion of a central venous line or pulmonary venous catheter;

- in patients with bullae in the lung (congenital or acquired with emphysema); Marfan's syndrome, chest trauma or rib fracture, and barotrauma;
- after thoracic surgery if the tubing on a chest drain becomes kinked or occluded in some way. If the drain tube stops bubbling exclude this cause first;
- following nephrectomy, where the pleura has been accidentally breached or a rib resected for easier surgical access;
- as a complication of laparoscopic surgery.

If the escaped air or gas collects under pressure it causes a tension *pneumothorax*. The collection of air progressively grows in size to squash the lungs, heart and major blood vessels. Blood vessels get kinked and the cardiac output falls. In the recovery room the patient may suddenly panic, collapse, blue in the face, struggling to breathe, with almost undetectable pulses. Sometimes the neck veins will be grossly distended. The displaced heart and lungs push the trachea to the opposite side. No breath sounds can be heard on the affected side, and if you percuss the chest the note will be booming (similar to what you hear if you percuss a pillow). Listening with the stethescope at the same time as the percussion improves the your ability to diagnose a pneumothorax.

In neonates sometimes simply holding a bright light behind the chest will sometimes reveal the pneumothorax.

A tension pneumothorax is a medical emergency.

INITIAL MANAGEMENT
- Call for help;
- sit patient up;
- give high concentrations of oxygen;
- attach pulse oximeter and ECG.

FURTHER MANAGEMENT
If the patient has collapsed with a suspected pneumothorax, and you are unsure what side is affected, then aspirate each side with 23 G needle through the second intercostal space in the mid-clavicular line on either side. If you freely aspirate air on one side then you will need to insert an intercostal catheter on that side. While preparing to insert the catheter push a 14 G cannula through the same spot you found free air when you aspirated. This will relieve the pneumothorax immediately. For the emergency insertion of a pleural drain see page 96.

EMBOLISM

Various substances can pass in the blood stream and lodge into the lungs obstructing blood flow and causing an inflammatory response. The most common are air, blood clots, fat, and amniotic fluid. It is a useful rule to regard any patient in recovery room who becomes abruptly breathless to have had either a pulmonary embolis or a pneumothorax.

Air embolism

Air embolism can cause sudden collapse. It usually occurs during the insertion, or with the accidental disconnection, of a central venous line. It is thought that between 20 - 50 mls of air entering a vein is sufficient to cause a cardiac arrest. With a 5 cm H_2O negative pressure gradient 100 mls of air can be sucked through a 14 G needle in one second! Despite these alarming facts most episodes of air embolism are minor, and over almost as soon as they are diagnosed.

> *Suspect air embolism if a patient collapses*
> *while a central venous line is being handled.*

If a sufficient bolus of gas enters the right ventricle it makes the blood froth. This churning mass of bubbles blocks the flow of blood to the lungs. The patient, unable to achieve a cardiac output, rapidly becomes hypoxic and hypotensive.

Reports of gas embolism are becoming more frequent, because of the increasing use of carbon dioxide to inflate the abdomen during laparoscopic procedures. Carbon dioxide was chosen as the inflating gas because it is less likely to cause stable emboli than other gases.

In 11 per cent of Caesarean sections detectable air embolism occurs during the operation[11]. If the patient is under epidural or spinal anaesthesia they may become breathless, fearful, hypotensive and show arterial oxygen desaturation. These effects may continue into the recovery room.

Other procedures associated with air embolism include: laminectomy, head and neck surgery, total hip replacement, hysterectomy, and epidural catheterization. The common factor in all these procedures is that it is possible for the patient's right atrium to be lower than the operative site favouring air entering the venous system.

Signs of less severe air embolism include: brassy dry cough, wheeze, chest pain, and dyspnoea.

Signs of potentially fatal air embolism include: collapse, cyanosis, hypoxaemia, hypotension, feeble pulse, tachycardia, engorged neck veins, cardiac arrest. If you listen over the posterior chest you may hear the characteristic *mill-wheel murmur*. It sounds like water squelching around inside a rubber gum (Wellington) boot.

Occasionally bubbles of gas will pass through a patent foramen ovale, or through a ventricular septal defect to enter the left ventricle and embolize to some other vascular bed. If the gas enters the cerebral circulation the patient will have a stroke.

IMMEDIATE MANAGEMENT
Stop further air entering the circulation; if necessary put your finger over the hole where the air is getting in. Call for help. Give high concentrations of oxygen. Tip the patient head down and turn him on to his left side so that the froth in the right ventricle is carried away from the entry into the pulmonary artery (*Durrant's manoeuvre*). If you can not feel a carotid pulse then treat as a cardiac arrest, and begin external cardiac massage this may help break up the froth.

FURTHER MANAGEMENT
If the patient has a central line, then try to suck up the froth. This is not usually a fruitful manoeuvre and only worth trying in the first few moments after the incident. If the patient is moribund the surgeon may attempt to aspirate the air from the right ventricle using a large bore needle.

ONGOING MANAGEMENT
The patient should stay on high flow oxygen for at least 6 hours to help wash out the nitrogen from his blood. Where available, consider hyperbaric oxygen therapy as an option.

Pulmonary embolism

Pulmonary embolism (PE) occurs when venous thrombi break off, pass to, and obstruct the arteries of the lungs. During surgery fibrin blood clots (deep vein thrombosis) can form in large veins, mostly in the calf veins and these do not generally embolise. When the clots form in the ileofemoral or pelvic veins pulmonary embolism is far more likely. Pulmonary embolism occurs uncommonly in the recovery room. It usually presents in the ward a few days later.

Pulmonary embolism causes a series of events ranging from cough, pleuritic or other chest pain, wheeze, dyspnoea, haemoptysis, to catastrophic circulatory collapse.

IMMEDIATE MANAGEMENT
Call for help, lay patient flat, give high concentrations of oxygen, attach pulse oximeter, ECG monitor and automated blood pressure machine. Establish intravenous access.

FURTHER TREATMENT
Heparin is the mainstay of treatment, and should be started immediately. Normally the thrombolytic agent streptokinase is used to dissolve the clots, but this is no use after scalpel surgery because the patient will bleed. In the operating suite with life threatening pulmonary embolism open pulmonary embolectomy under cardiopulmonary bypass is an option.

Fat embolism

Orthopaedic, and trauma cases are at risk from fat emboli. (Sometimes called *fat emboli syndrome*, or FES.) It occurs in up to 10 per cent of bone trauma, and in the past has been a major cause of death. It is thought that fat from the bone marrow is released into the circulation. In the blood stream enzymes change some of it to free fatty acids. These are toxic to alveolar cells in the lungs, resulting in pulmonary oedema and disturbance in oxygen diffusion into the body. The fat may also trigger disseminated *intravascular coagulation* (DIC). The syndrome usually occurs 12 - 72 hours after injury; but more acutely, may present in the recovery room, especially in cases of trauma admitted the day before.

Signs of fat emboli seen in the recovery room may include:
- a respiratory rate increasing to more than 20 breaths per minute, with a developing respiratory alkalosis;
- fine moist sounds especially in lung's bases;
- hypoxia;
- headaches;
- disorientation, confusion, and deteriorating conscious state;
- possibly fitting;
- fever;
- scattered petechiae, seen on the chest wall;
- retinal petechiae.

Prevention of fat emboli includes early immobilization, and stabilization of fractures. Treatment may require ventilation for a few days in intensive care unit.

Amniotic fluid embolism

Amniotic fluid embolism usually occurs after a difficult delivery, and causes severe hypoxaemia. This is followed by disseminated intravascular coagulation with bleeding. The mortality rate is high.

HYPOXIA, HYPOXAEMIA AND HYPOVENTILATION

Hypoventilation and hypoxia are separate but inter-related problems.

SIGNS OF HYPOVENTILATION	SIGNS OF HYPOXIA
• High $PaCO_2$; • drowsiness; • coma; • bounding pulse; • vasodilation.	• Low PaO_2; • confusion; • restlessness; • agitation and aggression; • deterioration of mental state; • hypertension and tachyardia; • coma; • pallor and cyanosis; • bradycardia and hyotension.
TREAT BY IMPROVING BREATHING	TREAT WITH OXYGEN
A restless person is a hypoxic person until proven otherwise	

HYPOXIA

There are many causes for this, and only one of them is hypoventilation. Hypoxia occurs when there is not enough oxygen to supply the metabolic needs of the tissues. Initially hypoxic tissue switches to anaerobic metabolism causing lactic acid to be released from the cells (metabolic acidosis)

The treatment for hypoxia is oxygen, oxygen and oxygen.

Causes include airway obstruction and increased tissue demands, such as shivering. Loss of lung function, for all the reasons outlined above, plus others relating to the surgery and the patient's obesity can all contribute, singly or together, to some degree of hypoxia.

Over half of all patients, and most of the elderly patients have a reduced blood oxygen saturation when they arrive in recovery room. All patients should receive supplemental oxygen for the first ten minutes after arrival. *Diffusion hypoxia* is a very common problem. It occurs as nitrous oxide washes back from the circulation into the lungs and displaces the inspired air containing oxygen. Severe hypoxia can occur, but the patient need not necessarily become cyanosed.

Elderly patients require oxygen for days
rather than hours after major surgery.

INADEQUATE BREATHING ("HYPOVENTILATION")

If a patient is not breathing deeply enough or has a respiratory rate of less than eight breaths per minute, then give oxygen while you think logically about the problem.

IS SOMETHING DEPRESSING THE RESPIRATORY CENTRE?

All opioids depress respiratory rate and depth, even short acting ones like fentanyl, and especially in babies or elderly patients. Look for the side effects of the opioids, small pupils, drowsines, pallor. Patients affected by excessive opioids will take a deep breath and cough adequately when you ask them to, but then simply resume their shallow, slow breathing.

ARE THE RESPIRATORY MUSCLES WEAK?

This is usually due to residual paralysis from the muscle relaxant drugs. This weakness is sometimes called *post operative residual curarization* (PORC). Patients with PORC move like a jerky, floppy rag doll. Test the patient's muscle strength. He should be able to lift his head from the pillow and maintain this for at least five seconds. Test his grip by putting two (but no more) of your fingers in his hand, and ask him to squeeze as tightly as he can. Patients with PORC can only cough weakly.

Do not use a nerve stimulator
on an awake patient, because it hurts!

If the patient has PORC then gently ventilate him with a bag and mask. Repeated doses of neostigmine and atropine usually make the situation worse. Never attempt to stimulate breathing with other drugs such as tacrine or doxepram in patients with PORC. Occasionally you will need to sedate the patient, re-intubate him and then ventilate him until the muscle relaxant has worn off.

All muscle relaxant drugs wear off, eventually.

Causes of hypoxia include:
- diffusion hypoxia;
- hypoventilation - inadquate breathing;
- airway obstruction;
- shivering which increases oxygen requirements seven fold;
- collapse of many small sections of the lung during long general anaesthetics;
- obesity which reduces the lung's oxygen stores in their functional residual capacity.

The treatment for hypoxia
is oxygen, oxygen and oxygen.

RESPIRATORY FAILURE

By definition respiratory failure occurs if either the PaO_2 falls below 60 mmHg (7.9 kPa) *hypoxaemia,* or the $PaCO_2$ exceeds 50 mmHg (6.6 kPa) *hypoventilation.* That is, if either hypoxia and hypoxaemia, advance to a point where the oxygen in the blood is so low, below 60 mm Hg, or hypoventilation becomes so profound that carbon dioxide in the blood rises above 50 mm Hg.

Respiratory failure is made up one or both components: Hypoxaemia is treated with oxygen, and hypoventilation is treated by improving ventilation. Hypoventilation may require assistance with intermittent positive pressure ventilation.

1. Cottam S, Eason J, (1991). *Anaesthesia Review,* 8 (ed by Kaufman L) p 71.
2. Hartley M. Vaughan RS, (1993). *British Journal of Anaesthesia,* 71:561-8.
3. Barin ES, Stevenson IF, et al. (1986). *Anaesthesia and Intensive Care,* 14:54-7.
4. Bareka M, (1978). *Anesthesia and Analgesia,* 57:506-7.
5. Gefke K, Andersen LW, et al. (1983). *ACTA Anaesthesiology Scandinavica,* 27:111-12.
6. Burgess GE, Cooper JR, et al. (1979). *Anaesthesia,* 51:73-7.
7. Child CS. (1987). *Anaesthesia,* 42:322.
8. Engelhardt T, Webster NR, (1999). *British Journal of Anaesthesia,* 83 (3) 453-60.
9. Bannister WK, Sattilaro et al. (1961) *Anesthesiology,* 22:440-3.
10. Karuparthy VR, Downing JW, et al. (1989). *Anesthesia and Analgesia,* 69:620-3.

18. THE BLEEDING PATIENT

The recognition of HIV and other diseases transmitted by blood transfusion have altered the way we use blood during, and after surgery. Anaesthetists are more reluctant to give blood during operations, and patients are more afraid to receive it. Advances in understanding the physiology of tissue oxygenation have made it possible to reduce the amount of blood transfused. Keep the risks in perspective. Transfusion is a life saving therapy, and when properly screened, is safe. When blood is needed to save a life, do not withhold it because of unrealistic fears of transfusion transmitted disease.

*The blood pressure
does not necessarily fall early
in haemorrhagic shock.*

Signs that blood transfusion may be needed are:
• continuing bleeding;
• persistent tachycardia;
• cold extremities;
• postural hypotension, where the blood pressure falls when you sit the patient up;
• angina;
• dyspnoea;
• decreasing urine output;
• deterioration in conscious state, associated with confusion or anxiety;

Patients who will not tolerate a low haemoglobin include those with:
• coronary artery disease;
• myocardial ischaemia;
• congestive heart failure;
• haemodynamically significant valvular heart disease, such as aortic stenosis;
• a history of transient ischaemic attacks, or suspected cerebral ischaemia;
• a history of previous thrombotic stroke.

PHYSIOLOGY OF BLOOD LOSS[1]

To understand the rationale for blood transfusion, you must understand the physiology of oxygen transport and its use by the tissues (see page 296).

Most young fit adults can withstand a haemoglobin of 60 - 70 gm/l, providing they have no lung, or heart disease, and their vascular volume is normal. Elderly people respond to a low haemoglobin in a more inconsistent way, depending on their ability to increase their cardiac output, the health of their lungs and whether they have diseases which impede tissue blood flow. During anaesthesia, where the patient can be ventilated with high concentrations of oxygen, and the blood gases and physiological parameters can be monitored minute by minute, it is possible for the anaesthetist to precisely manipulate oxygen delivery to the patient's tissues. In recovery room, where the patient's metabolic requirements are high, the monitoring is not as intense and oxygen therapy less controllable, an equivalent haemoglobin level may not be sufficient to meet the oxygen requirement of tissues.

Neonates and infants are at risk after losing only 10 per cent of their blood volume (25 ml in a 2.5 kg baby). A haemorrhaging infant can neither increase his cardiac output, nor adequately vasoconstrict his circulation to maintain his blood pressure and tissue perfusion. On the other hand, healthy young adults can tolerate up to a 30 per cent loss of blood volume (about 1500 mls) before haemorrhage becomes life threatening. In younger patients the blood pressure may actually rise in early haemorrhagic shock, because of a brisk neurohumoral response to the stress. Elderly patients drop their blood pressure earlier than younger patients, and have a lower pulse rate.

An adult responds to haemorrhage in two stages.

1. Arterial stretch receptors (baroreceptors) in the carotid sinus and aortic arch detect a fall in arterial pulse pressure, and send messages to the hypothalamus and cardiovascular centres in the brainstem which, in turn, stimulate the secretion of adrenaline from the adrenal medulla, and noradrenaline from sympathetic nerve endings. These catecholamines cause vasoconstriction in the arterioles, especially in the gut, kidney, muscle and skin. They also cause the heart's rate and force of contraction to increase. The heart attempts to push blood against the constricted arterioles and the blood pressure rises, or is maintained, ensuring blood flow through the vital structures of the coronary arteries and the cerebral circulation.

2. When about 35 per cent of the blood volume is lost (about 1600 ml in an adult), the reflex sympathetic drive switches off. The blood pressure drops rapidly, the cardiac output falls, and blood bypasses oxygenated areas in the lungs. The supply of oxygen to the tissues starts to fail. Ischaemic gut and pancreas release shock factors (cytokines and leukotrienes) into the circulation, and these depress the heart, and damage capillaries. The results are a progressive circulatory collapse, with profound tissue hypoxia, leading to ischaemia, and then death.

CLINICAL SIGNS IN A 70 kg YOUNG ADULT MALE				
Severity of shock	Mild	Moderate	Severe	Critical
American College of Surgeons' Class[3]	Class 1	Class 2	Class 3	Class 4
Blood loss (ml)	< 750	750 – 1500	1500 – 2000	> 2000
Pulse rate	80–110	> 110	> 120	> 140
Blood pressure	Normal	Normal	Decreased	Decreased
Pulse pressure	Normal	Decreased	Decreased	Decreased
Respiratory rate	12 – 20	20 – 30	30 – 40	> 40 (gasping)
CVP (cm H$_2$O)	2 to 5	-2 to +2	-2 to -5	< -5
Urine output ml/hr	> 30	15 – 30	5 – 15	minimal
Perfusion	cool hands	pale hands	cold hands	sweating
Psychological status	anxious	agitated	confused	lethargic/coma

Causes of on-going bleeding

In order of frequency, these are:

- hypothermia;
- inadequate surgical haemostasis;
- drug therapy such as warfarin, heparin or aspirin;
- platelet deficiencies;
- venous congestion particularly in head and neck operations;
- plasma clotting factors deficiency;
- dilutional coagulopathy;
- disseminated intravascular coagulation;
- citrate toxicity;
- hypofibrinogenaemia;
- fibrinolysis;
- blood transfusion reactions;
- lupus anticoagulant.

HYPOTHERMIA (see also page 145)

Temperatures of 36°C or less inhibit the enzymes in the clotting cascade which form the platelet plug and finally the thrombin clot.

Hypothermia also:

- slows the production of clotting factors in the liver;
- inhibits platelet function;
- retards platelet release from bone marrow, and the count falls;

- slows the circulation leading to intravascular clot formation;
- increases fibrinolytic activity.

In the recovery room hypothermia
is the main reason patient's blood will not clot.

INADEQUATE SURGICAL HAEMOSTASIS

Bleeding from the surgical incisions may occur as the patient's blood pressure rises in the recovery room. Watch wounds and especially drain bottles. If they drain blood more than 100 ml in 30 minutes inform the surgeon. If the bleeding is coming from a wound, apply direct pressure on the bleeding site. Put on a pair of gloves, pad the site and press firmly. Pressure dressings are not effective, and cause venous congestion aggravating the problem. Limbs can be temporarily isolated by applying a blood pressure cuff and inflating it above systolic pressure.

DRUGS

HEPARIN: Some patients are given heparin in theatre, especially during vascular surgery. It normally has a clinical life of about 50 minutes, but this is prolonged after blood loss or hypothermia. Check whether the heparin has been reversed with protamine before the patient came to the recovery room. An additional dose of protamine is sometimes needed. Protamine 1 mg will reverse the effects of about 100 units of heparin. Give the protamine slowly intravenously, no faster than 5 mg per minute because it is a potent cause of hypotension, and pulmonary vasoconstriction. Excessive protamine can aggravate bleeding by depressing platelet function.

LOW MOLECULAR WEIGHT HEPARINS are used in patients who are likely to form deep vein thrombosis, or throw off clots from a heart valve. The two most common are enoxaparin (Clexane®) and daltaparin (Fragmin®) The normal preoperative dose of enoxaparin for high risk patients is 40 mg, but doses as high as 1.5 mg/kg are used to achieve an anticoagulated patient.

WARFARIN: Some patients are taking warfarin for the long term treatment of deep vein thrombosis, atrial fibrillation, or because they have a prosthetic heart valve. Warfarin interferes with the ability of vitamin K to activate factors II, VII, IX, and X of the clotting pathway (see fig. 18.3). Warfarin is usually stopped 3 clear days or more before surgery, and the INR is checked on the day of surgery to make sure it is within acceptable limits. It is rarely necessary to reverse the residual effects of warfarin with fresh frozen plasma.

Do not use vitamin K, or its analogues to reverse the effects of warfarin, because it takes 4 - 8 hours to work and makes it difficult to restabilize the patient on their oral anticoagulant regime after surgery.

PLATELET DEFICIENCY

All non-steroidal anti-inflammatory drugs (NSAIDs) inhibit clotting, and patients who have taken them preoperatively are more likely to bleed in the recovery room. Aspirin in particular, has an antiplatelet effect which lasts for up to 10 days after the patient's last dose. The effect of these drugs, which interfere with prostaglandin synthesis, in causing postoperative haemorrhage, is probably not as great as previously thought; although many surgeons are uncomfortable with these drugs. It is significant in operations where bleeding could be a problem, such as neurosurgery, eye surgery, inner ear surgery, some facio-maxillary surgery and delicate plastic surgery. The bleeding tendency can only be reversed by a platelet transfusion.

CLOTTING FACTOR DEFICIENCY

After about a week in storage blood is deficient in platelets, factors V and VIII. Fresh frozen factor contains factor V (labile factor), and factor VIII (antihaemophilic globulin).

CLOTTING FACTORS			
Factor	Name	Half-life	Stability
I	fibrinogen	4 days	stable
II	prothrombin	2 - 5 days	stable
III	thromboplastin		
IV	calcium		
V	proaccelerin	12 hours	7 days
VII	proconvertin	5 hours	stable
VIII	antihaemophilic	17 hours	7 days
IX	Christmas	40 hours	stable
X	Stuart-Prower	40 hours	7 days
XI	plasma thromboplastin antecedent		
XII	Hageman		stable
XIII	fibrin stabilizing	12 days	stable

VENOUS CONGESTION

Venous congestion will cause bleeding. The most common causes are tight bandages or plasters. Typically the blood is dark, and the skin is purple. Notify the surgeon.

DILUTIONAL COAGULOPATHY

Most bleeding in massive blood transfusion is due to hypothermia or platelet deficiency. Occasionally dilutional coagulopathy occurs after replacing more than twice the blood volume. If the patient is warm they can make clotting factors swiftly. If bleeding becomes a problem, treat it initially as a platelet deficiency, coagulation factor depletion occurs later.

Giving platelets or fresh frozen plasma in anticipation of bleeding is not useful during massive blood transfusion. The older notion of giving these components after 6 (or 8 or 10) units of blood should be abandoned. Wait for the onset of clinical coagulopathy, oozing from the operation site and around intravenous cannulas before giving the appropriate components. The coagulation system shows great tolerance to a low platelet count, and clotting factor depletion.

DISSEMINATED INTRAVASCULAR COAGULATION (DIC)

DIC is a hypercoaguable state where fibrin plaques out along vessel walls. So many of the clotting factors and proteins are consumed in the process, that if bleeding occurs there are not enough to form a clot. The mortality exceeds 50 per cent. It is caused by many things including:

- head injury;
- multiple trauma;
- severe sepsis;
- massive tissue damage;
- incompatible blood transfusion;
- any severe illness;
- a dead foetus.

The signs are the same as for a coagulation defect and include:
- uncontrollable bleeding from wound edges;
- excessive blood draining from the operating site;
- oozing occurs from old venipuncture sites and drip sites;
- blood stained urine;
- bleeding mucosal surfaces;
- a sudden fall in urine output.

Prevention includes early stabilization of fractures and debridement of wounds, early adequate resuscitation, and early use of antibiotics to control infection.

Laboratory confirmation of the clinical diagnosis of DIC includes:
• falling platelet count;
• elevated fibrin degradation products;
• falling fibrinogen;
• prolonged prothrombin ratio;
• prolonged partial thromboplastin time;
• a blood film that shows microangiopathic haemoglobinaemia.

Management of disseminated intravascular coagulation:
• replace blood loss;
• replace clotting factors with platelets and fresh frozen plasma;
• seek expert help.

CITRATE TOXICITY

Citrate toxicity is rare. Citrate phosphate dextrose (CPD) is the anticoagulant in packs of stored blood. It is readily metabolized by the liver, however if the patient is hypothermic, or receiving more than a litre of blood every ten minutes, then blood levels of citrate rise. Citrate toxicity may cause hypocalcaemia with hypotension and continued bleeding despite an adequate blood volume. Awake patients may complain of tingling around the mouth and muscle twitches. The ECG may show a prolonged QT interval, and cardiac arrhythmias. Treat hypocalcaemia with 10 ml of calcium gluconate 10% and then a further 2 ml with each successive 500 ml unit of blood. Each mole of citrate is eventually metabolised in the liver to three moles of bicarbonate, which explains the metabolic alkalosis seen a day or so after massive blood transfusion. Serum calcium levels will not help with the diagnosis because they do not distinguish between free calcium ion and bound calcium.

HYPOFIBRINOGENAEMIA

Hypofibrinogenaemia (fibrinogen less than 100 mg per cent) occurs as a complication of:
• haemorrhage;
• abortion;
• intrauterine foetal death;
• amniotic embolism;
• hydatiform mole.

Treat it with fresh frozen plasma, or more specifically 10 - 20 units of cryoprecipitate.

FIBRINOLYSIS

Fibrinolysis may complicate prostatectomy where the patient continues to bleed from the prostatic bed. Use tranexamic acid, which inhibits plasminogen activation, 0.5 - 3.0 gm slowly intravenously. Epsilon aminocaproic acid (EACA) is sometimes used as an alternative.

BLOOD TRANSFUSION REACTIONS (SEE PAGE 362)

LUPUS ANTICOAGULANT

Lupus anticoagulant is a cause of prolonged bleeding. It was first associated with systemic lupus erythematosis, but is mostly found in patients with other disorders.

Associated with:
• HIV/AIDS;
• chronic inflammatory disorders;
• infectious diseases;
• antibiotic or drug exposure;
• strokes;
• spontaneous abortions;
• lymphoproliferative disorders.

Presents with:
• a prolonged aPPT, and a normal INR;
• a tendency to clot, causing perioperative DVTs;
• with significant bleeding during or after surgery.

THERAPEUTIC PRINCIPLES FOR BLOOD TRANSFUSION[3]

1. Give blood to prevent tissue hypoxia. Do not use blood to expand plasma volume, or in the absence of anticipated tissue hypoxia. One unit of blood will raise the patient's haemoglobin by about 10 gm/l.

2. Restore blood volume as quickly as possible to preserve renal function and organ blood flow. If blood is not immediately available use polygeline (Haemaccel®), or normal albumin solutions. If these are not available use 0.9% saline or Hartmann's solution. Titrate volume until you see the jugular venous pressure (JVP) start to rise.

3. Avoid automatically giving a blood transfusion because the haemoglobin is less than 100 gm/l. Patients do very well maintained at 70 - 90 gm/l.

4. Increasing the haemoglobin does not, in itself, improve tissue healing. Wound healing requires an adequate tissue oxygen and nutrient supply. There are many factors involved including: cardiac output, haemoglobin concentration, tissue blood flow, blood viscosity, lack of tissue oedema and the pressure at which oxygen is presented to the tissues[4].

5. Patients receiving a transfusion should receive supplemental oxygen.

6. Use autologous blood where possible. Homologous blood increases the risk of infection, transfusion reactions, and immunosupresses the patient.[5] Most patients are reassured by receiving their own blood back.

7. Even one unit of blood may be enough to improve tissue oxygenation. Make a decision to give blood on a unit-by-unit basis.

8. During a transfusion the therapeutic goal is to keep blood pressure, and pulse rate within normal limits.

9. If at all possible use Rh negative blood for the 15 per cent of the population who are Rh negative. If you give Rh positive blood to an Rh negative woman in the child bearing years, give anti-Rh antiglobulin to prevent maternal antibodies damaging future babies. Rh negative blood can be given to Rh positive patients provided the ABO blood group is compatible; but Rh positive blood cannot be given to Rh negative people.

10. In an emergency uncross-matched, but appropriately grouped blood, may be given. The chance of a severe reaction is less than one per cent. Many operating suites keep a few units of low antibody titre group O negative blood for use in an emergency.

Management of the bleeding patient

MONITOR: Pulse rate, blood pressure, urine output, ECG, oximetery, core temperature, perfusion status and jugular venous pressure, conscious state and patient well being. Consider monitoring central venous pressure, direct arterial pressure.

ADMINISTER: high flow oxygen.

Low titre O negative blood can be used as a first resort while waiting for blood to be cross matched. During an emergency transfusion you can give up to 10 units (ie. 100 ml/kg) of low titre O negative packed cells and still return to the patient's blood group. However beyond this point you will need to continue with O negative blood. If you are using low titre O negative whole blood you can only return to the patient's own blood group if you have used two units or less. After this you should adopt the blood group of the donated blood.

PRACTICAL ASPECTS OF BLOOD TRANSFUSIONS

Taking blood for cross match

Send 8 ml of blood in a plain tube to the laboratory. If further blood is needed for cross-matching, do not to take the blood sample from a vein above the site where a drip is running, because the blood will be diluted with the contents of the drip, and furthermore the puncture wound will ooze.

Transfusing blood?
- watch for transfusion reactions.

Most problems with blood transfusion occur because of clerical errors. You must be scrupulous labelling blood samples and their accompanying cross matching slips. Take and process blood for cross-matching from one patient at a time. Be especially careful if there are two patients booked on the day's operating lists with the same surname.

Storing blood

Get the blood from the hospital blood bank as it is required. Blood is a living substance and must not be stored in an ordinary household refrigerator even for a short time. Frozen blood cells are dead. If thawed and then transfused into a patient the red dells will immediately haemolyse and the released haemoglobin will clog the kidneys causing renal failure. Blood should either be dripping into a patient or stored correctly in a dedicated blood fridge at 4°C. Do not leave packs of blood lying around at room temperature for more than a few minutes.

Checking blood

Human error is responsible for nearly all deaths due to incompatible blood transfusion. Every hospital has a routine procedure for checking blood before infusing it into a patient. Know your hospital's routine. To prevent errors, two trained staff at the bedside should independently check the patient's identification: hospital number, name and initials with those on the blood pack and the laboratory's cross-matching form. Be absolutely sure the patient's identification exactly matches the one on the blood pack, and the cross matching form.

Cross-matching

The blood bank *types* (or groups) donor and recipient blood in the *ABO and Rh (rhesus) systems*, and then screens for other antibodies to red cell antigens. During the cross-match procedure the patient's serum is mixed directly with donor's red cells to make sure that undetected antibodies in the serum don't haemolyse the red cells.

If further blood is needed for cross-matching, do not to take the blood sample from a vein above the site where a drip is running, because the blood will be diluted with the contents of the drip, and furthermore the puncture wound will ooze.

> *Blood for cross-matching?*
> *- send 8 ml of blood in a plain tube.*

Take and process blood for cross-matching from one patient at a time. Be especially careful if there are two patients booked on the day's operating lists with the same surname.

Cross-matching usually takes 20 – 60 minutes. It can take longer if the patient has been receiving dextran 70, or the antihypertensive drug methyldopa. Tell the laboratory about these drugs.

In an emergency you can give type-specific, but uncross-matched blood. The chance of a severe reaction, although still possible, is less than one per cent.

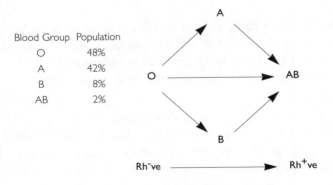

Blood Group	Population
O	48%
A	42%
B	8%
AB	2%

fig 18.1 Blood or platelet groups theoretically safe to give

Type O red cells lack both A and B antigens and consequently cannot be haemolysed by anti-A or anti-B antibodies in the recipient's plasma. Many operating theatres keep a few units of low plasma antibody titre type O negative blood. Use packed cells rather than whole blood. This is because type O plasma may contain anti-A or anti-B antibodies, which could cause haemolysis in an A, B, or AB patient. In desperate circumstances type O positive blood can be used in males, or post-menopausal females where Rh sensitization can never cause a threat to a foetus.

If more than two or three units of uncross-matched blood has been used without signs of an adverse reaction, then continue transfusing the same blood group rather than switching to properly cross-matched blood. This precaution is necessary because the already transfused uncross-matched blood may contain antibodies to any properly cross-matched blood.

Presentation of blood

Blood is supplied from the blood bank usually as 200 - 250 ml of packed cells in plastic containers called a *unit*. Packed cells are viscous and do not pass through filters easily. Units of whole blood, 400 - 450 ml, may be supplied under special circumstances.

Do not vent plastic blood containers. Be careful not to put your finger on the needle introducer of giving set in such a way that it carries your skin flora into the bag.

Do not mark any intravenous bags with marking pens because the ink may penetrate through the plastic and contaminate the solution.

Giving blood

It is preferable to give blood as quickly as possible because it starts to deteriorate as soon as it is removed from the refrigerator. A unit of blood should be given in less than 60 minutes if possible. Transfusion over 3 - 4 hours causes undue haemolysis and increases the risk of contamination.

Filtering blood

Blood is transfused through giving sets with standard 170 μm filters. Consider using a new giving set after four units of blood. Stored blood contains microaggregates, and the longer it has been stored the more there are. If you anticipate you are going to give more than 2 units of blood quickly then use a 20 - 40 μm microfilter which removes much of the cell debris in the bag of blood. Microaggregates contribute to the development of adult respiratory distress syndromes, non-haemolytic febrile reactions, and thrombocytopaenia.[6] Microfilters cause blood to flow more slowly. To overcome this re-expand packed cells before infusion with either human albumin solutions, or normal saline (but not calcium containing solutions such as Hartmann's solution). Use a Y-infusion set with blood on one arm and saline on the other. Run the saline into the blood bag and then transfuse the mixture through the filter.

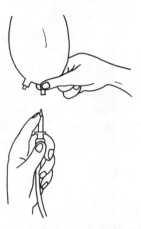

A common mistake when setting up a drip. Note the forefinger contaminating the sterile needle as it is being inserted into the bag of intravenous fluid.

fig 18.2 Introduction of skin flora into a bag of blood

Warming blood

If you anticipate giving more than more than 100 ml/min, or more than 2 units of blood in an hour use an *in-line blood warmer* to warm the blood to 37°C. Also, warm blood for the very young, the elderly and the infirm. If you give cold blood at 4°C, each unit will decrease the patient's core temperature by about 0.25°C. Cold blood is painful to infuse through peripheral veins. It may trigger red cells to clump impeding flow through the microcirculation. Do not transfuse cold blood rapidly through a central venous line, it is likely to cause arrhythmias and a fall in cardiac output. Never warm blood by heating the pack in warm or hot water because it can cook and haemolyse the blood cells and destroy the clotting factors. Never warm blood in a microwave oven!

In-line blood warmers are essential for massive blood transfusions. Warming blood from 48°C to 37°C decreases its viscosity 2.5 times, and dilates the patient's veins allowing the transfusion to run faster. Blood transfusions run slowly through standard blood warmers. To overcome this difficulty, there are two expensive systems available, the Level 1™ delivers 500 ml/min, and Rapid Infusion System™ 1500 ml/min.

Cannulas

Blood requires a large, preferably 14 gauge, intravenous needle to get an adequate flow rate. Maintain sterility when inserting a drip; wear sterile gloves, swab the site with poviodine (Betadine®) and allow it 90 seconds to work before breaching the skin. To get a rapidly running drip, use the shortest, widest bore cannula, and the highest drip stand.

For massive transfusions, following a large acute haemorrhage, wide bore catheters as large as 10 gauge are placed in central veins. If you cannot find a vein anywhere consider cannulating the femoral vein, which lies immediately medial to the femoral artery, using a Seldinger wire technique and an 8.5 F sheath.

Compatibility

Use 0.9% saline to prime the drip set. Do not prime lines with calcium containing solutions such as Hartmann's or Haemaccel®, because the calcium will neutralize the citrate anticoagulant forming blood clots. Fluids compatible with blood include: 0.9% saline, and blood products such as 5% normal serum albumin (NSA) and fresh frozen plasma (FFP). When the blood is finished put up a new drip set. Do not follow blood with 5% dextrose, polygeline, Hartmann's solution, parenteral nutrition fluids, or anything else. Do not add medication to units of blood because it may cause haemolysis, and it is difficult to tell whether any reaction is due to the blood or the drug.

> *Most blood transfusion disasters*
> *are due to human errors.*

Watch for transfusion reactions

These are discussed in more detail on page 362, but any one or more of the following may indicate this complication: tachycardia, fever, chills, wheeze, dyspnoea, anxiety, rashes, hypotension, cyanosis, mottled skin, blood in the urine, chest pain, headache, nausea.

Massive Blood Transfusion[7]

The normal blood volume is 70 - 80 ml/kg. The most generally accepted definition of massive blood transfusion is replacement of the patient's blood volume within a 24 hour period. This is not a helpful definition. In practice a massive transfusion causes problems if you are giving more than 5 units of blood per hour.

Management

MONITOR: Pulse rate, blood pressure, urine output, ECG, oximetery, core temperature, perfusion status and jugular venous pressure, conscious state and patient well being. Consider monitoring central venous pressure, direct arterial pressure. Laboratory: Clotting studies including haemoglobin; platelet count; partial thromboplastin time (aPPT); prothrombin time (INR). Also blood gases, electrolytes especially potassium, bicarbonate and anion gap.

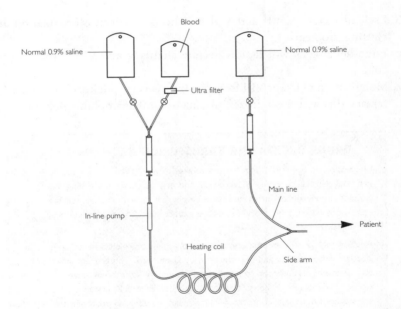

fig 18.3 Set up for massive blood transfusion

ADMINISTER: high flow oxygen. After six units of blood have been given notify the haematologist-on-call. If you are giving five units, or more, of blood an hour, coagulopathy becomes a problem.

Useful facts are:

1. Hypothermia is the most important cause of bleeding. In the laboratory aPPT and INR are measured at 37°C. So if your patient is cold these reassuring results will be misleading. Hypothermia enhances thrombolysis and inhibits platelet function.
2. Blood clotting factors are lost in an exponential manner. This means that if you exactly replace the patient's blood volume as it is lost, then 63 per cent of the patient's blood will be transfused blood, and 37 per cent the patient's own blood.
3. Clotting disturbances do not become a problem until clotting factors are reduced by at least 50 per cent.
4. Lack of functioning platelets is the first thing to cause problems.

Keep your patients warm, use platelets first,
and then, only if necessary, use fresh frozen plasma.

5. Lack of factors V, VII and VIII are the first to cause coagulation and clotting problems.
6. Endothelial cells will rapidly secrete factors V and VIII if they are not cold.
7. Mobilization of factor VIII from the liver is very quick and so no need to replace this with fresh frozen plasma or antihaemophilic globulin.

DRUGS DECREASING TRANSFUSION REQUIREMENTS

Desmopressin (DDAVP®) induces the release of von Willebrand's factor and pro-coagulant components of factor VIII and may be useful in bleeding due to platelet abnormalities occurring with uraemia. It is sometimes used during operations where large blood losses are expected such as the insertion of Harrington's rods.

Antifibrinolytics. Tranexamic acid and epsilon-aminocaproic acid (Amicar®) stabilize existing clots, and prevent primary fibrinolysis. These drugs inhibit the conversion of plasminogen to plasmin, so preventing fibrin breakdown. Aprotinin (Trasylol®) inhibits fibrinolysis, and also inhibits kallikrein-induced activation of the coagulation cascade. It appears to diminish postoperative blood loss. Antifibrinolytics occasionally promote pathological thrombosis.

Techniques of last resort

In cases of uncontrollable haemorrhage consider using fresh whole blood, and drugs that may reduce transfusion requirements such as aprotonin and desmopressin. *Nearly fresh whole blood*, less than 7 days old, is remarkably effective in all forms of coagulopathies and bleeding patients. We believe it is an under used resource.

Other problems arising during massive transfusion

STORAGE LESION

The term *storage lesion* is used to refer to all the changes that occur in a bag of stored blood in the refrigerator, and includes:

* loss of function of platelets and granulocytes;
* loss of lymphocytes;
* loss of some coagulation factors;
* for the first 12 - 18 hours there is a reluctance for haemoglobin to release oxygen in the tissues;
* haemolysis;
* formation of microaggregates;
* potassium ion leaves the red cell, and sodium ion enters;
* increasing acidity.

NON-CARDIOGENIC PULMONARY OEDEMA

Transfusion related acute lung injury occurs if there is an infusion of antibody to leucocytes inducing complement activation. Septicaemia is the most common cause. The patient becomes dyspnoeic after a small volume of blood has been received. It may be accompanied by fever, chills, cyanosis, and hypotension. A chest X-ray will reveal interstitial pulmonary oedema.

CIRCULATORY OVERLOAD

Pulmonary oedema from too rapid infusion will present with a wheeze, dyspnoea, coughing, cyanosis, tachycardia, added heart sounds and raised jugular venous pressure. Neonates, infants, and patients with heart disease are at greater risk.

RENAL FUNCTION

Urine output is a sensitive index of tissue perfusion. Insert a urinary catheter. An output of less 30 mls an hour is a sign of poor tissue perfusion. Support renal perfusion with low dose dopamine infusion 3 - 5 microgram/kg/min, give oxygen, maintain blood pressure and consider using frusemide.

HYPERKALAEMIA

The concentration of extracellular potassium in stored blood rises by about one mmol per day, so that by its expiry date blood may contain up to 30 mmol/l. This can cause cardiac arrythmias especially in children, or patients with renal failure, acidosis and hypothermia. The ECG will initially show signs of peaked T-waves, and finally broadening of the QRS complex, leading to asystole. In an emergency give 0.1 ml/kg calcium gluconate 10% slowly intravenously to counteract the effects on the heart.

METABOLIC ACIDOSIS

Haemorrhagic shock causes a low PaO_2, usually a compensatory low $PaCO_2$, and a metabolic (lactic) acidosis. Do not correct a metabolic acidosis unless the pH is less than 7.12 and or you suspect myocardial function is compromised. The acidosis will resolve in under an hour, providing tissue oxygenation is adequate, and the blood pressure and liver perfusion are restored. A moderate acidosis improves tissue oxygenation, so hesitate before using bicarbonate to correct it. If you do decide to use sodium bicarbonate use slow injections of small doses of intravenous bicarbonate 0.2 mmol/kg into a central vein, and monitor the response. Wait at least 5 minutes between increments.

Use bicarbonate with extreme caution.

INFECTION AND BLOOD TRANSFUSION

Immunosuppression

Although immunosuppression is not an immediate concern in the recovery room, it can become a problem to the patient later. It has long been known that kidneys transplanted from a donor survive longer if the patient has previously had a blood transfusion. It is probable that in cancer patient's blood transfusions are associated with a greater risk of tumour recurrence, than in non-transfused patients. Blood transfusion is associated with a very real risk of wound or chest bacterial infection following surgery. Transfusion poses a greater risk than other factors such as wound contamination, shock, or duration of surgery. Whole blood seems to suppress the immune response, more than packed cells; and fresh frozen plasma is the worst offender.[8]

Infected blood

Blood can be contaminated during collection from the donor. Some bacteria particularly pseudomonas species, will grow in a blood pack in the refrigerator. Examine every unit before infusing it. Contaminated blood is often a chocolate brown colour with bubbles in it, and the pack may be distended with gas. Do not even think of opening the pack, return it to the laboratory or blood bank. Contaminated blood, if transfused, can kill a patient almost instantly, or cause high fever, shock, haemoglobinuria, intravascular coagulation, renal failure, abdominal cramps, and generalized muscle pain.

Since they are stored at room temperature, platelets are more likely to incubate bacteria than other blood products. Bacteria contaminated platelets have a similar effect to a transfusion of contaminated whole blood; they may cause massive cardiovascular collapse. After platelets have been given a rise in temperature during the next 6 hours is an infection until proved otherwise. Platelets are now the most likely cause of infection.

Blood transfusions and blood products can transmit many disease from the donor to the recipient these include:
- hepatitis B, C, and D;
- human retroviruses: HIV (AIDS), HLTV-1 and 2,
- cytomegalovirus;
- hepatitis A, and E, (oro-faecal hepatitis);
- herpes virus 6;
- influenza;
- malaria
- Epstein -Barr virus
- slow virus (eg Creutzfield Jakob Disease). These prions cannot be destroyed by any known means short of heating to red heat, and may very rarely be transmitted by transfusion.

HEPATITIS VIRUSES
Screening of donated blood eliminates most, but not all, post transfusion viral hepatitis. The risk varies from place to place but is thought to be between 1:3000 to 1:15 000 units. Hepatitis G has been recently discovered, and may be transmitted by blood. There is no practical means of screening blood for hepatitis G virus at this time.

HIV VIRUS
Although the risk of transmitting hepatitis is much greater than any other disease, it is the transmission of HIV which troubles potential recipients. Recent advances in detection and prevention of disease transmission have reduced the risks greatly in the past few years. A new test called the *nucleic acid test* (NAT) can detect virus before antibodies developed and should be available soon. The risk of acquiring HIV from repeat donors at the Victorian Red Cross Blood Bank has been estimated at 1.31 per 100 000 person years.[9]

CLOTTING STUDIES

Clotting studies enable you to work out the cause of bleeding and the adequacy of the clotting mechanisms. Order clotting studies in the bleeding patient after major surgery. If possible collect the blood from an established arterial line, take 5 ml of blood and discard it before collecting your sample. Be sure there is no heparin, or other contamination, in your sample. If taking venous blood, collect it with a fine needle, or you may not be able to stop the bleeding from the venipuncture site. Do not take blood samples from veins in which a drip is flowing.

USE THE RIGHT TUBE FOR CLOTTING STUDIES		
Test	Abbreviation	Laboratory tube
Cross match	X-match	8 ml in plain tube
Haemoglobin	Hb	5 ml in heparin tube
Platelets	Plat	5 ml in EDTA tube
Activated partial Prothrombin time	aPTT	5 ml in citrate tube
also called INR	PT INR	5 ml in citrated tube
Fibrin degradation products	FDP	5 ml in special FDP tube
Fibrin D-dimer	XDP	5 ml in EDTA tube

Blood clotting is a complex series of biochemical reactions involving clotting factors (see table on page 345), platelets, calcium ions and the microvasculature. Once triggered it progresses like the chain reaction that occurs when you knock over a row of dominoes. Prothrombin and coagulation factors VII, IX, and X are made in the liver with the help of vitamin K. The coagulation factors circulate in an inactive form in the blood ready to help form a clot.

When a blood vessels is breached, the circulating *platelets* (little plates) come into contact with exposed collagen, either in the vessel wall, or in nearby tissue. The platelets adhere to the exposed collagen. They then change to a burr-seed shape, and become sticky. Other platelets became tangled (or *aggregated*) with them. A long stringy plasma protein called *fibrinogen* also gets stuck to the platelets as it floats by. The aggregated platelets then release a number of factors (such as adenosine diphosphate, prostaglandins, and 5-HT) that are needed for the chain reaction known as the coagulation cascade. In the presence of calcium ions the coagulation factors then convert circulating prothrombin into thrombin. The thrombin causes the fibrinogen, already stuck to the platelets, to turn into a loose *fibrin* mesh. This fibrin mesh snares passing platelets, red cells, and white cells. Factor XIII then shrinks the mesh, to form a tight fibrin plug that blocks the hole in the blood vessel.

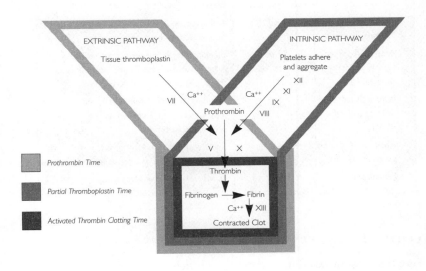

fig 18.4 Clotting diagram

Fortunately blood does not clot unless it needs to. Factors preventing this are:
• a good blood flow through vessels;
• rapid removal of activated clotting factors by the liver;
• a circulating enzyme called *plasmin* that dissolves clots.
This *fibrinolytic system* involves a precursor called plasminogen which is activated into plasmin in the vicinity of clots. Plasmin breaks down fibrin into fibrin split products, and prevents the fibrin mesh being formed.

FIBRINOLYSIS can be measured using fibrin D-dimer levels. Fibrinolysis is usually secondary to *disseminated intravascular coagulation* (DIC). Primary fibrinolysis; occurring after amniotic embolism, resection of carcinoma of the prostate, cardiopulmonary bypass, and with cirrhosis of the liver; is treated with tranexamic acid.

NORMAL VALUES IN HAEMATOLOGY

Blood volume	70 - 80 ml/kg	Established shock if < 50 ml/Kg
Haematocrit Hct men women	0.4 - 0.55 0.35 - 0.47	
Haemoglobin men women	130 - 170 gm/l 120 - 160 gm/l	Haemoglobin levels were formerly quoted in gms% now they are standardized to gms/l
Platelet count	150 - 400 x10⁹/l	Bleeding unlikely if > 60 000 x 10⁹/l
Whole blood coagulation time	3 - 12 min	Although seldom used it is a useful basic test for the recovery room.
Activated partial thromboplastin time (aPPT)	25 - 37 sec	Bleeding may occur if rises to > 45 secs. A preoperatively raised aPPT may indicate the presence of lupus anticoagulant.
International normalized ratio (INR)	1.0	Bleeding unlikely if INR < 1.5. INR was formerly known as the prothrombin time.
Fibrin degredation products (FDP)	< 40 microgram/l	Rises with DIC and massive trauma, especially if there are crush injuries.
Fibrinogen	1.6 - 5.0 gm/l	Low levels indicate a coagulopathy.

BLOOD TRANSFUSION REACTIONS[10]

Severe transfusion reactions are rare[11] and include:

1. Acute haemolytic reactions transfusion reactions occur in about 1:6500 transfusions;
2. Febrile non-haemolytic reactions occurs in about 1 - 3 per cent of transfusions;
3. Anaphylaxis and anaphylactoid reactions occur in about 1:20 000 transfusions.

1. Acute haemolytic transfusion reaction (HTR)

HTR is caused by red cell incompatibility. These occur in about 1:6500 transfusions. It is characterised by fever, chills, hypotension, nausea, headache, dyspnoea, chest pains, back pains, shock, and uncontrolled bleeding; sometimes leading to death. The diagnosis is made on clinical signs, but can be confirmed later by: a blood film showing signs of abnormal red cells and haemolysis; with accompanying haemoglobinaemia, and haemoglobinuria. If renal failure occurs, then the mortality is high.

MANAGEMENT:

MONITOR: Pulse rate, blood pressure, urine output, ECG, oximetery, core temperature, perfusion status and jugular venous pressure, conscious state and patient well being.

Initial management

1. Turn off the transfusion, but do not remove the intravenous cannula.
2. Give oxygen at 10 litres/min via face mask.
3. Change drip set and continue infusion with 0.9% saline.
4. Re-identify patient and blood pack.
5. Inform blood bank and return unused blood and pack.

Further management:

1. If there has been major fall in blood pressure, associated with dyspnoea, treat for anaphylaxis (see page 462).

2. Treat wheeze with nebulized salbutamol, and hypotension with a plasma expander. Take care as patients may be allergic to the plasma expanders too.

3. If haematuria occurs, or urine output falls below 0.5 ml/kg/min, give mannitol 1.5 gm/kg IV to promote a diuresis. Mannitol works within minutes and lasts for about 3 - 4 hours. Commence a dopamine infusion through a central line at 3 - 5 microgram/kg/min.

4. Be prepared to manage disseminated intravascular coagulopathy (see page 346).

2. Febrile non-haemolytic reactions (FNH)

Febrile non-haemolytic reactions are caused by sensitivity to donor granulocytes. They occur in about 5 - 7 per cent of transfusions, and are characterised by febrile, non-haemolytic reactions. Usually fever begins within 30 - 60 minutes of commencing the transfusion, but may occur at any time up to two hours after the transfusion has started. These reactions are seldom dangerous, and are treated by stopping the transfusion. Only one patient in eight who has an FNH reaction will have a similar reaction to the next blood transfusion. Consult a haematologist. Use leucocyte-poor blood if the patient has had two previous FNH reactions.

3. Urticarial reactions

Urticarial reactions are usually caused by antibodies to the donor plasma proteins. They occur in 1 - 3 per cent of transfusions. An urticarial reaction is characterized by local erythema, urticaria (hives) itching, but seldom fever. Treat it by stopping the transfusion. The urticaria will resolve in a few hours.

4. Anaphylaxis can be fatal

Anaphylaxis is rare, and the incidence is estimated to be about 1 in 20000 transfusions. Its usual cause is an antibody reaction to donor IgA. Suspect anaphylaxis if features occur after only a few millilitres of blood have been transfused. Coughing is usually the first sign, followed by acute wheezing, respiratory distress, hypotension, abdominal cramps, vomiting, diarrhoea, shock and collapse. (See page 462 for treatment).

BLOOD PRODUCTS

Blood issued by the Blood Bank is different from blood in the body. Unlike normal red cells, banked blood is deficient in 2,3 diphosphoglycerate (2,3 DPG). These banked red cells pick up oxygen readily, but in the absence of 2,3 DPG are bound strongly to the haemoglobin, and not released to the tissues. The banked red cells are rigid, and circulate in clumps like stacks of plates. They do not easily deform to flow through the microcirculation. It takes about 18 - 24 hours for the banked red cells to regain their normal function.

Whole blood

Whole blood contains red blood cells, and plasma components. It comes as a 450 ml pack of blood from one donor.

Indications are:
• acute blood loss following trauma, where the patient is volume depleted patient;
• ongoing haemorrhage in a patient with a coagulopathy.

Blood will keep for about 35 days in a special refrigerator held between 2 - 6°C. Clotting factors and immunocytes deteriorate more slowly than previously thought, but after 10 days of storage the clotting properties of whole blood are gone. Fresh whole blood which has been stored for less than 7 days, is most useful in the management of some coagulopathies especially during massive blood transfusion.

Packed cells

Units of packed cells contain 350 ml of red cell concentrate, but little plasma, and no clotting factors. Packed cells are useful where it is necessary to increase the oxygen carrying capacity of blood and there is a risk of fluid overload.

WHOLE BLOOD	**PACKED CELLS**
used for massive haemorrhage	used for correcting anaemia
easy to transfuse quickly	more difficult
450 mls of blood +	350 mls of red cell concentrate +
60 mls of CPD-AI anticoagulant	60 mls of CPD-AI anticoagulant
contains clotting factors	no useful clotting factor
large immune suppression	smaller immune suppression

Indications are:
- replacement of blood loss in a patient where ongoing bleeding is not a problem;
- correction of anaemia;
- in patients where red cells are needed, but volume is not, for instance cardiac failure, and renal failure.

Platelets

Platelets comes in packs of 70 - 100 ml at room temperature.

Indications are:
- first line management of continued bleeding after acute haemorrhage where the platelet count is less than 80 000/mm^3;
- patients with known thrombocytopaenia who haemorrhage after surgery (Platelets are ineffective in autoimmune thrombocytopaenia and haemolytic uraemic syndrome.)

Apart from hypothermia, platelet deficiency is the most probable cause of bleeding during a massive blood transfusion. Platelets can be deficient in numbers or in quality. The normal range of platelets is 150000 - 400000/mm^3. Bleeding time increases if the level is less than 100000/mm^3. Surgical bleeding may be hard to control if the level is below 40000 - 60000/mm^3. Life threatening spontaneous haemorrhage can occur if the level is below 20 000/mm^3. A platelet transfusion of 100 ml will raise the platelet count by about 10 000/mm^3. If platelet deficiency is the cause of bleeding give 6 units of platelets and reassess the situation.

Platelets are issued in O, A and B blood groups only. If Rh positive platelets are given to an Rh negative women, then give anti-D immunoglobulin. Platelets are damaged if they are sucked up into a syringe and injected through a fine needle. Do not filter platelets with a microfilter, they will all be removed. If you are keeping them for more than two hours before use they should be gently agitated on a special shaker. Store platelets at room temperature, and not in the refrigerator.

Indications for platelet transfusion does not rest solely on the platelet count. Drugs such as aspirin, NSAIDs, calcium channel blockers, ß-blockers and local anaesthetics inhibit platelet function. Peristaltic blood pumps, used during cardiac surgery damage the platelets. In these circumstances the platelet count may still be normal, but the platelets are not working. Consider platelet transfusion after neurosurgery, or operations on the eye or ear, because slight bleeding, or even ooze, can cause serious damage.

Use platelets before fresh frozen plasma in surgical induced bleeding. Bleeding is unlikely to occur until the platelet count has been diluted to less than 40 000/mm³ [12]. Because pooled platelet concentrates expose the patient to many donors, try to use single donor packs where available.

If platelet concentrates do not stop the bleeding,
then try fresh frozen plasma.

Fresh frozen plasma (FFP)

Fresh frozen plasma comes as packs of beige ice; 180 ml for adults and 60 ml packs for infants. FFP contains all the clotting factors, including Factor V, Factor VIII and fibrinogen; but its usefulness is limited by the need to give high volumes. Its major function is to replace Factor VIII. The liver rapidly synthesizes Factor VIII in response to injury but is reluctant to do so if the patient is hypothermic. Do not use FFP for volume expansion or to reconstitute packed red cells. Its routine use in massive blood transfusions is controversial. If you do need to use it aim to keep the INR between 1 - 1.4. Normally the body contains about the equivalent of 12 units of FFP, thus 12 units, or less, should full restore normal coagulation.

Indications for the use of fresh frozen plasma include :
• the patient is not hypothermic;
• the patient is bleeding and you are waiting on coagulation studies;
• if the INR is greater than 1.4;
• if the aPTT is grater than 44 seconds;
• active oozing or bleeding after at least a 20 per cent blood loss;

- correction of a coagulopathy in a bleeding patient;
- reversal of the effects of warfarin.
- if the patient has a damaged liver, or has disseminated intravascular coagulopathy.

When giving fresh frozen plasma administer the appropriate ABO blood group. It is stored at -18°C, and deteriorates at warmer temperatures, so it is often delivered packed in dry ice. Many hospital blood banks will thaw it for you. Otherwise place the pack of fresh frozen plasma in a watertight protective bag, and thaw it under running cold water. This takes about 20 minutes. Never thaw it in a microwave oven. Microwave or hot water will cook it, destroying its enzymes. Use it within six hours of thawing.

To reduce the infectivity of fresh frozen plasma use the same donor for all the units. FFP can be washed with a solvent detergent to make it safer.[13]

5% Normal serum albumin (NSA)

5% Normal serum albumin is similar to HPPD (Human Purified Protein Derivative) and PPF (Plasma Protein Fraction). Useful facts about this colloid are:
- store it at 5°C;
- it is stable for about 6 months at room temperature and many years at 4° C;
- the plasma half life is about 16 hours;
- it has been heated to 60°C for 10 hours and so it carries no risk of hepatitis or HIV;
- chills and fever occur in about 1:150 recipients.

It can be used to support blood pressure in a bleeding patient while waiting for blood to be cross matched. A recent meta analysis showed adverse outcomes when albumin was used for resuscitation following blood loss it was associated with a 4 per cent increase in mortality.[14] There is, however, insufficient evidence of harm to warrant withdrawal of albumin products from the market.[15]

BLOOD SUBSTITUTES AND PLASMA EXPANDERS

Colloid solutions are used to expand plasma volume in cases where blood is, either not available, or not needed. They do not contain any clotting factors.

Polygeline

The polygelines are suspensions of gelatin in saline ('Haemaccel®', 'Gelofusin®').

Useful facts are:
- it comes in 500 ml plastic bottle of clear solution of polymerized gelatin;
- it is a useful substitute for plasma proteins and much cheaper;
- it is cleared from the circulation in 8 - 12 hours, the half life is about 5 hours;
- allergic reactions occur in about 1 in 1500 patients;
- use it with care in atopic patients such as those with asthma;
- do not infuse polygeline with blood because the calcium ions will cause the blood to clot;
- it does not interfere with haemostasis or cross matching.

Esterified starches

Hetastarch ('Hespan®'), and pentastarch ('Pentaspan®') are esterified amylopectin solutions. Hetastarch causes allergic reactions in about 1 in 1200 patients and may damage the kidneys.[16] Pentastarch is better than hetastarch, because it does not interfere with clotting, is cleared from the plasma in half the time (12 hours), and is completely degraded by circulating amylase. Pentastarch has a higher colloid osmotic pressure, and produces an initial plasma volume expansion of 1.5 times the administered volume.

Synthetic blood

This is currently being developed and is possibly the way of the future:
- there is no risk of infection;
- no need for typing;
- good shelf life (one year);
- economical;
- no need for chemical modification;
- can be carried in dry form.

Disadvantages are:
- renal problems;
- the oxygen dissociation curves shifts to the left;
- potassium is easily lost due to the shape of the artificial haemoglobin;
- red eye syndrome (small blood vessel irritation).

VARIANT CREUTZFELDT-JACOB DISEASE (CJD)

Human prion disease is an accumulation in the brain of an abnormal, partially protease resistant, isoform of a host-encoded glyoprotein known as a prion protein. There are four main types of CJD identified, but only one has been shown to be transmitted in hospitals. There is a risk that the disease can be cross transmitted by surgical instruments, especially those used during neurosurgery or eye surgery (see page 108), because routine autoclaving or chemical sterilization do not inactivate the protein.

Up to now, individuals who have contracted prion disease are not those who have had excessive exposure, such as abbattoir workers, or those ingesting high titre diets. So far prion disease has been transmitted only to human beings who have a susceptible homozygous genotype.

There is concern that blood and blood products could incubate variant CJD and pose a risk to patients. Beta lymphocytes are required for the prions to invade nerves after peripheral inoculation. Tonsil biopsies will show prions and beta lymphocytes in the preclinical stage, but this test is impractical. At present there is no test sensitive enough to detect prions in the blood.

TERMINOLOGY

ABO groups are the major blood group in humans which is clinically important because of naturally occurring antibodies present in the patient's serum to ABO incompatible red cells These antibodies are high in titre, and capable of inducing intravascular haemolysis and acute haemolytic transfusion reactions

Agglutination is the clumping of particles that have antigens on their surface caused by antibody molecules that form bridges between the antigens on the red cell membrane.

Allergic transfusion reaction. A reaction clinically presenting with an itchy urticarial rash and wheeze caused by an immune reaction with soluble constituents of donor plasma

Alloantibodies are immunoglobulins produced in response to exposure to foreign antigens of the same species

Autologous blood refers to the patient's own blood. Blood is collected from the patient before surgery and given back later as an autologous blood transfusion

Cross match. This is, in effect, a mini-transfusion in a test-tube. In the lab the donors red cells are mixed with the patient's plasma and incubated for a time at body temperature to see if they are compatible.

Extravascular haemolysis. The phagocytosis and destruction of red cells by the reticuloendothelial system, commonly occurring in a delayed haemolytic transfusion reaction

Fibrinolytic system. The fibrinolytic system breaks down clots that form in the blood. It involves a series of enzymes including plasmin, protein C, and protein S.

Haematocrit (Hct) or packed cell volume (PCV) is determined by spinning a sample of blood in a centrifuge and measuring the volume the precipitated red cells as a ratio of the total volume of the blood cells.

Homologous blood refers to blood taken from a donor.

International Normalized Ratio (INR) is a test of the activity of the clotting factor prothrombin.

Intravascular haemolysis is where red cells burst open within the vessels of the circulatory system and release free haemoglobin into the circulation.

Jugular venous pressure (JVP). The internal jugular veins serve as useful clinical manometer of right atrial filling pressure. Examine them with the patient's head on a low pillow and the head rotated slightly. They are more easily seen if the light shines across instead of directly on the neck.

Massive blood transfusion occurs when the patient is given more than his total blood volume in any 24 hour period. In practice problems arise if you transfuse more than five units a blood per hour. It is, in effect, an organ transplant.

Rh factor is a blood group antigen, monkey, originally identified because the antibody agglutinated the red cells of all Rhesus monkeys and 85 per cent of blood donors. Rh incompatibility may cause haemolytic disease of the newborn and haemolytic transfusion reactions

Scavenged blood is collected from the patient as it is lost during surgery. It is filtered, washed and returned to the patient. It requires expensive equipment and is only practical in patients who are expected to lose more than 1500 ml during the operation. Some Jehovah's witnesses will accept scavenged blood, but others will not.

1. Van Leeuwin AF, Evans RG, *et al.* (1989), *Anaesthesia and Intensive Care*, 17:312-19.
2. 'American College of Surgeons' Committee on Trauma.' (1989). *Shock in Advanced Trauma Life Support Program*. Chicago. 57-73.
3. Audet A, Goodnough LT. (1992). *Annals of Internal Medicine*, 116: 403-6.
4. Johnson K, Jensen JA, Goodson WH, *et al.* (1991). *Annals of Surgery*, 214: 605-613.
5. Blumberg N, Heal JM. (1992). *Australian Anaesthesia*, pp. 159-163, published by Australian and New Zealand College of Anaesthetists, Melbourne.
6. Bareford D. Chandler S. (1987). *Journal of Haematology*, 66:574 - 6.
7. Kruskall MS, Mintz PD *et al.* (1988). *Annals of Emergency medicine*, 17:239-331.
8. Blumberg N, Heal JM. (1992). *Australian Anaesthesia*, pp. 159-163, published by Australian and New Zealand College of Anaesthetists, Melbourne.
9. Whyte, Savoia (1997). *Medical Journal of Australia*, 166:584-586.
10. McClelland DB. (1992). *Clinical Anaesthesiology*, Vol 6, No. 3, pp. 539-60, published by Baillères, London.
11. Duffy BL, Harding JN, *et al.* (1994). *Anaesthesia and Intensive Care*, 22:90-2.
12. Phillips TF. (1987). Journal of Trauma, 27:903-6.
13. MMWR JAMA (1997) 296:196 look this up.
14. Cochrane Injuries Group Albumin Reviewers (1998) *British Medical Journal*, 317:235-240.
15. Woodman R, (1999) *British Medical Journal*, 318:1643.
16. Cittanova ML, Leblanc I. (1996) Lancet 348:1620-2.
17. Ljungström KG. (1988). Acta Scandinavia Chirugae, S43:26-30.
18. Berg EM, Fasting S, *et al.* (1991). Anaesthesia, 46:1033-3.

19. MOTHERS AND BABIES

Pregnant women come to theatre for all the usual operations as well as those associated with their pregnancy. The surgery may be either elective or emergency surgery; and may, or may not be related to their pregnancy. Because their physiology is altered they present special challenges to those who look after them in recovery room.

PHYSIOLOGICAL CHANGES DURING PREGNANCY

Blood volume increases by up to 40 per cent reaching a peak at 37 weeks. Red cell mass also rises, especially if the patient is given supplemental iron, but the rise in plasma volume is proportionately greater, which accounts for the relative anaemia seen during pregnancy. The lowered viscosity increases blood flow through the tissues, improving tissue oxygenation and removing the waste products of cell metabolism more readily.

During pregnancy the heart is elevated by the diaphragm and rotated forward. Its muscle fibres lengthen and myocardial contractility increases. The ECG frequently shows left axis deviation, and a flattened or even inverted T-wave. These changes may imitate those seen in ischaemic heart disease. Extra systoles are common, and sometimes provoke a supraventricular tachycardia.

In early pregnancy the peripheral vascular decreases resistance. To compensate for this the cardiac output begins to rise. Increased stroke volume accounts for 40 per cent of the increase, but the heart rate also increases by about 15 beats per minute thus blood is pumped around faster. By the 17th week of gestation the cardiac output reaches 6 l/min, which is about 40 per cent greater than normal (4.5 l/min), this increase peaks at 32 weeks of gestation.

Systolic blood pressure changes little from the non-pregnant state, but the diastolic pressure falls as the peripheral vessels dilate. It is lowest at mid term and rises towards the non-pregnant level at term.

During the physical and psychological stresses of labour blood pressure fluctuates, but in most patients it rises. About 11 per cent of patients who lie on their backs experience a fall in systolic blood pressure of up to 30 mmHg. This *supine hypotensive syndrome* is caused by the pregnant uterus preventing blood from flowing back to the heart. This is dangerous to the mother and the unborn child. The supine hypotension may be severe enough to cause unconsciousness. If a pregnant woman feels uncomfortable lying on her back, tilt her gently to the left side to relieve the pressure of the pregnant uterus on her veins.

The work of breathing increases as the uterus grows larger. Both mother and foetus require extra oxygen. Higher levels of progesterone, and to a lesser extent, oestrogen stimulate women to breathe more deeply during pregnancy.

Because the diaphragm is pushed up by the pregnant uterus, functional reserve capacity decreases in pregnancy. By full term the functional residual capacity is reduced so much that most completely healthy women experience some dyspnoea. This will be aggravated if the patient has an epidural during labour because the relaxed abdominal wall muscles allow the abdominal contents to push up the diaphragm further. At this point any increased demand for oxygen, such as shivering or severe agitation, will rapidly cause hypoxia that will compromise the foetus.

The effective renal plasma flow and the glomerular filtration rate increase with the rise in cardiac output. The increase in blood flow and glomerular fitration rate enhances excretion, secretion and reabsorption of substances during pregnancy. Wastes are eliminated more efficiently so that plasma urea and creatinine concentrations decrease by 40 to 50 per cent. Rising aldosterone secretion causes the reabsorption of more water and sodium. Tissues tend to become oedematous as pregnancy progresses.

As the uterus enlarges it pushes up the stomach displacing the oesophageal sphincter so that gastro-oesophageal reflux occurs, causing heart burn. Gastric emptying is delayed. All pregnant patients should be regarded as having a 'full stomach'. Nausea and vomiting is common. Because there is a delay in gastric emptying it takes longer for drugs to reach the small bowel, and the onset of action of the drugs which are absorbed there, such as paracetamol, will be delayed. Opioids such as pethidine further delay gastric emptying.

Serum albumin concentration is reduced, due to dilution, and free fatty acids are increased.

Pregnancy enhances coagulation, predisposing women to thromboembolic events such as deep vein thrombosis and pulmonary embolism (see page 336).

SURGERY FOR OBSTETRIC CONDITIONS

In many hospitals the obstetric operating theatre is in a different part of the hospital to the main operating suite. If this is the case in your hospital, the obstetric recovery room needs to be scrupulously maintained, equipped, and staffed, with the same standards as the main operating suite. Resist the temptation to relegate older equipment to this area.

Surgery in obstetric patients can be grouped as follows:
- before 20 weeks gestation;
- between 20 and 30 weeks gestation;
- after 30 weeks gestation.

In each of these groups there will be emergency, as well as elective operations.

BEFORE 20 WEEKS GESTATION

Before 20 weeks the most common operations are a dilatation and curettage, and clercage.

Dilatation and Curettage (D&C)

D & Cs are performed for spontaneous, incomplete or missed abortions. Under these circumstances no attempt is made to save the foetus. Blood loss is sometimes enormous, and the mother may need resuscitation to treat haemorrhagic shock before reaching the operating theatre.

In the recovery room watch for persistent vaginal bleeding. If the woman continues to bleed, give ergometrine 0.25 mg intravenously; or in less serious haemorrhage insert four prostaglandin 200 microgram suppositories. Both these drugs cause nausea and you will probably need to give an antiemetic such as metoclopramide 10 mg intramuscularly. Some women are very emotionally distressed by the loss of their pregnancy. If practical, allow her partner or mother to come in and sit with her.

Clercage

Another common procedure in the first trimester of pregnancy is cerclage for cervical incompetence. If the patient starts to bleed in the recovery room it may be because either she is aborting, or the suture site is bleeding. Notify the the obstetrician immediately.

Painful uterine contractions often occur following clercage. These do not necessarily indicate premature labour, but they will worry the patient. Treat them with hyoscine (Buscopan®) 20 - 40 mg IV slowly, and repeat it after 30 minutes if necessary. Hyoscine is an anticholinergic drug which relieves spasms, it also causes tachycardia and sedation. If the pains are severe, give pethidine. As a precaution against sepsis developing, make sure that antibiotics are given.

20 TO 30 WEEKS GESTATION

After 20 weeks and before 30 weeks the possible conditions requiring surgery are:
• antepartum haemorrhage;
• severe early onset pre-eclampsia requiring urgent delivery by Caesarean section;
• premature labour with breech or twin pregnancy and unavoidable delivery.

Antepartum haemorrhage

Patients who experience an antepartum haemorrhage may be shocked, or have coagulation problems. If they are shocked from blood loss a coagulopathy is more likely. In recovery room keep a close watch on the vaginal pads, and the bed sheet below the woman's buttocks. Report any significant loss to the obstetrician.

MONITOR: Blood pressure, pulse rate, ECG, oximetry, urine output, perfusion status and external blood loss.

LABORATORY: Haemoglobin, packed cell volume, platelet count, aPPT, prothrombin time, fibrinogen and fibrinogen degradation products. Cross match at least 4 units of blood.

Suspect disseminated intravascular coagulation (DIC) if:
• the platelet count less than or 70 000 mm³;
• increased prothrombin time and partial thromboplastin time;
• fibrinogen levels less than 150mg/l;
• increased fibrin degradation products.

Make sure the patient has a large bore, freely flowing, infusion in place. Be prepared to give a massive blood transfusion (see page 355) if DIC develops. These patients will be highly anxious as it is probable that their baby has died, or will die. They need a lot of emotional support.

Pre-eclampsia and eclampsia

In severe, early onset, pre-eclampsia some form of coagulopathy is always present. It most commonly presents with thrombocytopenia (a platelet count less than 100 000/mm³). Pre-eclamptic patients behave as if they are severely volume deplete, with excessive adrenergic drive pushing up their blood pressure. The decreased blood volume is associated with a decreased renal blood flow and a decreased glomerular filtration rate. This may progress to renal failure.

Before coming to theatre this patient should have been stabilized with magnesium sulphate. An intravenous infusion of magnesium sulphate acts as a central nervous system depressant. It reduces the probability of convulsions, controls hypertension and improves cardiac stability and renal function. The usual infusion rate is about 0.5 mg/kg/hr. Other drugs used to reduce the chance of convulsions are phenytoin, or occasionally diazepam. Make sure you have detailed written protocols about how to care for these infusions.

Even after an epidural anaesthetic for her Caesarean section vomiting is a risk. Because magnesium is sedating, the woman will be drowsy and at high risk of aspiration pneumonitis. Never turn your back on these women. They should be nursed in the recovery position and not on their back. Make sure that you know how to tilt the bed head down if necessary.

Pethidine is a suitable analgesic if she does not have an epidural in place. Check that anti-epileptic drugs have been prescribed before she leaves the recovery room.

The woman should have a urinary catheter in place. Keep a careful note of the hourly output, and report a decrease below 30 ml/hr. Monitor the blood pressure every five minutes for the first 30 minutes, and watch for vaginal bleeding.

Patients who fit, or lose consciousness have progressed from pre-eclampsia to eclampsia. Pre-eclamptic patients run the risk of convulsions for up to 48 hours after delivery. Women who already show signs of toxaemia such as hypertension, proteinuria, oedema, hyper-reflexia, and muscle twitching, headache, confusion, or thrombocytopaenia may deteriorate in the recovery room. These patients need close monitoring for 48 hours, and usually longer.

Delivery of the foetus is not the
terminating event in eclampsia and pre-eclampsia.

Haemolysis, elevated liver enzymes and a low platelet count (HELLP syndrome) are all signs that the eclampsia is progressing. A diastolic blood pressure greater than 110 mmHg needs immediate treatment. Hydralazine, labetalol, or even nitroprusside may be required (see page 264). Use intra-arterial pressure monitoring to guide your therapy.

The onset of pulmonary oedema usually follows excessive intravenous fluid overload, or less commonly is due to cardiac failure. Monitor oxygenation with a pulse oximeter, check the lungs for crepitations, listen to the heart for added heart sounds. The best signs that pulmonary oedema may be developing are increasing respiratory rate, and the progressive onset of shortness of breath. A chest X-ray will confirm your diagnosis. (See page 283 for management.)

Premature labour

If the patient comes into premature labour, whether it is a single or multiple birth, there is a great deal of anxiety associated with the smallness, and vulnerability of the baby or babies. Be supportive.

These patient may have been on tocolytic agents, such as salbutamol, terbutaline and ritodrine, prior to delivery. These drugs increases the risk of post partum haemorrhage which, if it occurs, may involve a massive blood transfusion (see page 355).

FROM THIRTY WEEKS TO DELIVERY

After 30 weeks of gestation obstetric surgery will be Caesarean delivery or forceps delivery. This may also involve patients in obstructed labour.

Obstructed labour

Patients are usually well behind with their fluid replacement. During their fruitless labour, hyperventilation, sweating, vomiting, nausea and the inability to hold down oral fluids have caused big fluid losses. Furthermore, in a less than perfect world, especially in an isolated region, they may have been like this for hours. By the time they come to recovery room after delivery this fluid deficit should have been corrected. The patient must have a urinary catheter and it is important that she has a urine output greater than 60 ml/kg .

MONITOR: Pulse, blood pressure, oximetry, perfusion status, JVP and urine output.

Keep a good free flowing intravenous line in place. The urine output is an excellent guide to fluid balance.

Caesarean delivery

Traditionally Caesarean sections are only performed to deliver a neonate who is in jeopardy, or because the mother has an intercurrent medical or physical problem that makes it impossible to deliver the child safely. In some parts of the developed world however, Caesarean sections are performed in otherwise healthy women who are capable of normal vaginal delivery, for reasons of convenience, or fear of medical litigation.

Both the mothers and their babies undergo massive physiological changes in the first few hours following delivery. For this reason they require one-on-one nursing care.

Establish the reason for the Caesarean delivery. Are there any medical problems which may require special attention in the recovery room? Common intercurrent diseases in the mother include: obesity, diabetes, asthma and anaemia. Life style illnesses such as drug, alcohol and nicotine addiction affect both mother and baby and may cause problems to both patients in the recovery room. Sometimes religious beliefs or social pressures impinge on the care of the woman; for instance post partum haemorrhage requiring transfusion, which normally is relatively easy to manage, becomes a life threatening disaster for a Jehovah's witness patient who refuses blood transfusion.

Let the mother have her baby as soon as she is fully conscious. Lie the mother on her left side with her baby beside her.

MONITOR:

1. Perfusion status including pulse, blood pressure, oximetry, JVP, and urine output.
2. The uterus. Feel the fundus, it should be firm like a large orange and be located just below the umbilicus. If it feels soft like a loaf of bread, consult the obstetrician. It may firm up with gently massage. A soft uterus is in danger of haemorrhaging.
3. Check that the intravenous line runs well. Oxytocin (Syntocinon®, Syntometrine®) is given to contract the uterus after delivery. Normally, an oxytocin infusion 30 units in 500 ml of saline will be running. Control the rate to 80 ml/hr or as prescribed. The vaginal contractions, caused by oxytocin are painful. You may need to give intravenous pethidine 25 - 50 mg to control these. Oxytocin can sometimes drop the blood pressure because of its action to reduce the peripheral vascular resistance so check this every five minutes. If more oxcytocin is required because the uterus is soft, it can be given as a slow bolus. If the uterus

remains soft, the obstetrician may decide to give ergometrine 5 - 10 mg intravenously. Always give an antiemetic such as metoclopromide 10 mg I/M with ergometrine as it frequently stimulates nausea and vomiting.

4. Prostaglandin F_2 alpha, called *carboprost*, (Hemabate®) is used for severe postpartum haemorrhage that does not respond to ergometrine or oxytocin. The dose is 250 microgram, and it is injected by deep intramuscular injection. It has nasty side effects including: bronchospasm, nausea, vomiting, diarrhoea, and flushing. Excessive doses can cause the uterus to rupture. Check the dose, and administration with another member of staff before giving it.

5. When you look at the perineal pad, check for blood pooling under the buttocks as well. The normal vaginal loss is about 100 ml, or one and a half pads. If more than this occurs while the woman is in recovery room, report it to the obstetrician immediately.

6. Record the blood pressure every five minutes for the first 30 minutes, and then every 10 minutes. If the pulse rate rise to more than 100 beats per minute, or the systolic blood pressure falls below 100 mmHg, then assume the cause to be haemorrhage and treat it. If bleeding persists the patient will have to go back to the operating theatre for an examination under anaesthesia to find out whether the bleeding is coming from the cervix, or the uterus.

Prolonged labour

If the woman has been in labour for some time before coming to theatre she may have been given a variety of pain relief ranging from multiple doses of intramuscular pethidine, to sophisticated epidural infusions of dilute anaesthetic and opioid. Her requirements for post operative pain relief and the liveliness of the new born child will be influenced by this preoperative medication.

If an epidural infusion is in place it may be possible to continue this as *patient controlled epidural anaesthesia* (PCEA - see page 223). Preferably this option will have already been discussed with the patient, but if not wait until the patient is sufficiently awake and talk about this with her. Make sure clear instructions have been written for continuing epidural infusions, and the lines are clean and well secured, with no uncovered injection ports.

Patient controlled analgesia (PCA - see page 484) is another option which is popular with the nurses in the post natal ward. This can have troublesome side effects of nausea and itching, and many mothers later say these were worse than the pain. Do not add antiemetics to the PCA infusion for mothers who intend to breast feed their babies. Many women would rather be free of all drips and catheters as soon as possible so that they can attend to their infant. Respect the wishes of your totally sentient and competent patients.

Breech deliveries

Premature breach presentations and footling presentations usually require Caesarean section. With vaginal breech delivery there may have been a period in the ward of great urgency, which the mother may interpret as panic. If general anaesthesia was administered rapidly she might wake in a state of extreme anxiety. Have all the information about the baby ready for her. In some units it may be possible to have the baby ready to show her. If the result of her delivery is not good, it is the obstetrician's duty to explain what has happened directly to her. Do not attempt to explain yourself.

OTHER POST OPERATIVE PROBLEMS

These include:
- air embolism;
- aspiration pneumonitis;
- amniotic fluid embolism;
- pulmonary embolism (see page 336);
- spinal headache (see page 380).

Air embolism

Air emboli occur surprisingly often during Caesarean sections. These emboli seldom seem to do much harm. These may account for the feelings of alarm, and restlessness that occur in a patient with an epidural or spinal anaesthetic, directly after delivery of the baby. Occasionally they are severe enough to cause hypotension, breathlessness and chest pain which persists into the recovery room.[1]

Aspiration pneumonitis[2]

Pregnant patients are at high risk from aspiration pneumonitis. Aspiration pneumonitis (*Mendleson's syndrome*) in obstetric patients is particularly fulminant and often fatal. The anaesthetist should personally supervise her care until she is fully awake. Keep her on her side until you are sure she has complete control of her reflexes. Patients who have had their operation under epidural or spinal are also at risk, especially if their blood pressure drops and they experience nausea. Keep them on their side postoperatively.

If aspiration has occurred on induction the patient will remain intubated, and should be transferred to intensive care unit for further management. If it occurs on extubation, the patient will have to be re-intubated, sedated and ventilated. You will need a smaller than normal endotracheal tube, a 7.0 or 6.5, as there will be tracheal oedema. In a fully resourced unit the patient may be given a trial without intubation and ventilation. This has the advantage that she will be able to deep breath and cough on her own. She will require high oxygen flows and if she cannot maintain a PaO_2 over 90 mmHg she will probably need ventilating. It is generally accepted that steroids, bronchial lavage, and prophylactic antibiotics are not warranted in the early stages of aspiration pneumonitis. If lumps of food have been vomited up then consider a bronchoscopy to eliminate blockage of a major airway. Chest X-ray changes will not show up for 2 - 3 hours.

Amniotic fluid embolism[3]

This is an uncommon complication (1:50 000), and is characterized by sudden collapse at the time of delivery, with hypotension, cyanosis, haemorrhage, and disseminated intravascular coagulation. There is no consistent specific test to confirm the clinical diagnosis, even though foetal cells can sometimes be isolated from the maternal circulation. The patient will require ventilation in the intensive care unit, with ionotrope support, antibiotics, and management of their coagulopathy. The outcome is poor, with a mortality of 80 per cent.

Pulmonary embolism (PE - see page 336)

This dreadful condition uncommonly occurs in the recovery room, and is more likely to occur in the ward 2 - 14 days postoperatively. However it can and does occur after Caesarean section. Consider pulmonary embolism if a patient becomes abruptly short of breath, has pleuritic chest pain; or collapses.

Spinal headaches

This complication occurs in 1 - 2 per cent of patients. It is as likely to occur after either epidural or spinal block. Excessive cerebrospinal fluid leaks into the epidural space and causes traction on the meninges in the brain. Modern *pencil point needles* lessen the risk. Good hydration helps prevent spinal headache and eases the symptoms if they do occur. Most patients, however will require a *blood patch* (see page 216). Give psychological support until this can be arranged.

SURGERY IN PREGNANT PATIENTS FOR NON-OBSTETRIC CONDITIONS

The incidence of surgery in the pregnant patient is between 0.75 and 2.2 per cent.

The most common operation performed during pregnancy is appendicetomy. The incidence varies from 1:350 to 1:10 000 and most occur in the third trimester.

Less common are cholecystectomy, ovarian cystectomy and a procedure for strangulated haemorrhoids. These operations are normally performed electively between the 14th and 24th week of gestation. Obstetric patients are most often young, and healthy and their recovery should be straightforward if their physiology, outlined above is understood. Nurse the unconscious patient on her side, because there is an increased risk of aspiration. Give plentiful oxygen, for the foetus as well as the mother. Make sure that any drugs you give are safe to use in pregnancy.

Particular problems can arise from the carbon dioxide insufflation during laparoscopic cholecystectomy. Carbon dioxide embolism is more likely in a pregnant patient due to the increased vascularity of the vessels in her abdomen. Carbon dioxide also dilates capillaries. increasing risk of haemorrhage.

Antibiotics must be given to patients having appendicectomies, a combination of a cephalosporin and metronidazole is suitable. There is a real risk of sepsis harming the foetus.

After major surgery consider foetal monitoring. This detects signs of foetal distress secondary to hypoxaemia. Bradycardia, or persistent tachycardia are signs of foetal distress. If foetal distress or signs of early labour are detected do everything possible to improve the perfusion and oxygenation of the uterus, the placenta and the foetus. Keep the mother on her side, give her oxygen. increase her circulating blood volume with fluids. Use colloids if her blood pressure is low.

About 22 per cent of patients having surgery in the second or third trimester will go into labour in the following week[4]. Prevent preterm labour by giving salbutamol. Dilute 10mg in one litre of Hartmann's solution and run this at 10 to 45 microgram/min. Avoid a maternal tachycardia over 140/min. Ritodrine 50 to 150 microgram/min is an alternative treatment to salbutamol but it also causes tachycardia.

Ritrodrine is the only drug passed by the Federal Drug Authority in the USA. Elsewhere salbutamol is widely used. Terbutaline* is another alternative.

Check the blood sugar of the pregnant patient in recovery room, this may be elevated in those suffering from gestational diabetes.

If the patient coming for incidental surgery is also preeclamptic extra sedation may be required. Magnesium sulphate is often prescribed 5mls of 49.3% solution = 10 millimols. Give 10 millimols intravenously slowly over 5 minutes.

Take special care to shield pregnant patients from any X-rays that might be being taken in recovery room.

Septicaemia
Pregnant patients with their high metabolic rate and increased blood volume are very susceptible to infection. Take care with sterile procedures.

Breast feeding mothers[5]
Breast feeding women produce between 500 - 1000 ml of milk daily. If more than 6 hours elapse between feeds the mother becomes uncomfortable. Allow the mother to express her milk. A well timed anaesthetic avoids most of these problems.

Following a minor operation, the mother may safely breast feed within a few hours of surgery. After major surgery the mother should express the first postoperative feed and discard it.

Avoid drugs with high lipid solubility, such as diazepam and morphine, because they readily enter breast milk and sedate the baby. A single dose of pethidine is less likely to do this.[6] Avoid NSAID drugs because they enter breast milk. Indomethacin has been reported to cause neonatal convulsions, and aspirin carries the theoretical risk of Reye's syndrome (see page 209). Paracetamol causes no problems in full term babies, but avoid it if the mother is breast feeding a premature baby. All antiemetics are contraindicated because they may cause dystonia and sedation in the infant.

---

* Problems with tocolytic drugs
All these drugs cause tachycardia, hypertension, hypokalaemia, especially if potassium depleting diuretics have been used, aggravate tachyarrhythmias, and cause hyperglycaemia. Use them with utmost caution in pre-eclampsia. You will need to monitor the pulse rate, which should not exceed 135-140 beats per minute, and the blood pressure. Fatal pulmonary oedema has been reported with ritodrine, and although the cause is multifactorial, fluid overload is probably the most important factor. Tocolytic therapy can cause post-partum haemorrhage; counteract this with ß-blockers.

Stress and fluid restriction depresses breast milk production. To help a breast feeding mother keep up her milk supply make sure she is well hydrated. Even after minor surgery she should have a litre of normal saline as she will have fasted preoperatively.

Blood group

Check the maternal blood type of all obstetric patients in recovery room. If the mother is Rh negative, and the baby or the father is Rh positive, RhoGAM® must be administered by I/M injection within 72 hours of delivery. This will prevent Rh isoimmunisation by preventing the mother forming antibodies to the Rh positive factor and protect her subsequent babies from haemolytic anaemia.

Drug Addicts (see page 420)

Legal Aspects

Be very careful what you say to obstetric patients and also what you say to each other within their hearing. Young women are very well informed about their rights and privileges. The birth of their baby is a very emotional time. Some babies will not, even with the best of care, be normal. Sometimes patients misunderstand or misinterpret what they have heard. If there has been anything untoward in the delivery of the baby there may be legal repercussions. Take care of what you say, and do not pass comments about the practice of your colleagues. or the circumstances of the delivery.

Obesity (see page 426)

Gynaecology (see chapter 62)

CARE OF THE NEWBORN

After delivery, or Caesarean section, neonates sometimes come to the recovery room with their mothers. You should be familiar with the immediate care of the newborn. In emergency situations you could be called right into theatre to assist with immediate neonatal resuscitation. This is especially likely if there are multiple births. For a list of requirements when preparing for resuscitation of the newborn see page 566.

Resuscitation

1. Minimize heat loss. Cold stress leads to hypoxia, hypercarbia and acidosis and these prolong the persistence of the foetal circulation and delay resuscitation. Take the newborn baby in a drape or towel from the surgeon, wipe him quickly and place him on the special trolley which is high and slopes towards you, under radiant light.

2. Gently suck out the nose and pharynx and if necessary remove meconium.

3. Assess the baby's respiration, if this is gasping give *positive pressure ventilation* (PPV) 40 - 60 breaths/min with 100% oxygen. This oxygen flow should not be above 4 sl/min. Do not simply offer the green tubing in front of his face. Use the Ambu® or Laedal® bag, a small airway, and an appropriate mask; lift his face into the mask and puff oxygen into his chest. You must see the chest rise or you are not doing it correctly.

   Over 90 per cent of babies will scream and turn bright pink. Wrap him warmly and securely and put him into his crib.

4. In some cases, the baby stays, quiet, blue and flaccid. Do not panic. Do not spend too much time with suction. Oxygen is what the baby requires. If the baby does not respond to positive pressure ventilation prepare to intubate. This is not difficult if you have the correct equipment. Measure the distance from the babies lips to the sternal notch with the tube so you have an approximate idea of the length required. Once the tube is in place you should have no trouble oxygenating him. Check your position with a stethoscope. You should hear breath sounds on both sides of the chest. Fix the tube in place with tape. Ask the anaesthetist to help you. If intubation fails a size one laryngeal mask can be used.

5. Assess the heart rate, if there is bradycardia commence chest compression at 120/min, use only your thumb or 2 fingers. Do not wait for assessment scores, nothing is lost by beginning early. Apply the pulse oximeter to the right hand, feet are unreliable in the newborn.

6. If the pulse rate remains below 80/min after a minute of full rescuscitation give naloxone 0.1 mg I/M to reverse the effect of opioids given to the mother during labour, which is one of the common reason why babies do not breath well at birth. Do not give atropine as bradycardia of the newborn is not vagal. Adrenaline 1:10 000 can be used 0.2 ml/kg.

7. Intravenous access is best achieved in the newborn via the umbilical vein. Use sterile techniques and insert a 3.5 F catheter, with one hole, into the cut end of the vein until it lies just under the skin. Do not slide it in too far or it will enter the liver. Free blood should flow back into the catheter.

Other problems with distressed infants

These include:

- hypoglycaemia;
- hypothermia (see page 145);
- cardiorespiratory problems that arise at birth;
- congenital abnormalities;
- meconium;
- oxygen toxcity.

HYPOGLYCAEMIA is possible if the birth has been stressful, or the mother is diabetic, or the mother has received a large glucose load within a few hours of delivery. Check the glucose level of any lethargic baby. It should be at least 2.5 mmol/l. If necessary give 2 - 3 ml/kg of 10% dextrose by mouth. An IV infusion should give 8 mg/kg/min.

NEONATAL RESPIRATORY PROBLEMS arise because the lungs are immature in preterm babies, and from the aspiration of meconium, or amniotic fluid. Sometimes mild respiratory distress or *transient tachypnoea of the newborn* (TTN) occurs. The signs are nasal flaring, grunting respiration, indrawing of the sternum, and cyanosis. If any of these signs occur, arrange for the baby to be assessed by a paediatrician, and consider transferring him to a neonatal intensive care unit.

OXYGEN TOXICITY. If exposed to high oxygen concentrations, premature babies and neonates (less than 1500 grams) are at particular risk from retrolental fibroplasia (also called *retinopathy of prematurity* or ROP), and will go permanently blind.

OPTIMAL PAO₂ FOR THE NEWBORN			
Babies age	PaO₂ (mmHg)	PaO₂ (kPa)	Hb saturation %
Pre term	40 - 60	5.3 - 8.0	70 - 90
Full term	50 - 70	6.6 - 9.2	84 - 92

1. Fong J, Gadalla F, et al. (1990). *Canadian Journal of Anaesthesia*, 37:262-4.
2. Sage DJ. (1993). *Current Opinion in Anesthesiology*, 6:471-5.
3. Clark SL. (1991). *Critical Care Clinics*, 7:877-82.
4. Mazza RI, Kallen B. (1991). *Obstetrics and Gynaecology*, 77:835-840.
5. Lee JJ,Rubin AP. (1993). *Anaesthesia*, 48: 615-6.
6. Bond GM, Holloway AM. (1992). *Anaesthesia and Intensive Care*, 20: 426-30.

20. PAEDIATRICS

Children and babies frequently have operations and come to recovery room. Their anatomy and physiology pose special problems.

For the purposes of this book:
- premature babies are those born before 37 weeks of gestation;
- neonates are babies in the first month of life;
- infants are under the age of one year;
- babies include neonates and infants;
- children are between the age of one year and twelve years;
- adolescents are between the age of 13 and 16 years.

PREMATURITY

The age of premature babies is calculated in post conceptual weeks. A baby born at 28 weeks, and now 4 weeks old, is 32 weeks post conception.

Premature infants are less able to maintain body temperature, suck, swallow or even breathe properly. Asphyxia during birth predisposes them to brain damage. If they are given 100% oxygen they are at risk of developing *retinopathy of prematurity* (ROP). They also risk intraventricular haemorrhage, respiratory distress syndrome, bronchopulmonary dysplasia, anaemia, apnoeic episodes, patent ductus arteriosis and necrotising colitis.

Premature babies can consume oxygen up to 8 ml/kg/min (compared with full term 7 ml and adult 3.5 ml). Their respiratory rate can be as high as 60 breaths/min with tidal volumes of 110 - 160 ml/kg/min.

Compared with full term babies, premature babies are more sensitive to anaesthetic agents. The volatile anaesthetics prevent their heart rate from increasing, and their baroreceptors and chemoreceptors do not trigger responses, so they do not compensate for hypoxia or falling perfusion. They are also particlarly intolerant of hypothermia.

Fully monitor premature babies
all the time they are in recovery room,
even when they are fully awake.

RESPIRATORY SYSTEM

Neonates have a high metabolic rate. Their oxygen consumption is about 7 ml/kg/min. This is twice that of the adults 3.5 ml/kg/min, and is another reason why neonates desaturate more rapidly than adult.

The dead space volume of the neonatal airways is proportionally the same as an adult, so they must breathe twice as quickly to meet their high oxygen demands. Children become hypoxic and cyanosed frighteningly fast.

Neonates cannot alter their volumes
so they alter their rates instead.

Although neonates, and to a lesser degree, infants have pliant chest walls, their lungs are stiffer (less *compliant*) than an adults. Events such as pneumonia, or neonatal respiratory distress syndrome, make the lungs even stiffer. When the neonate attempts to breathe in, instead of the lungs filling with air, the chest wall tends to cave in. This results in a reduced amount of air entering the lungs. Furthermore at the end of expiration there is proportionately less air left in their lungs, than in an adult. This means that neonates do not have a big reservoir of air (*functional residual capacity*) left in their lungs at the end of expiration, and without this store they become hypoxic very quickly. After anaesthesia they are sometimes literally too tired to breath. Babies should be completely awake before the anaesthetist leaves them.

While the hearts of babies and children
are relatively resistant to hypoxia,
their brains are not.

Airway obstruction

Factors that contribute to an obstructed airway in infants and children are:
• big floppy tongues;
• large tonsils and adenoids;
• a large epiglottis;
• a high larynx, with a small opening which is prone to oedema if it is traumatized, or the infant is over hydrated; the narrowest part of a child's airway is at the cricoid cartilage;
• the ribs are flexible making forceful coughing difficult;
• neonates, and infants less 2 - 3 months old, cannot breath through their mouths.

Airway problems seen in the first postoperative hour include:
• airway obstruction caused by the tongue obstructing the pharynx;
• laryngeal spasm;

- croup following extubation;
- respiratory depression;
- aspiration;
- apnoea.

Signs of an obstructed airway in an infant or child are:
- supracostal, intercostal, and subcostal retraction;
- inspiratory stridor or crowing;
- nasal flaring;
- decreased, or absent air entry.

Prevent airway obstruction, caused by the tongue falling back into the pharynx, by routinely nursing children in the recovery position. If this fails, gently extend the head to relieve the obstruction. If the obstruction is still not relieved then insert a nasal airway. Nasal airways are better than oral airways in children because they are less likely to stimulate gagging, vomiting or laryngospasm. Give 100% oxygen until the airway is completely clear. Use gentle suction and if this is not successful have a proper look at the pharynx with a laryngoscope.

If a spontaneously breathing baby cannot sustain a PaO_2 greater than 60 mmHg (7.89 kPa) or a $PaCO_2$ less than 60 mmHg it should be reintubated. Intubation in babies is not difficult. An emergency trachestomy is almost never required.

Keep nasal airways available
when recovering children.

Laryngeal spasm[1]
Stimulation of the pharynx causes the intrinsic muscles of the larynx to reflexly contract, closing the glottis. Laryngeal spasm is the body's emergency response to prevent foreign material entering the lower respiratory tract. Spasm can be triggered by mucous, blood or other material in the pharynx; and sometimes just by suction of the upper airway. Be gentle when using a sucker.

The incidence of laryngeal spasm is higher in children under the age of 9 years, and reaches a maximum between the ages of 1 - 3 months. Patients with Down's syndrome are particularily susceptible. If the child has a respiratory tract infection the problem is more likely to occur. Laryngeal spasm is a frightening event. It may not resolve spontaneously, until the child has become deeply and dangerously hypoxic. Seek help early. Have your protocols on how to manage it worked out, and practised beforehand.

Acute pulmonary oedema is an uncommon complication of laryngospasm.[2] It is probably caused by the violent swings in intrathoracic pressure generated as the child attempts to overcome the obstruction. In young children the oedema responds to oxygen and diuretics, but older children may require assisted ventilation for some hours.

INITIAL MANAGEMENT

1. Give oxygen by mask.
2. Call for help.
3. Bring the emergency paediatric trolley.
4. Attach a pulse oximeter.
5. Attach an ECG monitor and non-invasive blood pressure monitor.
6. Relieve the spasm by firm pressure applied behind the angles of the jaw which lifts it forward. Initially try ventilating the child using firm positive pressure from a mask. This may fail. Attempts to strenuously ventilate the patient by forcing air into the pharynx will worsen the obstruction.

FURTHER MANAGEMENT

1. If the above measure fails to relieve the obstruction within 30 seconds try 1% lignocaine 1.5 mg/kg intravenously[3] and flush this through the intravenous line.
2. If this is unsuccessful an anaesthetist should give a small dose of suxamethonium 0.5 - 1 mg/kg intravenously together with atropine 20 microgram/kg. You may need to intubate the patient and support his breathing until he is able to look after his own airway.

Croup

A hoarse voice, or a barking cough are signs of croup. These signs tend to resolve spontaneously. Rarely it progresses to stridor, a far more serious problem, heralding complete airway obstruction and respiratory arrest. Croup is due to oedema of the airway just below the larynx. It occurs in 1 - 6 per cent of children who have been intubated. Oedema fluid easily accumulates in the loose submucosal tissue, where the cricoid cartilage forms a complete ring around the trachea. Intubation is the most probable cause of croup immediately postoperatively. Infants are more susceptible than older children, because they have a smaller larynx (4 mm in diameter compared with 8 mm in an adult).

The signs of croup or stridor usually occur within the first hour after extubation, but it can be much later.

The signs are:
- stridor;
- rib and subcostal retraction;
- hoarseness;
- croupy cough;
- distress.

MANAGEMENT
1. Sit the patient up, give humidified oxygen, and nebulized adrenaline.
2. Take 2 ml of 1:1000 solution of adrenaline and make it up to a total of 5 ml in normal saline.[4] Give it in a nebulizer using a flow rate of oxygen of 5 l/min. It is believed to act by inducing vasoconstriction in the inflamed mucosa thus reducing oedema. The effects are short lived, lasting about 2 hours. If the child is a day case then it is safer to admit him.

Respiratory Depression

Children recover readily from muscle relaxants so look for other reasons for postoperative respiratory depression. If an infant is pulling up his legs up when he cries he is unlikely to have residual muscle relaxants as the cause of his respiratory depression.

Hypothermia, hypocalcaemia or acidosis delay recovery from muscle relaxants. Under these circumstances do not hesitate to reintubate the

---

ASSISTED VENTILATION IN THE NEONATE AND INFANT UNDER 10 kg

Aim for:

- respiratory rate 30 – 40 per minute;
- inflation pressure of up to 25 cm H_2O;
- fresh gas flows of 4 litres per minute;
- positive end expiratory pressures of 5 cm H_2O.

---

infant and transfer him to intensive care for observation and ventilation. Opioids also contribute to respiratory depression. Use naloxone dose up to 4 - 5 microgram/kg to reverse the effects of the opioids. It only lasts for 30 - 60 minutes, and when it wears off the respiratory depression may recur. Fentanyl is very slowly metabolised in babies, and should not be used in the recovery room.

Aspiration

Suspect aspiration if the child suddenly develops a wheeze or a cough. Infants are more susceptible to aspiration because: they have a shorter oesophagus, their cough reflex is not well developed, and their laryngeal competence is decreased for 6 - 8 hours following extubation.[5]

Apnoea in the newborn

Apnoea in the newborn and premature infant is defined as a respiratory pause of 20 seconds or longer, or a briefer episode if it is associated with bradycardia, cyanosis, or pallor.[6]

Infants who have been born prematurely, or have a history of respiratory distress syndrome or bronchopulmonary dysplasia, are susceptible to apnoea following anaesthetics even for minor operations such as hernia repair. This susceptibility persists for the six months of life and usually occurs within 12 hours of surgery. It is more common if muscle relaxants have been used. For this reason all infants who have been premature babies, and all infants who are less than three months (52 postconceptual weeks) are unsuitable for day case surgery. They need hospital admission and respiratory monitoring for the first 24 hours. Monitor infants of less than 45 conceptual weeks for 18 hours post anaesthesia. Monitor all infants under 6 months of age (64 postconceptual weeks) with a pulse oximeter, and if possible a respiratory monitor for at least two hours postoperatively.

Factors contributing to episodes of apnoea in the recovery room are:
• immaturity of the central nervous respiratory control centres;
• depression of the chemoreceptor response to hypoxia by residual anaesthetic agents;
• and residual effects of muscle relaxants.

Pneumothorax in infants

Pneumothorax is not uncommon. It occurs if their little lungs are over inflated. It can easily happen if the baby coughs during intubation or extubation. Physical signs, such as absence of breath sounds, are difficult to detect, but the apex beat may be displaced with the shift in the mediastinum. Shine a light through the chest wall from behind and you may see the outline of the collapsed lung. Cyanosis and bradycardia are late signs. Think of pneumothorax if there is any sudden deterioration in a baby postoperatively. Have the necessary equipment, sterilized and ready, to drain a pneumothorax.

THE CARDIOVASCULAR SYSTEM

As soon as you have the baby settled, check his notes to find out his preoperative pulse rate. This is an excellent guide to progress in recovery room. Although you can read averages from charts such as the one below, individual readings are preferable as they do vary. A return to the preoperative pulse rate is a very good sign that all is well.

NORMAL PAEDIATRIC HEART RATES AND BLOOD VOLUMES		
AGE	HEART RATE beats/min	BLOOD VOLUME ml/kg
1 day	95 – 150	100
1 week	90 – 160	90
1 month	120 – 180	85
6 months	110 – 170	80
12 months	90 – 150	75
6 years	70 – 135	70

The cardiac output in children is rate dependent. This means a bradycardia will cause hypotension. The heart's sympathetic innervation is not as well developed as its parasympathetic nerve supply. This makes children prone to bradycardia, which is not as well tolerated as a tachycardia. Bradycardia and apnoea may follow suctioning the pharynx. In a child the heart is relatively resistant to hypoxia, so by the time hypoxia is severe enough to cause a bradycardia cardiac arrest is near and severe brain damage will have already occurred.

Hypoxic bradycardia in children
is a grave sign.

Hypovolaemia

Hypovolaemia is a grave threat to neonates and infants. While an adult can lose 10 per cent of his blood volume without noticeable effect, a 10 per cent loss in a neonate is life threatening. A 2.5 kg neonate, with a normal a blood volume of about 250 ml, is severely shocked by a blood loss of only 20 - 25 ml.

As soon as possible acertain the fluids given in theatre. Up to 15 kg the baby should have received approximately 20 ml/kg. From 15 to 30 kg approximately 15 ml/kg and older children 10 ml/kg. Signs of hypovolaemia are a low blood pressure, a rising pulse rate (small infants may not get a tachycardia) a sunken fontenelle and poor peripheral capillary perfusion. The baby may have a mottled blue appearance.

Check the urine output if this is possible. It should be greater than 0.5 ml/kg/hr. Hypotension in older children is a disasterously late sign of hypovolaemia. It only becomes evident when the blood loss is more than 30 ml/kg. To test this diagnosis give a fluid challenge of 10 ml/kg of saline or a colloid. Signs of hypovolaemia are a falling systolic pressure with a rising diastolic pressure and a muffled apex beat when you listen with a stethoscope.

> *Do not be afraid to give fluids to neonates,*
> *hypovolaemia is a greater threat*
> *than fluid overload.*

If hypovolaemia is suspected check the drains and catheters for continuing loss. Check the haemoglobin and cross-match blood. Hypovolaemia will reduce cardiac output leading to metabolic acidosis. Liver ischaemia can result in a coagulopathy. Tissue hypoxia can cause disseminated intravascular coagulopathy can occur in babies.

Fluid replacement

1. In the operating theatre infants lose blood, and there is evaporation from the surgical site. For some hours after the abdomen has been opened isotonic fluid will transudate into bowel. These losses need to be replaced appropriately. Use potassium free fluid for this initial replacement. Use 4% dextrose with 1/5 normal saline for babies under 7 months of age, or less than 10 kg in weight. For older babies and children normal 0.9% saline can be used as the replacement fluid. Use a microdrip set with a burrette to ensure accuracy.

2. The usual intravenous maintenance fluid to used in the recovery room is 4% dextrose with a 1/5 normal saline.

3. Do not use 5% dextrose for replacement or maintanence. Even a small rise in blood glucose to 8 mmol/l can cause an osmotic diuresis so that excessive water will be lost in the urine.

If you use 5% dextrose to replace isotonic fluid lost during surgery the infant's serum sodium concentration will fall, and water will move into the cells. This shift causes cerebral oedema, and the infant will develop signs of irritability, restlessness, a mew-like cry, drowsiness, vomiting and in severe cases, convulsions.

4. Oliguria is usually temporary, and reverses when fluid losses are replaced. If it persists after adequate fluid replacement a diuresis can often be induced using frusemide 1 mg/kg or dopamine 3 microgram/kg. If urine output is not readily achieved then consult a specialist paediatrician.

Fluid maintenance (see page 120)

INJECTION TECHNIQUE AND DRUG DOSE

Children under 12 years do not respond to drugs like small adults; this particularly applies to neonates. Children's doses may be calculated from adult doses by body weight, or more reliably, by body surface area. The upper outer lateral aspect of the thigh is the only safe intramuscular injection site in children (see fig 1.3 on page 15).

IDEAL BODY WEIGHT IN CHILDREN

A well nourished child's approximate ideal weight

Age less than 9 years Weight in kg   = (2 x age) + 9

Age more than 9 years Weight in kg = age x 3

$$\text{Approximate dose for a child} = \frac{\text{surface area of child (m}^2\text{)} \times \text{adult dose}}{1.8}$$

Keep a 'weight-for-age' nomogram available in case you do not know the child's weight. Having determined the correct dose of a drug you may need to convert this into millilitres of drug as supplied by the maker. Under a stressful situation it is easy to make mistakes. So make up charts to convert directly from body weight to millilitres of solution. Tie these charts to your paediatric resuscitation trolley.

It is still common practice to give drugs to children based on their body weight. This can cause unexpected reactions; for instance, a fat child would receive a higher than appropriate dose. In such a case the dose should be

calculated from an ideal weight based on height and age. If you need to
calculate doses on weight alone, never give more than you would to a
50 kg patient. Be careful of sedatives, which may cause hallucinations, and
antiemetics. Which can cause dystonic reactions.

It is better to use a table such as the one below to calculate approximate
drug doses. Even using this table does not ensure safety, because some
drugs, such as digoxin, have a small margin between the therapeutic dose
and the toxic dose. If you have any doubts about the safety of a drug, or
how to use it in children, then consult the literature, or a paediatric
specialist. Be especially careful when giving drugs to babies in their first
thirty days of life.

PAEDIATRIC DRUG DOSES		
AGE	**AVERAGE BODY WEIGHT (kg)**	**PERCENTAGE OF ADULT DOSE**
Neonate*	3.5	12.5
1 month*	4.2	14.5
3 months*	5.6	18
6 months	7.7	22
1 year	10	25
2 years	12	28
3 years	14	33
4 years	16	35
5 years	18	40
6 years	20	46
7 years	22	50
8 years	25	54
9 years	28	59
10 years	31	66
11 years	35	70
12 years	39	75
13 years	43	80
14 years	50	100
Applies to full term, but not to premature infants.		

Venous access is difficult in chubby infants. Try the external jugular or
cubital veins. If this fails the intraosseous route is a valuable access for

drugs and fluid. Use a short thick needle and screw it through the anteromedial surface of the proximal tibia, just below the level of the tibial tuberosity.[8] The results of drugs given is similar to that with intravenous administration.

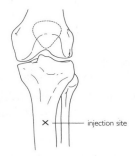

fig 20.1 Tibial site for intraosseous injection

Endotracheal administration of drugs

Patients in recovery room usually have intravenous lines. If for some reason this has come out, or is not working, bear in mind that in an emergency lipophilic drugs such as adrenaline, atropine, lignocaine and naloxone can be given into the trachea. The doses are variable, give the intravenous dose, diluted in 2 ml of normal saline, and if necessary, give it again.

Transfusion in infants

Blood volume is higher in the neonate being 90 - 100 ml/kg compared with the 70 - 80 ml/kg in the adult. Replacement of blood should be to the nearest 10 ml above the loss. It is safer to slightly overload neonates and infants than to have them plasma volume deplete.

Arrhythmias

If a child has had a respiratory tract infection within the last two weeks, elective anaesthesia should be deferred. Viral respiratory tract infections are not uncommonly associated with mild viral myocarditis, and children may develop a tachyarrhythmia during or after anaesthesia.

TACHYCARDIA: Abnormal arrhythmias are uncommon in children. The most common is a supraventricular tacycardia. Treat this with a rapid intravenous bolus of adenosine 0.05 mg/kg up to 0.25 mg/kg. In an emergency this can be given through an intraosseous needle.

BRADYCARDIA: Bradycardia is one sign of dangerous hypoxia. Do not symptomatically use atropine without improving the child's oxygenation by ensuring a clear airway, supporting breathing and if necessary, external cardiac massage.

Hypertension

Hypertension in babies is probably related to fluid overload. Check this first.

Anaphylaxis (see page 462)

Anaphylaxis can occur at any age. Intubate, ventilate and give adrenaline in a dilution of 1/10 000. The dose is 0.02 - 0.1 ml/kg up to 1 ml. Also give hydrocortisone 0.4 mg/kg. Lift the legs and give adequate fluids.

CEREBRAL PROBLEMS

Intracranial haemorrhage

Circumcision or even intubation of a neonate, without an anaesthetic, causes a sudden surge in blood pressure. This may rupture intracranial, especially intraventricular, vessels. If a neonate deteriorates for no obvious reason in the recovery room, consider this possibility.

Emergence phenomena

Otherwise healthy children are often restless after anaesthesia, especially children who have had their entire anaesthetic with sevoflurane. Sometimes these children are unable to recognize their mothers when they wake up.[9]

Never turn your back on a child.
They get into trouble quickly.

METABOLIC PROBLEMS

Hypoglycaemia

Hypoglycaemia is uncommon. It sometimes occurs after operations that involve long periods of starvation. Hypoglycaemia is difficult to diagnose as signs and symptoms vary. It is defined as a blood glucose of less than 2.2 mmol/l, at a level of 1.7 mmol/l brain damage is imminent. It usually presents as muscle twitching, an obtunded conscious state, convulsions or just a reluctance to breathe. Most at risk are those weighing less than 15 kg.

Hyperthermia

Hyperthermia can occur. Babies do not sweat, they vasodilate and look red. Consider the following causes:

- an overdose of atropine - the baby will have a racing pulse;
- an infection;
- CO_2 retention.

Hypothermia

Hypothermia causes profound problems for babies. Unless they have been well wrapped or under special lights in theatre nearly all have cooled to a certain extent. Compared to an adult, infants have a much bigger surface area in relation to their body weight. Neonates lose heat rapidly, because they have little subcutaneous fat to insulate them.

Measure the temperature of a baby
as soon as possible
after arrival in recovery room.

Considerable amounts of heat can be conducted to cold mattresses and blankets. Infants under the age of about 6 months do not shiver. If there is sufficient oxygen available babies generate heat by metabolizing specialized fatty tissue called brown fat. Brown fat can, at the best, only provide energy for a few hours. Once used, it is gone and it is not replaced.

An increasingly drowsy
infant may by hypothermic.

Keep small infants warm. Cover their heads with a woollen or gamgee hat, because infants lose heat through their bald heads quickly. Ideally they should go straight into an incubator after surgery. To prevent heat loss, and provide a neutral thermal environment, full-term babies require an incubator temperature of 32.5°C, and premature babies require 35°C. Their oxygen requirement is high; so make sure that 28% oxygen flows into the incubator.

In small infants hypoventilation and hypothermia cause drowsiness. If the infant becomes lethargic and floppy, and its respiration, and pulse rate are slow, assist his breathing with a Cardiff™ or small Ambu™ Bag, and summon someone to help you. You will need to warm the baby, and check his blood sugar.

Vomiting

Although children frequently vomit after anaesthesia they are not usually distressed. Clean the mouth and pharynx carefully and allow the child to sit up. Initially withhold antiemetics as they can cause severe dystonic reactions.

DYSTONIA

Dystonia causes the child to become stiff with their arms held rigidly at their sides and their teeth clenched. Their eyes may turn up or flick from side to side (nystagmus). This can be reversed by benzotropine (Cogentin®) 0.02mg/kg as a bolus intravenously. If necessary repeat this dose after 15 minutes.

If vomiting persists in older children give metoclopramide 0.3 mg/kg slowly intravenously. Droperidol is sometimes given preoperatively is effective, but it causes postoperative sedation.

Salivary gland enlargement[10]

Sometimes acute engorgement of the parotid, submaxillary or sublingual glands occurs during anaesthesia and persists during the recovery room stay. The face appears to be bloated, as if the child has mumps, and the glands are felt as firm masses. It usually subsides with an hour, and is not dangerous unless it causes airway obstruction.

PAIN RELIEF

Assessment of pain (see page 178)

Children waking from anaesthesia are often distressed, frightened, disoriented and in pain. Small children quickly respond to the warmth of a cuddle. It may not be possible to pick the child up, but touch is very reassuring. A toddler out of his routine is anxious and upset; but a toddler out of his routine, and in pain, is inconsolable, and very, very angry.

Ideally pain relief should be established in theatre. Depending on the site of the surgery a combination of regional techniques, such as caudals; with opioids, and/or paracetamol (Panadol®, Tylanol®) suppositories can be used to suit most circumstances. Never let a baby or child cry in pain. Incremental small doses of opioids, especially pethidine are ideal for quickly settling small patients.

Do not use aspirin in children. It may cause Reye's syndrome (see page 209).

Diazepam suppositories 0.1 mg/kg are useful to relax the painful adductor spasms which occur when babies have plaster splints applied.

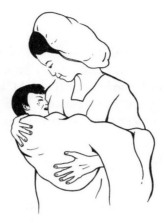

fig 20.2 Cuddle crying children

Opioids (see page 180)

Both morphine and pethidine are effective forms of pain relief in children, the onset of action of pethidine is quicker than morphine. Opioids are metabolized in the liver. Pethidine metabolites are active and occasionally cause twitching and even seizures. All the side effects of opioids seen in adults also occur in children. The duration of action of opioids is unpredictable up to 3 months of age. Never use fentanyl in neonates or babies. It has a very long action, causes respiratory depression and is slowly metabolized. Avoid all opioids in babies after neurosurgery.

Oral codeine takes about 40 minutes to relieve pain. In the recovery room such a delay is only acceptable where alternative drugs cannot be used, such as paediatric neurosurgery. Codeine lasts for 2 - 3 hours. The dose is 0.5 - 1 mg/kg. Codeine can be given intramuscularly, but not intravenously, because it causes hypotension and histamine release.

Continuous morphine infusions are useful after major surgery though they require the patient to be closely supervised in a high dependancy unit. The loading dose is 0.1 mg/kg before the end of surgery then 0.5 mg/kg added to 500 ml of lactated Ringers solution and given via an infusion pump or burette at 10 - 40 ml/hr. Side effects include respiratory depression, itching and nausea.

Continuous epidural, with or without narcotics, can be successfully used if the child is going to a supervised area, such as intensive care. Use 0.5 ml/kg of 0.25% bupivicaine and infuse at a rate of 0.1 - 0.15 ml/kg/hr.

VISITORS FOR CHILDREN

A child is comforted by seeing his mother as he emerges from the anaesthetic. Thoroughly brief the mother on what to expect beforehand, so that she does not convey her anxiety to the child. It is wise to keep other visitors and relatives away from patients who are recovering from anaesthesia. They may become upset to see someone vomiting or in pain.

ADOLESCENTS

Privacy

Young people are very shy, keep them well covered and do not embarrass them.

Restlessness

Teenagers and young adult patients can become very restless while waking up. They roll about, and may try to climb off the trolley before they can be reasoned with. Those who have had nasal surgery are the worst. Make sure the trolley sides are raised, and there is a strong person to help restrain the patient. Secure the intravenous lines, nasogastric tubes and other drains, otherwise they may be pulled out during this restless phase.

Shivering and shaking

When emerging from any of the volatile agents, younger patients may get the *halothane shakes* with muscle rigidity and violent shaking. When this happens they use considerable amounts of energy so try and keep their oxygen masks on and cover them with warm blankets.

Drugs

From their early teenage years through young adulthood, many patients seem surprisingly resistant to sedative and analgesic drugs. An alarmed young person will divert most of his blood supply to his muscles, (a part of the fight or flight response). When drugs are given intravenously they are more likely to be pumped to his muscle, rather than to his brain.

Nausea and vomiting

See chapter 13.

CARDIAC ARREST

Cardiac arrest in children is usually caused by a lack of oxygen to the heart. The most common cause of this is a respiratory arrest. Another cause is blood loss (see below).

Children under the age of 1 year of age are most at risk. There is less time to respond to apnoea in children, because they become hypoxic fast. Children nearly always (95 per cent) have asystole or bradycardia as the initial rhythm.

Cardiac arrest is usually preceded by:
- respiratory distress with tachypnoea, cyanosis, distress, and decreased breath sounds;
- poor perfusion with tachycardia, poor capillary return, cool or mottled peripheries;
- deterioration in conscious state, flaccidity.

Cardiac massage

When performing cardiac massage remember the heart is positioned under the lower third of the sternum in all children.[7] Place the index finger of the lower hand just under the line between the nipples. The area of compression is at the junction between the middle and ring finger. Compress the heart with either two fingers or the heal of your hand, depending on the size of the child. Use about 80 compressions per minute.

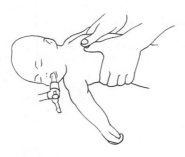

fig 20.3 Position of thumbs on baby's chest for cardiac massage

The brachial pulse is easier to feel in chubby children than the carotid. Neonates, infants and small children have short necks. Do not hyper-extend them, just lift the head forward a little into a sniffing the morning air position. Insert a Guedal airway, use an appropriate mask, and ventilate at a rate of 40 - 60 per minute with puffs of 100% oxygen.

Cardioversion

Cardioversion is in the sequence 2, 4, and 4 joule/kg. Over use of energy will damage the myocardium. Use paediatric paddles. Most modern defibrillators have a preset maximum dose of 100 joule when the paediatric paddles are connected. Remember that small babies who have been stressed, or starved are at risk from hypoglycaemia.

To be successful it is far more important to restore vascular volume, maintain a clear airway, give adequate ventilation and oxygenation and use early cardioversion, than it is to use drugs.

When to stop?

The outcome of paediatric cardiac arrest is poor. Failure to achieve a return to spontaneous respiration after 15 minutes has a dismal outcome. The exceptions for this are arrests associated with hypothermia, hyperkalaemia, and bupivacaine toxicity. If in doubt phone a paediatrician for advice.

1. Roy WL, Lerman J. (1988). *Canadian Journal of Anaesthesia*, 35: 93-8.
2. Leek W, Downes JJ. (1983). *Anesthesiology*, 59:347-9.
3. Baraka A. (1978). *Anesthesia and Analgesia*, 57:506-7.
4. Child CS. (1987). *Anaesthesia*, 42:322 -35.
5. Burgess GE, Cooper JR, *et al.* (1979). *Anaesthesiology*, 51:73-7.
6. American Academy of Pediatrics Task Force. *Pediatrics* (1985) 76:129-31.
7. Orlowski JP. (1980) *Pediatric Clinics of North America*, 27:495-512.
8. Spivey WH. (1987) *Lancet*, 2:1235-6.
9. Davis PJ, (1999) *Anaesthesia and Analgesia* 88:34-8.
10. Bonchek LI. (1969). *Journal of the American Medical Association*, (JAMA) 209:1716-8.

21. ELDERLY PATIENTS

It is generally accepted that *elderly* patients are those of 65 years or older. The *aged* are elderly patients of 80 years or older.

Ageing leads to a progressive impairment of all body functions. Even the healthy aging have a loss of organ functional reserve. They will have a more exaggerated reponse to surgical manipulation, anaesthesia, and drug therapy. If they are suffering from chronic diseases these problems are much worse. Age alone cannot be used as the sole predictor for the outcome of surgery, or the likelihood of problems in the recovery room.

The following factors will warn you to expect problems in the recovery room:
- surgery of over 45 minutes in duration;
- obesity;
- associated chronic illness, especially diabetes or hypertension;
- age greater than 70 years.

RESPIRATORY SYSTEM

Lungs

In the elderly the lungs are less elastic, the chest wall is stiff, the respiratory muscles are weaker, airways are floppy and collapse easily; and the alveolar surface area is reduced. This means gas exchange is less efficient. For these reasons the elderly rapidly become hypoxic, and are slow to respond to oxygen therapy. They are likely to develop sputum retention, their floppy airways and muscle weakness make it difficult for them to cough effectively.

Oxygen and the elderly

The arterial PaO_2 falls with age from around 100 mmHg (13 kPa) in a fit young person to about 80 mmHg (10.5 kPa) in an 80 year old. This fall is aggravated by smoking or lung disease.

Diffusion hypoxia is a significant problem in the elderly. For about 10 minutes after the end of the anaesthetic, nitrous oxide seeps out of the blood and enters the lungs. This nitrous oxide occupies lung space normally available for oxygen resulting in persistent hypoxia in the early recovery period.

After operations, such as hip replacements, haemoglobin oxygen saturations below 85% may persist for up to a week.[1] If this hypoxia is untreated, particularly in conjunction with a low haemoglobin, it will result in confusion, delirium, cardiac failure, infarction or death.

Oxygen is necessary, even after local or regional anaesthesia. Regional anaesthesia causes vasodilation which requires the heart to increase its output in order to maintain a blood pressure. This extra work increases the cardiac oxygen demands. If the oxygen supply is not adequate the heart either fails, or becomes ischaemic.

Oxygen demand is highest when the patient wakes up with severe pain, and is further aggravated if there has been a major blood loss. Here, a rise in cardiac output, and respiratory effort cannot meet the oxygen demand of the tissues.

Consider giving oxygen to elderly patients
at night following major surgery.

CARDIOVASCULAR SYSTEM

All forms of cardiovascular disease are more common in the elderly. Circulation time is slower; the blood volume is less and blood vessels are more rigid. This means the elderly are less able to compensate quickly, for sudden changes in blood pressure or blood volume. Monitor the ECG in recovery room and look for depression of the ST segment. This is a sign of ischaemia (see page 275).

RENAL FUNCTION

Kidney function declines in the elderly. By the time a patient is 70 years old, up to half his nephrons may not be functioning. This delays the excretion of water soluble drugs and may delay recovery. The glomerular filtration rate declines by 10 ml per minute every decade after 30 years of age, but the serum creatinine does not rise, reflecting the decline in muscle mass.

The ageing kidney is susceptible to
drug induced renal damage.

LIVER FUNCTION

Intestinal absorption and liver metabolism are altered. There is a fall in serum albumin and other drug carrier proteins that alter the availability of free drug. This delays the elimination of drugs and prolongs their effects.

CONNECTIVE TISSUE

Joints

Elderly patients have stiff and easily damaged joints, be careful how you position them. Take care not to injure stiff backs and hips. The recovering patient cannot report pain that would normally warn them that their joints are over stretched. Also they are unable to manoeuvre themselves around to relieve uncomfortable positions.

Skin

Skin is often very fragile and easily torn by simple things, such as turning the patient, or even removing the sticky ECG dots roughly. Check under the automated blood pressure cuff because the skin can be damaged by the cuff.

HYPOTHERMIA

The elderly cool down quickly on the operating tables, and have a poor tolerance to heat loss. Hypothermia delays the metabolism and excretion of drugs. This is an important factor if the operation has lasted more than an hour. During, and after their operations they have a greater fall in body temperature than younger patients. This loss is even worse if they are thin as well as old, because they have little subcutaneous fat to help conserve heat. Intraoperative hypothermia leads to a marked rise in post operative catecholamine levels, and energy requirements. Check the patient's temperature as soon as possible, and use warm blankets.

HYPOGLYCAEMIA

Many elderly people suffer from diabetes (see also page 416). Check their blood sugar, on admission to recovery room. If the elderly person is returning to the ward soon after minor surgery, a sweet drink is a far better remedy for low blood sugar than an intravenous bolus of glucose, which irritates the veins. Patients who have had major surgery will be on a regime set by physicians preoperatively, follow their instructions.

Confusion and Postoperative Delirium

Confusion is common postoperatively and approaches 50 per cent after fractured femurs[3]. Hypoxia, as always, must be the first suspect; and it comes in many disguises. Apart from obvious lung problems, heart failure is the major cause of hypoxia. The heart just cannot pump the blood around fast enough to deliver the oxygen to the tissues. This is made worse by anaemia (see page 411). It is difficult to over emphasize the importance of proper oxygenation in the elderly. Once an old person has been hypoxic, even for a few minutes, their brain is damaged. Confusion, restlessness, agitation and aggression are difficult to manage. Even if proper tissue oxygenation is restored promptly, it takes, at best many hours, and probably days to resolve the delirium. It is a far, far better thing, to prevent hypoxic brain damage, than to have to treat it.

Always look for hypoxia as the cause of confusion.

Other causes of postoperative confusion include:
- pre-operative dementia;
- hypotension during the anaesthetic;
- anticholinergic medication;
- stroke;
- depression;
- hypothyroidism;
- hypoglycaemia.

Poor eyesight and hearing add to an elderly person's disorientation. Despite their confusion they have an accurate perception of hurt and insult. Courtesy and respect for their dignity helps reduce feelings of alienation.

1. Fugere F, Owen H, *et al.* (1994). *Anaesthesia and Intensive Care*, 22:724-8.
2. Motamed S, *et al.* Metabolic changes during recovery in normothermic versus hypothermic patients undergoing surgery and receiving general anaesthesia and epidural local anaesthetic agents. *Anaesthesiology* 1998; 88: 1211-8.
3. Berggren D, Gustafson Y, *et al.* (1987). *Anesthesia and Analgesia*, 66:497-500.

22. PRE-EXISTING DISEASE

Unfit patients frequently undergo surgery. Their illness may be a result of their life style of smoking, drinking or over eating, or an acquired or inherited disease. In the 1940s the American Society of Anesthesiologists published a scale, known as the ASA classification, to grade the fitness of patients presenting for anaesthetics. Despite its deficiencies it is still widely used. This chapter includes many diseases that directly affect the care of the patient after operation. Cardiac diseases are dealt with in Chapter 15.

ASA GRADINGS	
ASA I	Patient is fit for age
ASA II	Patient has mild systemic disease which does not interfere with day to day activity
ASA III	Patient has severe disease which does limit day-to-day activity
ASA IV	Patient has severe disease which is a constant threat to life
ASA V	Patient is not expected to live 24 hours with or without surgery
An E is added if the surgical procedure is an emergency; for example ASA IV E	

ADULT RESPIRATORY DISTRESS SYNDROME (ARDS)

ARDS is a form of respiratory failure arising from a variety of insults on the lung, presenting with similar pathophysiological changes. It is characterised by respiratory distress, progressive refractory hypoxaemia, diffuse pulmonary infiltrates and increased stiffness of the lungs (reduced pulmonary compliance).

About one-third of the patients who die, following successful resuscitation after major trauma, succumb to progressive respiratory failure.

The lung responds to injury by becoming permeable to fluid from the circulation. This is sometimes called *low pressure pulmonary oedema*, to contrast it with the *high pressure pulmonary oedema* of cardiac failure.

Predisposing factors to ARDS include:

- aspiration of gastric contents;
- sepsis;
- fluid overload;
- multiple transfusions;
- prolonged hypotension;
- cardiopulmonary bypass;

- fat emboli;
- uraemia;
- burns;
- pancreatitis;
- lung contusion;
- massive adrenergic discharge, such as after head injury.

Patients with ARDS sometimes come to theatre from the intensive care unit for stabilization of fractures, laparotomies, or tracheostomies. They usually have a number of infusion pumps running, and many drains. Generally, they are transferred straight back to the intensive care unit, but they may come to the recovery room. Make sure all the tangle of infusion lines are properly connected as they sometimes become dislodged when transferring the patient from the operating table to their intensive care beds.

Recovery room management of ARDS
- Take care not to give excessive intravenous fluids. Monitor central venous pressure, or better, maintain their pulmonary artery wedge pressure to keep it less than 10 cm H_2O;
- filter and warm all blood transfusions;
- administer oxygen;
- turn the patient half hourly, because the dependent lung is the worst affected;
- to minimize the stress response give adequate analgesia.

AIDS

Those at high risks of HIV/AIDS include homosexual and bisexual men and their partners, haemophiliacs, intravenous drug users, and children of affected mothers. Problems are mainly confined to staff, because of the danger of *needle stick injury* (see page 103).

ALCOHOLICS

Alcoholics and regular drinkers are tolerant to some of the sedative drugs. As they emerge from anaesthesia they tend to be restless, often moving about in a semipurposeful manner before they wake properly. They may try to sit up, and open their eyes before spitting out their airway. Do not remove the airway, let them take it out themselves. Sometimes they appear dazed, will not respond when you talk to them, and occasionally become violent. If this happens call security personnal to help you.

Alcoholics are susceptible to spontaneous hypoglycaemia, especially when stressed after operations. If they remain obtunded, or become sweaty or restless check their blood sugar. It should be greater than 4 mmol/l. If it is less than 3 mmol/l give 20 mls of 50% glucose slowly through a freely running drip.

Thin alcoholics are often hypothermic in the recovery room and tolerate analgesics and sedatives poorly. Do not discharge them from the recovery room until their temperature is greater than 36.5°C.

ANAEMIA

Anaemia is defined as haemoglobin less than 100 gm/l (10 gm/dL). If there is not sufficient haemoglobin to transport oxygen then the tissues will become hypoxic. The pulse of an anaemic patient is both fast and very easily felt. This 'bounding' tachycardia reflects a high cardiac output that increases the amount of oxygen carried to the tissues. Should this compensation fail the patient will become hypoxic. Anaemic patients are pale, particularly on the mucosa of the cheeks and lips. In coloured patients check their fingernail beds which should be pink. White nail beds are sign of anaemia. Anaemia disguises the warning signs of cyanosis and the pallor associated with shock. Hypoxia develops rapidly in an anaemic patient, and will be made worse by bradycardia, reduced cardiac output, respiratory depression, or hypotension. In the tropics hookworm, malnutrition, malaria, and chronic tuberculosis cause severe anaemia.

A subtle cause of *relative anaemia* occurs in patients who have received a large blood transfusion in the operating theatre. Although the measured haemoglobin may be acceptable, the donated red cells are reluctant to release oxygen to the tissues. Transfused red cells take up to 18 - 24 hours to regain normal function.

MANAGEMENT:

1. Monitor the patient with a pulse oximeter and an ECG. Watch particularly for signs of cardiac ischaemia, or cerebral hypoxia.

2. Give high inspired oxygen concentration by mask. This needs to be continued in the ward for at least 24 hours, until the red cells are functioning properly again.

3. Replace blood loss early and adequately.

4. Do not allow the patient to become hypotensive, or allow his perfusion to fall. He may require dopamine to maintain his renal perfusion and cardiac output.
5. Initially assume confusion or disorientation is a result of hypoxia. Give oxygen and then look for other causes for the confusion.

ASTHMA

Asthma is characterized by non-specific irritability and inflammation of the respiratory tract. In some parts of the world asthma may affect up to one in ten in the population. Underlying the inflammatory reaction is the constriction of bronchial smooth muscle and mucosal oedema with mucus production. The airways are narrow causing obstruction of air flow, wheezing and coughing. Unlike chronic airway disease, asthma usually responds well to bronchodilators. Asthmatic patients are frequently apprehensive of anaesthesia, because community folk law dictates that it is dangerous for them to have an anaesthetic. Volatile anaesthetic agents are excellent bronchodilators and asthma is rarely a problem in theatre or the recovery room.

Before diagnosing asthma, eliminate other factors as a cause of wheeze and cough in the recovery room. First consider:
• anaphylaxis;
• allergic reactions to drugs;
• reactions to blood transfusions;
• aspiration;
• acute pulmonary oedema;
• emboli of fat, blood clot, amniotic fluid or air.

Listen to both lungs with a stethoscope. Wheeze confined to one lung, or part of one lung, indicates aspiration of foreign material, pulmonary embolism or partial airway obstruction. In contrast, asthma and pulmonary oedema will equally affect all zones of both lungs. A wide spread wheeze, especially if it is associated with a drop in blood pressure and changes in skin colour indicates anaphylaxis (see page 462).

NORMAL PEAK FLOW RATES

Approximate peak flow (L/sec) should be:

= 6 x height in metres (age < 50 years)

= 5 x height in metres (age > 50 years)

A peak flow less than their height in centimetres indicates critical airway obstruction.

Patients with unstable asthma, especially if their *peak expiratory flow rate* (PEFR) is less than 75 percent of normal, should be optimized the week before their operation. Tracheal intubation, insertion of a laryngeal mask, and some drugs such as thiopentone or methohexitone, can trigger bronchospasm which may persist after their admission to the recovery room. Other drugs which may precipitate asthma include: ß-blockers (eg. metoprolol, atenolol), or NSAIDs (eg. ketorolac, ibuprofen, aspirin). Treat the asthma if the patient is coughing or wheezing, or if he says his chest is tight.

Warnings of impending respiratory arrest in an asthmatic include:
• obvious respiratory distress;
• use of accessory muscles of respiration;
• indrawing of the suprasternal notch;
• difficulty in speaking;
• $PaCO_2$ rising to and exceeding 40 mmHg (4.26 kPa) in a wheezing patient.

Patients who experience an acute bout of asthma while in the recovery room, should be transferred to an intensive care unit as soon as they are stable, because of the risk that they may suddenly deteriorate.

Sudden abrupt collapse in an asthmatic patient?
- consider tension pneumothorax.

MANAGEMENT OF ASTHMA
High concentrations of oxygen through a close fitting mask may irritate the patient causing him to to keep taking it off. Compromise with a loose fitting mask and a high oxygen flow, then at least there is a chance of the mask staying in place.

1. Salbutamol (Ventolin®)
   Mainstay of the treatment of acute asthma is a ß-agonist bronchodilator. Salbutamol is preferred with terbutaline as second choice. (Terbutaline is a ß-agonist similar to salbutamol).

   Give salbutamol by nebulizer and face mask. Start with 1 ml salbutamol 0.5% in the nebulizer. This is equivalent to 50 puffs by a metered dose inhaler and is close to the optimal dose for an adult. In some nebulizers it is necessary to dilute the salbutamol with sterile water. Compared to the risks of severe asthma, the risk of toxicity of these agents is negligible. The secret is to give enough salbutamol. As soon as the effect of the previous dose has worn off, give the next. Never withhold salbutamol for fear of toxicity. Life threatening side effects of ß-agonists are almost unknown. Side effects include: muscle tremor, tachycardia; and after prolonged use hypokalaemia, hypomagnesaemia and hypophosphataemia. Unless respiratory arrest is imminent, it is rarely necessary to use intravenous ß-agonists. Never give salbutamol by an intramuscular injection.

Monitor all patients with an ECG
while they are receiving bronchodilators.

HINTS ABOUT ASTHMA

- Salbutamol is safe;
- If you are concerned about the wheeze, then use more salbutamol;
- Cyanosis, or an oxygen saturation < 90 per cent, is a sign of impending death;
- The confused, restless or agitated patient is hypoxic;
- Blood gases will reveal a low $PaCO_2$ and a low PaO_2. If the $PaCO_2$ starts to rise then it will probably be necessary to intubate the patient;
- Sedation is absolutely contraindicated in a wheezing patient.;
- In a severe asthmatic consider the possibility of a pneumothorax. This can occur unsuspected during the anaesthetic.

---

2. Hydrocortisone
   If the asthma is severe give at least 200 mg of hydrocortisone hemisuccinate intravenously. This takes up to 8 hours to reach its peak effect.

3. Aminophylline is toxic and rarely used. If you do decide to use then make sure the patient was not previously taking theophylline.

Aminophylline toxicity is hazardous
and difficult to treat.

4 Adrenaline and ephedrine are effective, but are rarely used because they cause hypertension and cardiac arrhythmias.

Chronic Obstructive Airways Disease (COAD)

Acronyms include: chronic obstructive lung disease (COLD), and chronic obstructive pulmonary disease (COPD).

This common disease is usually caused by smoking and is characterized by floppy airways where chronic inflammation has dissolved the supporting cartilage rings. These floppy airways collapse, trapping air in parts of the lungs, as the patient breathes out.

There are broadly two groups of patients with chronic obstructive airways disease: *blue bloaters* and *pink puffers*. Blue bloaters are chronically hypoxic with pulmonary hypertension and right heart failure; in contrast pink puffers are usually emaciated and have emphysema.

Blue bloaters may stop breathing if they receive more than 28 per cent inspired oxygen. However do not be afraid to give oxygen to patients with COAD. Remember hypoxia kills and their breathing can always be assisted. Monitor the respiratory rate meticulously and watch for a reduction. Measure it by putting your hand on their chest and counting the breaths for a full minute. If the respiratory rate decreases to below eight breaths a minute, or the patient becomes drowsy, assist his breathing with a bag and mask, until other measures can be taken. Inform the anaesthetist. Meanwhile, a dose of the respiratory stimulant doxapram (Dopram®) is useful. Give 1 - 1.5 mg/kg doxapram IV over 30 - 60 seconds. Repeat after one hour if necessary. Doxapram is contraindicated in patients with epilepsy or asthma and must be used cautiously in patients with hypertension. The patient should be admitted to the intensive care unit for further monitoring.

In patients which chronic bronchitis, even with the most diligent humidification and suctioning during an anaesthetic, sputum will collect in the airways and may obstruct them. If the sputum is not cleared there is a risk of the plugs causing segmental collapse and infection.

The patient must be able to sit up and cough without pain. This requires excellent pain relief. Respiratory depression may occur with even low dose opioids in these patients, so local anaesthesia or regional blockade is a better option. Once the patient is conscious sit him up, support his wounds, and encourage him to deep breathe and cough. To achieve this use a combination of a heated humidifier (such as an Aquapack® or Conchapak®) and nebulized salbutamol to loosen sputum. Postural drainage is sometimes necessary to help clear the mucus from the airway.

DIABETES[2]

Diabetes mellitus is a clinical syndrome characterised by raised blood glucose levels, caused by a deficiency, or lack of efficacy, of insulin. There are two broad groups of diabetics: Juvenile onset (Type 1) or *insulin dependent diabetes* (IDDM); and maturity onset (Type 2) or *non-insulin dependent diabetes* (NIDDM). Patient with NIDDM are usually elderly and obese. Check the blood glucose of all diabetics as soon as they are admitted to the recovery room.

Hypoglycaemia

Hypoglycaemia is a life threatening event which can cause permanent brain damage or even death. These life threatening events are unlikely to occur if the blood glucose concentration is greater than 2 mmol/l. Healthy patients experience symptoms when their blood glucose concentration is reduced below 2.5 mmol/l (30 - 45 mg/100 ml). Patients at risk of hypoglycaemia include: insulin dependent diabetics, alcoholics with liver disease, and neonates. Hypoglycaemia may also occur in non-insulin dependent diabetics, particularly if they are elderly or if they have been managed preoperatively with a long acting hypoglycaemic drug such as chlorpropamide.

Hypoglycaemia is more commonly seen in the recovery room if the patient has received a reduced dose of their morning insulin, and then been fasted for an afternoon operation.

Check the blood glucose,
in every patient at risk of hypoglycaemia.

Signs of hypoglycaemia include those of sympathetic stimulation: sweating, confusion, tachycardia, pallor and anxiety. These events may be difficult to detect in the patient recovering from anaesthesia. Untreated hypoglycaemia will progress, the patient will become difficult to arouse, then convulse, suffer irreversible brain damage and die. ß-blocking agents may mask the warning signs of hypoglycaemia by preventing the sympathetic discharge that accompanies a low blood glucose. They prevent the patient sweating, getting a tachycardia, or becoming anxious.

MANAGEMENT OF HYPOGLYCAEMIA

Every recovery room needs some means of measuring blood glucose, such as a portable glucometer. Measure the blood sugar with test strips or preferably a glucose meter. You must follow the manufacturer's instructions exactly to get accurate results. Also send a sample of blood to the laboratory for a formal measurement of blood glucose.

If the blood sugar is below 3 mmol/l give 20 mls of 50% glucose into a free flowing drip in large vein. Concentrated glucose irritates veins and will cause thrombophlebitis. You should see the patient's conscious state and well-being improve within 2 - 3 minutes. If you do not have concentrated glucose, then give 400 mls of 5% dextrose, initially. Repeat this in 5 minutes time. One litre of 5% dextrose contains 50 grams of glucose. Dextrose is the name used in the USA for glucose.

Hyperglycaemia

Hyperglycaemia is a blood glucose concentration raised above the normal range of 3.5 - 5.5 mmol/l. After an operation, a blood glucose concentration greater than 12 mmol/l is a sign of a physiologically stressed patient. Patients with hyperglycaemia are common in the recovery room. After major surgery a normal patient's blood glucose may rise to 15 - 18 mmol/l and remain at this level for 4 - 6 hours. In diabetics the blood glucose may rise much more. Uncontrolled pain can tip the balance in a diabetic patient causing hyperglycaemia and ketosis; this syndrome is called *diabetic ketoacidosis*. Diabetic ketoacidosis is a calamity after surgery because it can lead to hypovolaemic shock, arterial thrombosis, cardiac arrhythmias with pulmonary oedema, and even cerebral oedema.

A blood glucose concentration which is persistently elevated above 12 mmol/l may:
• cause an osmotic diuresis;
• delay wound healing;
• increase the risk of ischaemic brain damage and predispose to infection.

A carefully given anaesthetic, minimizing sympathetic stimulation, and a well planned recovery is unlikely to unbalance the diabetic. To prevent hyperglycaemia, a glucose and insulin infusion is usually started before the patient comes to the operating theatre.

MANAGEMENT OF HYPERGLYCAEMIA

If the patient's blood glucose is greater than 12 mmol/l then suspect a physiological stress; so control pain, check perfusion status and treat nausea and vomiting. In diabetic patients, give one unit of short acting insulin subcutaneously for every 10 kg of lean body mass. This dose can be repeated in 6 hours, but notify the physician so that control can be continued in the ward.

Sliding scales of insulin which depend on the amount of glucose in the urine are no longer recommended.

METABOLIC EFFECTS OF SURGERY IN A DIABETIC PATIENT

During and after surgery, a patient releases catecholamines including adrenaline in response to the stress. Adrenaline does four main things:

1. It breaks down glycogen in the liver and converts it to glucose, (glycolysis).
2. It accelerates the breakdown of fat tissue into free fatty acids, (lipolysis).
3. It increases the conversion of amino-acids to form glucose, (gluconeogenesis).
4. It inhibits the release of insulin from the cells in the pancreas.

Stress also causes the release of cortisol, growth hormone and glucagon; these hormones suppress the secretion of insulin. The overall effect is that glucose is released into the blood stream, while insulin secretion is being suppressed. As the stress subsides, a normal patient will secrete insulin. Insulin facilitates the transport of glucose into muscle cells. Diabetics cannot do this, and without insulin the blood glucose continues to rise; meanwhile the glucose starved muscle tissue breaks down protein to make more glucose.

INSULINS

Type	Brand	Onset (HOURS)	Peaks (HOURS)	Duration (HOURS)
Ultrashort	Humalog®	0.25	1	4 - 5
Short acting (regular)	Humulin R® Actrapid®	0.5	2 - 5	6 - 8
Intermediate acting	Monotard® Isophane® Protophane®	1 - 2.5	4 - 12	16 - 24
Mixed intermediate and short acting	Humulin® Mixtard 30/70® Mixtard 20/80®	0.5 - 1	2 - 12	16 - 24
Long acting	Humulin UL® Ultratard®	2 - 4	10 - 20	24 - 36

Hyperosmolar crisis

A complication of poor metabolic control of the diabetic patient is a non-ketotic hyperosmolar crisis. This can lead to coma in the postoperative diabetic patient. It presents as severe hyperglycaemia without ketoacidosis, which usually occurs in middle aged or elderly patients. As the blood sugar rises, serum osmolarity increases. The patient develops a high urine output. He becomes confused and obtunded. Signs appear when the blood glucose exceeds 25 mmol/l. You can check on the stability of the patient's diabetes over the last 2 - 3 months by the measuring the glycolysated haemoglobin level (HbA$_1$C). The normal value is 5 - 7.5 per cent; and a level of greater than 10 per cent indicates very poor control.

Aim to keep the blood glucose in the range of 5.5 - 11 mmol/l while the patient is in the recovery room.

USEFUL FACTS ABOUT DIABETES

- Dextrose is another name for glucose.
- Although insulin is adsorbed by glass, and some plastics, this is not significant enough to affect treatment when insulin is given in a intravenous infusion, or with a plastic syringe. It is not necessary to prime the IV tubing with glucose and insulin.
- One unit of regular insulin in a 70 – 80 kg stable diabetic lowers the blood glucose by about 1.5 mmol/l.
- 10 grams of glucose raises the blood sugar in a 70 – 80 kg patient by about 1.5 – 2 mmol/l.
- To convert mmol/l of glucose to mg/100 ml multiply by 18.
- The effects of subcutaneous soluble insulin starts in 30 minutes, reaches a peak in 2 – 4 hours and wears off in about 6 – 8 hours.
- Given intravenously soluble insulin has a half life of only about 5 minutes, and its effects disappears within about 30 minutes.

Long standing diabetics are at risk from many other problems including:
- renal vascular disease causing a decreased urine output;
- autonomic neuropathy causing postural hypotension, bradycardia and urinary retention;
- peripheral neuropathy may affect the pharyngeal muscles; and obstructive sleep apnoea is a particular hazard. Neither diabetics, nor any one else should be allowed to snore in the recovery room.

Autonomic neuropathy [2]

Diabetic patients are at great risk from coronary artery disease, hypertension, and *autonomic neuropathy*. Autonomic neuropathy may prevent the patient experiencing chest pain if the myocardium becomes ischaemic or infarction occurs. Monitor the ECG for developing ST depression, because this may be the only sign of myocardial ischaemia. Sometimes painless ischaemia makes the patient sweat, with nausea hypotensive and dyspnoeic.

A reliable sign that the patient has autonomic neuropathy is postural hypotension. Ask the patient if he normally feels unsteady when he stands up, or arising from his bed in the morning. In an affected patient, sit him up slowly and monitor his arterial pressure. If he becomes hypotensive or feels faint lie him down and check his perfusion status. He may require a colloid fluid load to restore his vascular volume.

DOWN'S SYNDROME [3]

Down's syndrome (mongolism is no longer an acceptable name) is a congenital disorder caused by the presence of three copies (trisomy) of chromosome 21, instead of the normal two. Patients have a lower intelligence than normal, and may become belligerent when frightened, especially if they are away from their usual surroundings and people they know and trust. Adult patients are often large and strong and may require restraint. The main risk is airway obstruction, particularly laryngospasm. Patients with Down's syndrome have large tongues, small mouths, and stiff necks. They tend to salivate excessively. Nurse them in the recovery position until they are conscious. They are at risk of extubation stridor, especially after long procedures. Give warmed humidified oxygen, and keep them in recovery room until they can deep breath and cough without distress. They sometimes have unstable atlanto-occipital joints. Be gentle when you extend their bull-necks, you could dislocate their cervical spine and render them quadraplegic. They are resistant to sedative drugs, but sensitive to opioids where a small dose can cause sedation. Forty per cent of these patients have associated congenital heart disease.

DRUG ADDICTS

Street addicts and intravenous drug abusers often have malnutrition and are in poor physical health. They have a high risk of carrying hepatitis and HIV. Universal precautions are your best protection against acquiring these diseases (see page 106).

Drug addicts often have thrombosed veins, and it is difficult to find sites to insert drips or take blood. Ask the patient where his best veins are, he will know.

Amphetamine and cocaine [4]

Amphetamine (Speed, Ecstasy or E), and cocaine stimulate the activity of the sympathetic (adrenergic) nervous system causing a state of hyper-alertness. because both these drugs displace nor-adrenaline from nerve ending, these patients are depleted of endogenous noradrenaline, and can become alarmingly hypotensive in the recovery room. They may require a noradrenaline infusion (see page 534) to restore and maintain their arterial pressure. Use phenylepherine or methoxamine as an interim measure if noradrenaline is not readily available.

Hypotension may also be a result of suppressed adrenal cortical function. If an addict becomes hypotensive, consider giving a dose of hydrocortisone to cover the stress of the period. Make sure the patient is volume replete, then give hydrocortisone succinate 100 mg intravenously. If the arterial pressure responds within a 5 - 20 minutes, maintenance hydrocortisone 100 mg 6 hourly will be needed. Refer them to a physician for further management.

Opioid addicts

Pain relief is best achieved with regional local anaesthetic techniques, but do not withhold opioids if pain relief is required. Recovering addicts may refuse an opioid. Active heroin addicts need higher than normal doses of opioid to achieve adequate pain relief. Be careful though, active addicts tend to overstate how much heroin they take. The street drugs are usually diluted with glucose or worse. Titrate morphine intravenously until the desired level of analgesia is achieved. Do not use partial opioid agonists such as pentazocine or nalbuphine which can precipitate acute withdrawal symptoms. Opioid withdrawal syndrome may occur for the first time in recovery room with sweating pallor and abdominal cramps. These signs can cause diagnostic confusion.

Some addicts are being treated with methadone. Check the methadone dose, and be prepared to substitute morphine if necessary. Initially give a quarter of their methadone dose, as morphine, slowly intravenously and watch for drowsiness and respiratory depression. For instance if a patient is taking 32 mg of methadone a day, start with 8 mg of morphine intravenously given over 10 minutes.

Opioid addicts may be slow to breathe postoperatively because their respiratory drive has been suppressed. This insensitivity to carbon dioxide persists for several months after their last 'fix'.

Benzodiazepines

Many, particularly elderly patients, have been taking one of the benzodiazepines such as nitrazepam (Mogadon®) or diazepam (Valium®) for many years. Sudden withdrawal of these drugs can cause unease, acute agitation or even convulsions. If the patient dependent on benzodiazepines becomes agitated while in the recovery room give a small dose of diazemuls.

Rarely, some patient are disinhibited by benzodiazepines, and may become aggressive, violent and confused. These patients are often aware of this problem from previous experience, and will have forewarned the medical staff. If this occurs, and either the patient or staff are at risk of injury as a result of the patient's rage, give ketamine 3 mg/kg into any available muscular area. This will rapidly render the patient catatonic. From then on you will need to manage the patient's coma as though they were under an anaesthetic. Give haloperidol 5 - 10 mg IV before the patient recovers from the ketamine.

EPILEPSY

Epilepsy is due to an unco-ordinated, spontaneous and uncontrolled discharge of neurones somewhere within the brain. The type of epilepsy on depends where in the brain the abnormality occurs. Epileptic patients may fit in the recovery room. This is more likely if they have not had their routine daily medication.

Drugs that can cause fitting are propofol, enflurane, methohexitone, pethidine and anticholinergic drugs. There have been a number of reports of patients developing fits within 48 hours of commencing pethidine infusions because of the toxicity of norpethidine, which is excreted only by the kidney. The total dose should not be more than 24 mg/kg/24 hr [5], and less if the patient has renal impairment. It is unwise to use pethidine in patients with renal failure.

Fitting may occur in a patient after a transurethral resection of their prostate (TURP) if water from the bladder irrigation enters the circulation.

Haemophilia

Haemophiliacs have generally been treated with *cryoprecipitate* (antihaemophilic globulin) before coming to the operating theatre. Fresh frozen plasma can be used as a substitute. They usually do not bleed immediately postoperatively, but may do so in the ward some hours later. Bleeding from superficial wounds although staunched by pressure, will resume when the pressure is released. Unfortunately many older haemophiliacs who were treated with blood products before 1985 have HIV, or before 1992 have hepatitis C, so take care with their body fluids.

Liver Disease

The liver is important for the metabolism of drugs and the maintenance of homeostasis. Hypoxia or acidosis is poorly tolerated in patients with liver disease, particularly if the patient is hypoglycaemic. Keep them well oxygenated, and maintain tissue perfusion if necessary with the support of an inotrope.

To avoid renal failure in jaundiced patients (*hepato-renal syndrome*) try to keep their urine output above 1 ml/kg/hr. Start with mannitol 1.5 gm/kg, and if needed add dopamine 3 - 5 microgram/kg/minute. Insert a urinary catheter to monitor the urine output.

Patients with liver disease metabolize most drugs slowly and their recovery may be prolonged. Use opioids with care as respiratory depression will aggravate their liver disease.

Spontaneous hypoglycaemia occurs without warning in patients with liver disease so check the patient's blood glucose on their admission to the recovery room. Suspect coagulation disorders in all patients with liver disease especially if they have prolonged bleeding from venous or arterial puncture sites.

Keep patients with liver disease warm. Shivering can rapidly deplete reduce muscle glycogen stores and predispose to hypoglycaemia.

Morphine can precipitate biliary pain in patients who have had a cholecystectomy. Use pethidine instead. NSAIDs, for example ketorolac gives good pain relief after laparascopic cholecystectomy but will be insufficient for an open operation.

Muscular Dystrophy[6]
and Musculo-Skeletal Disease

There are many types of muscular dystrophy, but dystrophia myotonica is the most common. It is inherited as an autosomal dominant trait. The symptoms first present in early adulthood with muscle weakness and the inability to release their grip quickly. Patients with muscular dystrophy are weak. They require smaller amounts of all anaesthetic agents than normal patients and because they have a low muscle mass they are very sensitive to muscle relaxant drugs. Keep a watch for signs of inadequate reversal of these drugs especially as neostigmine wears off after about 45 minutes (see page 441). You may need to give a second dose cautiously.

Neostigmine can make myotonia worse. Make sure the patient can sustain a head lift from the pillow for a minimum of five seconds, and that they have the capacity to deep breathe and cough before the anaesthetist leaves the recovery room. Where possible use regional blockade for pain relief. If opioids are needed use increments of about one-fifth of the estimated dose and watch for respiratory depression before repeating. Cardiomyopathy and cardiac conduction defects are common.

Patients with musculo-skeletal disease and myopathies are susceptible to malignant hyperthermia. This will present in the recovery room so monitor their temperature and watch for the signs of sweating, rising respiratory rate and tachycardia.

Thin atrophic skin and pressure sores or injuries are common. Be careful when moving these patients, not to drag them across the bed sheet, because of the risk of tearing their fragile skin.

Multiple Myelmatosis

Patients with multiple myeloma often have fragile vertebra and ribs. Be careful how you position and move them. The excessive protein they excrete can damage their kidneys, so keep their blood volume up, and do not allow them to become hypotensive or dehydrated. These patients have syrupy, protein laden plasma and are at risk from deep vein thrombosis. Prophylaxis depends mostly on adequate fluid replacement, and moving their legs around to prevent venous stasis. A low molecular weight heparin can be given and the use of compression stockings is recommended.

Neurofibromatosis
(Von Recklinhausen's Disease)

Patients with neurofibromatosis may have neurofibroma in their airway which cause stridor or upper airway sounds. Occasionally the patient also has undiagnosed phaeochromocytomas, and may become alarmingly hypertensive during anaesthesia or in the recovery room.

Neurological disease

The following neurological diseases all cause muscle weakness. This predisposes patients to respiratory tract infections, because they cannot cough effectively; and deep vein thrombosis, because they cannot move their legs readily. They are particularly susceptible to residual weakness following the use of muscle relaxants. Additionally their requirements for opioid drugs is about one-third less than unaffected patients.

Strokes

Patients with a history of stroke present a variety of problems in the recovery room. Depending on the type of dysfunction they may have:
- difficulty in coughing and deep breathing;
- problems in adjusting their position;
- inability to tell you if they are in pain, or have a full bladder.

It is helpful to make up a chart on a piece of white cardboard so that dysphasic patients can point to a symbol, or a picture which tells you they are in pain, want to empty their bladder, wish to move their position, would like to write something down, are too hot or too cold, and so forth.

Multiple sclerosis

The weakness of multiple sclerosis may be aggravated by regional anaesthesia[7]. These patients are predisposed to deep vein thrombosis and pulmonary embolism. Encourage stir-up exercises and leg movements in recovery room, as most thrombi start to form here. Compression stockings should have been fitted before their operation.

Myaesthenia gravis[8]

Patients with myasthenia gravis are at risk of respiratory difficulties in recovery room for two reasons. Firstly, their muscles are weak and they are not able to cough adequately enough to clear their mucus. Sputum blocks bronchi causing collapse of the lung. Secondly, neostigmine, used to improve their muscle power, may cause salivation, excessive bronchial secretions and bradycardia (the so-called *cholinergic crisis*). Treat these unpleasant side effects with atropine 0.6 - 1.2 mg intramuscularly.

Eaton-Lambert syndrome

Patients with carcinoma of the lung sometimes have *Eaton-Lambert syndrome* producing muscular weakness and causing respiratory distress. The patient may need to be re-intubated, supported on a ventilator and transferred to the intensive care unit. Other patients with dystrophica myotonia and familial periodic paralysis occasionally develop similar problems.

Diabetic neuropathy - see page 420

Quadraplegics

Pain and hypoxia may trigger autonomic hyperreflexia causing fulminating hypertension and cardiac arrhythmias. Once the hypertension is treated the arrhythmias usually resolve spontaneously.

OBESITY [9]

Obesity is a common health hazard, sufferers die early, and have many life threatening chronic diseases such as:

- peripheral vascular disease;
- heart disease;
- breathing problems;
- pulmonary disease;
- liver disease.

- diabetes mellitus;
- diaphragmatic hernias;
- hyperlipidaemias;
- polycythaemia;

Monitor the patient with an ECG, and pulse oximeter. Blood pressure cuffs rarely fit properly, consequently you cannot rely on their readings. Direct measurement of the blood pressure with an arterial line is useful if the patient has had major surgery. Oxygen consumption is increased, so give supplemental oxygen. Fat obscures anatomical surface landmarks and ECG dots are hard to place accurately. Intravenous lines are difficult to insert, so secure them well. Sometimes a central venous line will have been inserted in theatre. Make sure it is well secured, consider stitching the catheter to the skin.

> ## OBESITY
>
> Obesity is said to occur when a persons body weight is 10% over their ideal weight. The term morbid obesity applies to people more than twice their ideal body weight. Ideal height weight tables vary from place to place, so it is easier to calculate body mass index (BMI).
>
> $$BMI = \frac{weight\ (kg)}{height\ (m)^2}$$
>
> Normal   BMI < 25 kg/m²
>
> Overweight   BMI 25–30 kg/m²
>
> Obese   BMI > 30 kg/m²

Respiratory problems [10]

Large intrapulmonary blood shunts, poor compliance, and co-existing lung disease substantially increase the risk of hypoxia. Furthermore the muscular effort of just breathing is hard work, and uses lots of oxygen. These patient's breath with rapid short shallow breaths, characteristic of a restrictive respiratory disorder. Getting them to cough effectively is difficult. Incentive spirometry is a good way to help them expand their lungs.

Airway management is difficult in fat patients with bulky necks. There is a risk in using laryngeal masks in obese people, because they usually have hiatus hernias with oesophageal reflux, and may regurgitate and inhale (aspirate) their stomach contents. Do not wait until they start to vomit or regurgitate. Turn them on their sides as soon as possible. This is often difficult and you will need strong and capable help. If they come to the recovery room lying on their backs because there is no alternative, even if they are still intubated or with laryngeal masks, do not take out the laryngeal mask or tube until they are fully awake then sit them up at 45°.

Do not tilt obese patients head down. Nearly all obese patients have hiatus hernias. If they regurgitate or vomit while lying on their back and in a head down position they will almost certainly aspirate because you will not be able to move them on to their sides quickly enough.

Many anaesthetists give these patients prophylactic antacids and oral ranitidine 150 mg about 2 hours before the anaesthetic to lessen the risk of acid aspiration pneumonitis.

Nearly all obese patients have sleep apnoea syndrome. They get a bradycardia when they stop breathing and a tachycardia when they start again. These patients need constant attention to maintain an unobstructed airway. A nasopharyngeal airway often helps overcome obstruction caused by a floppy soft palate.

Severely morbidly obese patients may have the Pickwickian syndrome with chronic hypoxia and raised carbon dioxide levels causing pulmonary hypertension. Opioids will further depress their respiration so take special care if you give them.

Using drugs

Do not prescribe drugs on a dose per unit weight basis, because you will overdose the patient. Treat obese patients as thin people inside a fat body. Attempt to assess their lean body mass. An easy way to estimate this is to take the patients height in metres and centimetres and subtract the metres. For instance an average person 1.63 metres tall should weigh approximately 63 kg, while a patient of 1.84 metres tall would ideally weigh approximately 84 kg.

Avoid intramuscular injections in the grossly obese, because the needles may not be long enough to reach well perfused muscle, and the dose deposited in fat from where it will be poorly absorbed. Give analgesics intravenously. Pain relief is best achieved with regional blockade, but that is not always possible. Patient controlled analgesia with pethidine may be useful in these patients, but it is safer to avoid continuous opioid infusions.

Deep vein thrombosis

Obese patients are at risk from deep vein thrombosis and pulmonary emboli. Polycythaemia, immobility, heart failure, and increased intra-abdominal pressures which compress the vena cava make this risk worse. These patients should put on compression stockings before going to the theatre and be encouraged to move their legs in the recovery room. Low dose subcutaneous heparin is widely advocated to prevent deep vein thrombosis in obese patients. It does not require laboratory monitoring. The low molecular weight heparins such as dalteparin (Fragmin®) and enoxaparin (Clexane®) are as effective and safe as unfractionated heparin. In orthopaedic practice they are more effective than heparin.

Core hyperthermia

Although this is not a well known phenomenon, obese patients can become alarmingly hyperthermic. If they become stressed and a sympathetic discharge causes the blood vessels to the skin to constrict, they cannot dissipate heat from their hot core through the overlying fat. In the recovery room core hyperthermia may not be immediately obvious. The affected patient may have cool or cold skin, and poor peripheral perfusion. If his skin feels cold, but he is sweating slightly, or has a tachycardia suspect this problem. Check his core temperature. It requires vasodilator treatment in intensive care unit. The problem can be avoided with good analgesia.

Transport
Obese patients are best transported on their beds in a semi-sitting position (30° - 45°). This saves moving them on and off patient trolleys.

PAGET'S DISEASE

Paget's disease (osteogenesis imperfectans) is a slowly progressive disorder of unknown cause characterized initially by decalcification and softening of the bones in people over the age of 40 years. Paget's disease is easily missed on preoperative assessment. Classically the patients have a prominent forehead, and a prominent tibial ridge. The patients have a high cardiac output, which if depressed with ß-blockers, or other cardiac depressants jeopardises their tissue oxygen supply. Blood loss can be quite overwhelming after orthopaedic surgery, so be prepared for this. Their oxygen requirements are high, because they shunt blood from their arteries to their veins through sinuses in their bones, bypassing the tissues. Continue supplemental oxygen in the ward.

PARKINSON'S DISEASE

Parkinson's disease (paralysis agitans) is a neurotransmitter disorder of the basal ganglia characterised by muscle rigidity, tremor and slowness of intentional movement. These patients are often treated with L-dopa. As their sympathetic nerve endings are packed full of noradrenaline, which can be released by a trivial stimulus, they may develop arrhythmias or hypertension on emerging from anaesthesia. Monitor them with an ECG, and be prepared to use a ß-blocker, such as metoprolol, to control tachyarrhythmias. Use phentolamine intravenously in 1 mg increments to control a rapid rise in arterial pressure. This drug acts quickly and its effect lasts about 4 - 7 minutes. This will give time for you to set up either a nitroprusside or labetalol infusion.

Peptic Ulceration

Pre-existing peptic ulceration may be exacerbated by the stress of surgery. Over the perioperative period, use one or more of the following: prophylactic H_2 antagonists (for example ranitidine), a prostaglandin mediator (misoprostol), a surface covering agent (sucraflate) or a proton pump inhibitor (omeprazole). Avoid non-steroidal anti-inflammatory drugs (NSAIDs) for pain relief because they exacerbate ulcers.

Phaeochromocytoma

These tumours secrete catecholamines, and most secrete noradrenaline. The main problem in recovery room is hypotension secondary to an inadequate circulating volume. If the tumour has been active for more than a few months the continual adrenergic cardiac stimulation can cause a cardiomyopathy. Ventricular dysrhythmias are common and will respond to ß-blockers and lignocaine. The patient may require ionotropic support with dopamine or even noradrenaline in recovery room

Uncommonly, a patient may come to surgery with an unsuspected phaemochromocytoma. During the anaesthetic hypertension, sweating, pallor and palpations are the traditional signs. In the recovery room, the patient will require ß-blockade and nitroprusside to control his blood pressure.

Porphyria

These are a family of diseases of inborn errors in the synthesis of haem, the porphyrin unit of haemoglobin. The precursors of haem poison many organs causing: acute abdominal pain, vomiting, neuropathies, epilepsy, psychiatric disturbance and even coma. There are three acute hepatic porphyrias, all of which can be triggered by anaesthetic drugs especially barbiturates. Other drugs causing problems include anticonvulsants and alcohol. Porphyria is an unusual problem to present in recovery room, but consider it in patients who develop symptoms after receiving thiopentone.

Psychiatric Disorders

Some psychiatric patients become acutely disturbed in recovery room. If necessary sedate them with haloperidol 5 - 10 mg intravenously. Always exclude hypoxia and hypoglycaemia. For retarded or mentally handicapped patients it is helpful to have someone the patient trusts available to be with them when they awaken from their anaesthetic.

Many drugs used in psychiatry interact with analgesics and anaesthetic agents. These include selective seritonin re-uptake inhibitors (SSRIs), monamine oxidase inhibitors (MAOIs) and tricyclic antidepressant agents (TCAs).

The selective seritonin re-uptake inhibitors are used for major depressive illness. They are metabolized by the liver. SSRI drugs include: fluoxetine (Prozac®), sertraline (Zoloft®), venlafaxine (Effexor®), paroxetine, fluvoxamine, and citalopram. Pethidine and fentanyl may precipitate the seritonin syndrome by displacing the drug from its binding site in the brain.

Seritonin syndrome is characterized by progressive changes in mental state, motor activity and autonomic instability. Problems include agitation, disorientation, rigidity, myoclonus and hyperreflexia, tachycardia, sweating, hypertension, cardiac arrhythmias and even coma. Control autonomic instability with ß-blockers. Fortunately the problem usually resolves within a few hours. It is probably better to avoid benzodiazepines (eg. diazepam or midazolam), and butyrephenones (haloperidol, droperidol) in patients taking SSRIs and in particular fluoxetine, setraline and fluvoxamine.

Monoamine oxidase inhibitors (MAOIs) are used for life threatening depressive illnesses. These drugs delay the metabolism of seritonin (5HT), adrenaline, noradrenaline, and dopamine. They are not widely used because they interact dangerously with a wide variety of drugs and foods. Tranylcypromine (Parnate®) and phenelzine (Nardil®) are the most commonly used of the older long acting MAOI drugs. If you use pethidine within two weeks of the last dose of these drugs, you may precipitate the seritonin syndrome. A number of deaths have occurred from this complication. Indirect acting vasopressors, such as metaraminal and ephedrine will also precipitate fulminating hypertension.

Moclobemide (Aurorix®) is a newer short-acting MAO inhibitor which increases synaptic concentrations of seritonin, noradrenaline and dopamine, It has a short clinical action, and wears off after 18 hours. Provided the patient has stopped taking moclobemide 24 hours before surgery it should cause no problems in the recovery room.

PULMONARY DISEASE

(SEE ALSO ASTHMA PAGE 412 AND COAD PAGE 415)

The patient's position affects ventilation and perfusion of their lungs.[11] If the patient is on a ventilator, the non-dependent areas of the lung are better ventilated; but if the patient is breathing spontaneously, the dependent areas are better ventilated, which increases gas exchange. In recovery room sit patients up and lean them toward the side of their good lung.

Renal Disease (SEE PAGE 133)

Rheumatoid arthritis

Rheumatoid arthritis is a multisystem immunological disorder affecting joints and connective tissue in the body. It affects 2 per cent of men, and 5 per cent of women over the age of 65. Patients with rheumatoid arthritis are more susceptible to opioid induced respiratory depression than normal people.[12] They are more prone to respiratory obstruction in the recovery room, and especially to sleep apnoea. They have stiff necks and brittle bones, so be careful when turning them or transferring them from the trolley to the bed. They often have thin, atrophic skin which tears easily, and can rip off as you remove adhesive dressings. Similarly their veins are fragile, so make sure drip cannulas cannot move up and down in the veins. They often have joint destruction, so be careful, when inserting or removing airways. Take especial care not to over-extend their lower jaw.

Rheumatic joints means fragile cervical spine.
Take care when moving their head or neck.

Hypothermia may become a problem. Pulmonary fibrosis inflicts a restrictive lung disorder on these patients, so they tend to have a higher resting respiratory rate than normal people, and find it difficult to cough or deep breathe effectively. Chronic anaemia can contribute to tissue hypoxia.

Steroids

Some patients will be receiving long term steroid therapy for rheumatoid arthritis, polymyalgia rheumatica, Wegner's granulomatosis and a host of other chronic inflammatory diseases. These patients will require extra hydrocortisone support during the stress phase of their injury. Adrenal suppression caused by systemic steroids lasts for many months after the last dose of a long course of steroids. It is important to check if the patient has had long term systemic steroids therapy in the past.

Postoperative patients with adrenal suppression may need up to 500 mg hydrocortisone a day for the first 4 or 5 days after surgery, or as long as the stress phase of injury goes on. Use hydrocortisone 100 mg IV, 6 hourly.

Adrenocortical reserves are diminished in:
- Addison's disease either treated or untreated;
- after bilateral adrenalectomy;
- following steroid therapy in the past year or so;
- pituitary ablation.

> *No patient should be allowed to die of refractory hypotension without a large dose of hydrocortisone.*

SICKLE CELL SYNDROMES [13]

Sickle cell disease is a genetic disease characterized by abnormal sickle shaped red cells and caused by altered amino-acid sequences in the haemoglobin molecule. The abnormal red cells may clog capillaries causing tissue infarcts, and haemolyse releasing haemoglobin into the circulation. Suspect sickle cell trait in African negroid people. *Sickle cell trait (HbAS)* occurs in 25 percent of negroid patients and those from the malaria belt of Africa, Central America and around the Mediterranean Sea. *Sickle cell disease (HbSS)* occurs in 4 percent of negroid people.

At oxygen tensions below 60 - 70 mmHg (8 - 9.3 kPa) haemoglobin molecules deform and destroy the red cell. Multiple organ and tissue infarcts occur as the deformed red cells clog the microcirculation. Susceptible patients characteristically have large livers and spleens, but minimal jaundice. A *sickle cell crisis* can be triggered by a tourniquet or even applying an arterial blood pressure cuff. A *haemolytic crisis* can precipitate renal failure; particularly in the presence of sepsis.

Patients with the full disease (HbSS) usually undergo a series of exchange transfusions before their operation to reduce the number abnormal circulating red cells. Never let these patient become hypoxic or acidotic. Keep their inspired oxygen high, keep them warm and ensure their perfusion status is good. Beware if they show signs of poor peripheral perfusion. They require early replacement of blood loss and maintenance of a good cardiac output. Monitor them with a pulse oximeter while they are in the recovery room. To guarantee red cell oxygenation they should return to the ward and remain on oxygen for 8 hours, in the case of the sickle cell trait (HbAS), and for 48 hours in the case of the full disease (HbSS).

SMOKERS

Elderly smokers are usually arteriopaths with ischaemic heart, and peripheral vascular disease.

Adverse effects of smoking include:
- increased airways resistance making them wheeze;
- excessive sputum production;
- tracheobronchial ciliary paralysis delaying the clearance of sputum and predisposing to pneumonia;
- polycythaemia with increased blood viscosity increasing the work of the heart and predisposing to myocardial ischaemia;
- increased incidence of coronary heart disease predisposing to postoperative myocardial ischaemia;
- elevated carbon monoxide levels reducing the oxygen carried by haemoglobin andpredisposing the patients to occult hypoxia. The effect lasts many hours after their last cigarette;[14]
- An increase in heart rate, systolic and diastolic arterial pressure and peripheral vasoconstriction caused by nicotine predisposes to cardiac ischaemia.[15] The vasoconstriction can persist for up to 24 hours after the last cigarette;
- enzyme induction increasing analgesic requirements.

Monitor smokers closely in the recovery room. They often cough uncontrollably especially after bronchoscopy. The anaesthetist may have sprayed the throat during the procedure. Persistent cough can often be controlled by lignocaine 1 - 1.5 mg/kg intravenously as a bolus.[16]

On the other hand some older smokers will make no effort to cough postoperatively. They seem oblivious of the sputum rattling in their airways, or are unable to muster the lung reserve to cough it free. These patients are likely to suffer partial lung collapse and pneumonia. Encourage them to deep breathe and cough. Use a laryngoscope to clear the sputum from the upper airway. If possible use intercostal blocks or regional blockade for pain relief. Morphine will depress the desire to cough, and pethidine dries out the sputum making it thick, tenacious and difficult to expectorate.

THYROID DISEASE

Hypothyroidism
Up to 10 percent of elderly women are hypothyroid to some degree, and many will be already taking supplemental thyroxine (Oroxine®). Severe

hypothyroidism causes myxoedema, a syndrome that characteristically presents as an apparently oedematous, slow thinking, slow moving elderly person with coarse , dry hair, podgy features and a large tongue. They have low metabolic rates, some less than 60 percent of normal, and consequently feel the cold readily.

Not all hypothyroid patients have myxoedema, and the diagnosis can be easily be overlooked during the pre-anaesthetic work up. Patients with unsuspected hypothyroidism may undergo anaesthesia and return to the recovery room comotose, cold and bradycardic. They will emerge very slowly from the anaesthetic. Hypothyroid patients are often anaemic making them susceptible to postoperative hypoxia. Muscle relaxants are difficult to reverse. All drugs are metabolized slowly. Normal doses of opioids may profoundly depress respiration and consciousness Hypothyroid patients are best managed in intensive care following surgery.

Hyperthyoidism

Although not as common as hypothyroidism, excess production of thyroxine has a five fold greater incidence in females. Patients with an over active thyroid gland, presenting for elective thyroidectomy, must be well controlled with ß-blockers and anti-thyroid agents before coming to theatre Significant disease is invariably accompanied by a tachycardia, which may overflow into atrial fibrillation. Clinically, it is usually obvious. In the frail, elderly patient the diagnosis may be missed because many very old people are thin, demented, and have atrial fibrillation. Undiagnosed, these patients may develop uncontrollable tachyarrhythmias, myocardial ischaemia and die during or immediately after their operation. Treat the tachyarrhythmias with ß-blockers, and avoid catecholamines when treating hypotension.

Patients with undiagnosed hyperthyroidism can develop ventricular tachycardia or atrial fibrillation in the recovery room. Suspect this as a diagnoses if the patient has a pre-operative resting pulse rate greater than 100 beats per minute.

Von Willebrand's Disease (PSEUDO HAEMOPHILIA)

Patients with von Willebrand's disease (vWD) have defective platelet adhesiveness and a factor VIII deficiency. Excessive bleeding may be controlled by tranexamic acid which inhibits plasminogen activation and fibrinolysis. Desmopressin (DDVAP®) is often given before surgery and may make the patient pale and nauseated. Cryoprecipitate can be used to help control bleeding if necessary. Patients with von Willebrand's disease who are surgically stressed often have other changes in their blood that make them clot more readily than normal. In patients with vWD postoperative bleeding usually reveals itself in the recovery room, whereas patients with other clotting deficiencies bleed some hours later. Control superficial bleeding by direct pressure. When taking the arterial pressure do not to leave the cuff inflated, otherwise a shower of purpura will occur all over their arm.

1. Jones ME (1989). *Anaesthesia and Intensive Care*, 17:253-63.
2. Ravcoles M, Grimaud D, (1996). *Current Opinion in Anesthesiology*, 9:247-53.
3 Powell JF. (1990). *Anaesthesia*, 45: 1049-51.
4. Cheng DC (1996). *Current Opinions in Anesthesiology*, 9: 259-62.
5. Stone, McIntyre, *et al.* (1993). *British Journal of Anaesthesia*, 71:738-40.
6. Smith CL, Bush GH. (1985). *British Journal of Anaesthesia*, 57:1113-8.
7. Alderson JD. (1991). *Anaesthesia*, 45:1084.
8. Baraka A. (1992). *Canadian Journal of Anaesthesia*, 39:1002-3.
9. Shankman Z, Shir Y. (1993). *British Jopurnal of Anaesthesia*, 70:349-59.
10. Pasulka PS, Bistrian BR, *et al.* (1986). *Annals of Internal Medicine*, 104:540-6.
11. Gillespie D, Rehder K. (1987). *Chest*, 9: 25-9.
12. Gardner DL, Holmes F. (1961). *British Journal of Anaesthesia*, 33:258-64.
13. Galloway SJ, Harwood-Nuss AL. (1988). *Journal of Emergency Medicine*, 6:213-16.
14. Tait AR, Kyff JV, *et al.* (1990). *Canadian Journal of Anaesthesia*, 37:423-8.
15. Egan TD, Wong KC. (1992). *Journal of Clinical Anesthesiology*, 4:63-72.
16. Gefke K, Andersen LW. (1983). *Acta Anaesthesia Scandinavia*, 27:111-12.

23. PROBLEMS IN THE RECOVERY ROOM

This chapter covers the day to day problems encountered in recovery room,[1] and not covered elsewhere in the book. These may be major like uncontrollable emergence behaviour or minor like dry eyes. Some problems begin as minor like snoring, and become life threatening if not dealt with, like obstructed airway. Be prepared for problems to develop into emergencies. Have protocols for resuscitation up on your wall and practise life saving drills during your quiet times.

AGITATION AND CONFUSION

This section will also cover emergence delirium and the violent patient. Delirium is sometimes called *acute brain syndrome*. The patients become agitated or bewildered and need restraint on emerging from anaesthesia. The patient appears to have perceptual difficulties, not knowing where he is or what is going on. Incoherent speech, disorientation and a clouded consciousness are other features. He may well know his name and even respond to it but he remains confused.

The commonest causes of agitation and delirium are:
• hypoxia this can maim or kill so exclude it first;
• a full bladder in the presence of sedative drugs;
• hypoglycaemia;
• ketamine;
• pain.

Of all the causes of confusion, hypoxia, and hypoglycaemia are the most serious, they can irreversibly damage the brain within minutes. Assume all confused patients are hypoxic. Give oxygen while you attempt to diagnose the cause. Even transient hypoxia at some time in the perioperative period will later cause a prolonged period of postoperative confusion, especially in the elderly. Proving a patient is not hypoxic, or has not had a period of hypoxia, is very difficult. Blood gases and pulse oximetry, although reassuring my not be sufficient to provide this. Read more about hypoxia on (page 295).

> *The confused restless and agitated*
> *patient is hypoxic until proved otherwise.*

The cause of agitation may not be clear; but psychological factors, that occur with operations threatening body image (for example amputations) aggravate the problem.

Factors predisposing to agitation and delirium include:

- youth;
- drug or alcohol abusers;
- amputations;
- mastectomy;
- heart surgery;
- anxiety;
- intraoperative awareness;
- intraoperative hypoxia, hypotension;
- intraoperative cholinergic drugs;
- tricyclic antidepressants.

MANAGEMENT

1. Give 100% oxygen.

2. Give reassurance and orientation to time and place.

3. Restrain the patient as necessary. Be aware of hospital policy and if necessary consult security personnel.

4. Avoid sedation if possible.

5. Treat the cause, if identifiable.

6. Notify the anaesthetist.

THE VIOLENT PATIENT

Occasionally a patient will warn you that they have been violent on emerging from a previous anaesthetic. Take this warning seriously, because you could be confronted with a violent patient who is a danger to himself, or the staff. If you have no intravenous access give ketamine 1.5 mg/kg I/M. It is rapidly absorbed from most sites. This will rapidly bring the patient under control, making him comatose. Then support his airway, and treat him as a comatose patient. Allow him to emerge after giving him haloperidol 5 – 10 mg I/M.

ALLERGY

Give all intravenous drugs cautiously and slowly. Watch for signs of allergy, these are: urticaria, oedema, respiratory distress, nausea and vomiting, and hypotension. The treatment for allergic reactions is adrenaline. Give this immediately intramuscularly, subcutaneously or intravenously.

> < 50 kg give   0.25 ml   1/1000 adrenaline.
>
> 50 - 100 kg give   0.5 ml   1/1000 adrenaline.
>
> > 100 kg give   0.75 ml   1/1000 adrenaline.

Children: use 1/10 000 adrenaline and give 0.25 ml/year of age.

Penicillin allergy

Many patients state that they 'allergic to penicillin'. Often this statement is accepted without question by the medical and nursing staff. Once labelled as 'allergic to penicillin', they can be denied this life saving group of drugs in an emergency. Closer questioning often reveals that they do not have a true allergy, but that they felt 'sick after the tablet', or 'it upset their stomach', or 'the injection hurt' , or some other non-allergic response. True allergy is marked by urticarial rash, wheeze and tissue oedema.

Give all intravenous drugs cautiously and slowly. Use a test dose and watch for signs of allergic response. These are urticaria, respiratory distress, plushing and hypotension. The treatment for allergic reactions is adrenaline. Give this immediately intravenously, intramuscularily or subcutaneous.

Also give an antihistamine such as promethazine 25 - 50mg I/M (children 0.5 - 1.0 mg/kg) and hydrocortisone 100 - 500mg I/M or IV (children 2 - 4 mg/kg).

AWARENESS

Estimates of the incidence of awareness vary from 0.2 per cent to 0.9 per cent.[2] The experience of awareness varies from a fleeting impression of voices to an unpleasant sensation of real pain. Those who experience awareness also vary, from those who are mildly interested and not upset, to those who will go straight to lawyers and sue.

Awareness is especially common after Caesarean section. Patients who have been warned that their anaesthesia will be light in the best interests of the baby are usually calm and accepting. You will have the occasional patient who is distressed, crying and fearful. Some have been confused and unable to say what is wrong.

If the patient tells you she has been aware, do not dismiss her claim. Notify the anaesthetist and do your best to allay anxiety. Carefully record in the notes what you see and can measure, not your opinions. The anaesthetist and a senior colleague should take an accurate witnessed written record of the patient's claims and organise a series of consultations. The patient may need treatment for *post traumatic stress disorder* (PTSD).[3]

Patients who remember their stay in recovery room sometimes complain about this afterwards. The commonest complaint is "Something must have gone wrong, I woke up in pain and they had to give me oxygen" This *pseudo-awareness* can be avoided if patients are warned preoperatively that they will receive oxygen in recovery room.

BRUISING

If you do not apply firm pressure to a puncture wound after you withdraw the needle the patient will get a bruise. Venipunctures stop bleeding after one minute of firm pressure. Do not just tape a piece of cotton wool over the site and assume the job is done. Underneath the cotton wool a hidden painful haematoma will develop. Arterial punctures must receive firm pressure for at least 5 minutes, timed by the clock. It is worth checking the site again after another 5 minutes as well.

CHEST PAIN

Causes of chest pain include:
- angina (see page 277);
- pneumothorax (see page 333);
- air emboli (see page 335);
- pulmonary emboli (see page 336);
- trauma during surgery (in one case it was the assistant's elbow resting on the chest while holding a retractor).

CRYING PATIENTS

Occasionally patients sob when emerging from anaesthesia. Often they do not know why they are crying. It does not necessarily mean they are in pain. It is sometimes a sign that they have been aware during their operation. Unpremedicated patients and those who have been anaesthetised for a short procedure are more likely to cry, especially if the procedure is for a sad reason like an abortion. Patients with anxiety or depression are more likely to cry as well, as are children and elderly demented patients.

DEAFNESS

To help your deaf patients orient themselves put their hearing aids back even before they are conscious. Take your mask off so the patient can read your lips. Do not shout. Warn staff not to use painful stimuli if the patient does not respond to verbal stimuli. Sometimes a pen and paper can be useful.

If nitrous oxide was used during surgery patients with previous middle ear reconstruction may suffer from pressure changes causing transient loss of hearing. All patients with a bandage over their ear, will be relatively deaf, even after minor surgery.

Deafness has occured after spinal anaesthesia. A loss of 10 decibels or more has been recorded in 3.7 per 1000 cases.[4]

DEATH IN THE RECOVERY ROOM

From time to time a patient will die in the recovery room. Carefully document the events leading up to the death and the resuscitation attempts for medico-legal reasons. As these notes could be required by the coroner or in court it is important to record fact only. Give sufficient detail so there is no need to rely on memory, even years later.

Staff involved in a death will be upset, especially if the patient was young, or the death perceived as avoidable, they may require counselling. Have protocols ready to cope with the death of a patient. You will need guidelines about how to inform relatives, who is to be present at this interview and where the interview is to be held. It is important that senior medical staff initially tell the patient's relatives, telephone them and ask them to come to the hospital, simply informing them that there has been a problem. Suggest they bring someone with them. Many medico-legal and litigatory problems can be avoided if this difficult task is done in a humane, honest and sensible manner by the senior staff responsible for the patient. Litigation usually arises when the relatives believe they are being deceived.

DELAYED EMERGENCE AND REVERSAL

Sometimes patients take a long time to wake up and fully emerge from their anaesthetic. The reasons for this are:

1. Incomplete reversal of relaxant drugs.
2. Prolonged action of other anaesthetic drugs.
3. Metabolic causes.
4. Brain damage.

1. Incomplete reversal of relaxant drugs

Residual effects of muscle relaxants given during the anaesthetic sometimes persist to create problems in the recovery room. Check with the anaesthetist, he may not have given reversal. Signs of incomplete reversal are jerky floppy movements of the arms. The patient may have drooping eyelids, and use his eyebrows in an attempt to open his eyes. He will probably have double vision. His ventilatory effort will be poor, and his breathing rapid and shallow. He won't be able to cough effectively, and may panic because he feels that he is suffocating. *Tracheal tug* is seen when the patient does not have enough strength to breathe properly, and uses the strap muscles in his neck to assist the weakened respiratory muscles. You can feel his larynx jerk down every time he breathes in.

He will be unable to sustain a 5 second head lift. To test his grip, ask him to squeeze your hand, offer him two fingers. Postoperative residual curarization increases the risk of aspiration pneumonitis and contributes to postoperative respiratory failure. It can cause panic and cardiovascular stress, and may result in hypoxia and hypoventilation.

Causes of the prolonged effects of the muscle relaxants are:
- overdose of muscle relaxant drug;
- delayed metabolism or excretion due to hypothermia, renal or liver impairment;
- abnormal cholinesterase prolonging the effects of suxamethonium (*suxamethonium apnoea*);
- intercurrent disease, such as myasthenia gravis, motor neurone disease or myopathy;
- carcinoma or alcoholism giving rise to abnormal sensitivity to muscle relaxants.

Diagnosis
- If the patient is still unconscious, check the return of muscle power with a nerve stimulator;
- the other most useful test of adequate muscle power is the 5 second sustained head lift. If a patient can do this he will be able to look after his own airway.

MANAGEMENT
1. Reassure the patient. Remain beside his head at all times.
2. Give high concentrations of oxygen through a face mask, assist ventilation with a bag and mask if necessary.
3. Attach an ECG and pulse oximeter.

4. Notify the anaethetist.
5. Give one dose of neostigmine 1.25mg and atropine 0.3mg, or better, give this 'half dose' of neostigmine and atropine and wait for 5 minutes. It may be necessary to use the 'other half' but:

Consider the complications before using further neostigmine. Neostigmine can increase peristalsis and disrupt intestinal surgical anastomoses. It can also cause bronchorrhoea and bradycardia, and it has some muscle relaxing properties of its own.

Do not allow the patient to struggle on. The safest option, if simple measures do not reverse the relaxation, is to intubate, sedate and ventilate until the drugs have had time to wear off.

2. Prolonged action of other anaesthetic drugs

In some patients metabolism and excretion of drugs given during anaesthesia is slow. Do not use painful stimuli in an attempt to hurry the process. Droperidol and diazepam have a prolonged sedating effect, check the notes to see if these have been given in the preoperative period.

Drug interactions may be responsible, for example erythromycin prolongs the action of midazolam for many hours.[5]

Naloxone will reverse opioids. Proceed cautiously, consider the consequence of catapulting the patient into agonizing pain.

Flumazenil (Anexate®) will reverse the actions of benzodiazepines. It only works for about 35 minutes, so may need repeating. The dose is 3 - 5 microgram/kg over 15 seconds and repeat at 60 second intervals to a maximum dose of 40 microgram/kg. (In susceptible individuals this drug can cause convulsions.)

3. Metabolic causes

Hypothermia, hypoventilation, hepatic and renal dysfunction all delay the metabolism and excretion of drugs.

4. Brain damage

A serious complication and cause of delayed emergence from anaesthesia is neurological damage, caused by hypoxia, stroke, fat or air embolism, or intraoperative hypotension. Water overload after prostate surgery or uterine endoscopic procedures, can cause coma or hemiparesis. Consider occult head injury or alcohol poisoning in trauma patients who are slow to wake up.

Some of these conditions are treatable. Check the blood sugar and temperature. To treat water overload (see page 126). A stroke after carotid surgery requires immediate re-operation.

EXTRAVASATION AND ARTERIAL INJECTION

Some drugs are toxic to the tissues, and if they extravasate during an intravenous infusion they cause tissue death. If there is any pain at the site of an infusion, take it out and re-site it elsewhere.

Extravasated adrenergic drugs, such as adrenaline, dopamine, noradrenaline and isoprenaline cause intense vasocontriction. They should only be given centrally or into a large, rapidly flowing catheter. If they leave the vein during injection the surrounding muscle and skin become ischemic and die. The results can be horrific, with muscle, skin and tendon necrosis requiring disfiguring and destructive debridement.

Dilute phentolamine 10mg in 10ml of normal saline. Inject the dilute phentolamine in 1ml boluses around, and into the area of the extravasation. Watch the blood pressure because phentolamine causes hypotension.

Extravasation of drugs such as bicarbonate, potassium containing solutions, calcium chloride and some antibiotics cause similar problems. Keep the needle in place and inject saline into the area to dilute the drug. Apply warm (40° C) compresses to dilate the vessels serving the area. Block the nerves to the region with local anaesthetic to provide analgesia and improve tissue perfusion.

Accidental injection of a substance into an artery usually occurs when intravenous injections are attempted in the antecubital fossa, but it may occur anywhere, even on the back of the hand. After inserting a needle check to see that bright red blood does not pulse back. If something harmful has been injected down the line the patient will often complain of severe pain. In which case do not withdraw the needle, remove the syringe and replace it with a fresh syringe containing normal saline. Flush and then inject procaine 0.2 ml/kg. It may be necessary to perform a brachial plexus block, or a stellate ganglion block if the hand or arm turns white, although the results of these manoeuvres are disappointing. Phentolamine 1 mg made up to 10 ml in normal saline may be injected slowly to vasodilate the limb. This can be repeated, and the option of an continuous arterial infusion considered. Consult a vascular surgeon. For medicolegal reasons keep careful notes of what has happened, and what has been done, and by whom.

EYES

Red eyes

Unconscious patients do not blink. It only takes a few seconds for ulcers to form once the cornea drys out. Keep an unconscious patient's eyelids closed. Use a lubricating ointment such as methyl cellulose (Lacrilube®) to protect the eyes of a comatose patient. Do not use chloramphenicol ointment, because of the slight risk of bone marrow supression, and the nuisance of local irritation.

Sore, dry or gritty eyes occur if they have been open during the operation. If the patient complains of this, make a note about whether his eyes were taped shut during the operation, and which ointment, if any, was used. If you are concerned then stain the affected eye with fluorescein to reveal corneal or scleral damage. Irrigate the eye with saline, tape it shut and refer it to an ophthalmologist.

Foreign Bodies

When plaster of paris is used to splint fractured noses, fragments can easily enter the eyes. Gently wash these out.

Pupils

The oval pupil is a sign of early brainstem compression. The fixed unilateral dilated pupil is a sign of severe brainstem compression. If this develops after neurosurgery, notify the neurosurgeon and the anaesthetist immediately.

A unilateral contricted pupil on the affected side occurs in Horner's syndrome. *Horner's syndrome* is seen when the cervical sympathetic nerves are paralysed after surgery on the neck or thorax, or after spinal, epidural or brachial plexus anaesthetic blocks.

Dilated pupils occur with:
• hypoxia;
• severe head injury, a sign of poor prognosis;
• homotropine, used in eye surgery to dilate pupils.

Pin point pupils occur with:
• pilocarpine eye drops, used for the treatment of glaucoma;
• narcotic overdose;
• pontine (brainstem) haemorrhage.

Irregular pupils are sometimes seen for a few minutes after anaesthesia with volatile agents. If you test the patient's plantar reflexes at this time, you will find they are upgoing. This phenomenon lasts only about 10 minutes. These signs can also occur with hypoxic brain damage (low pressure cerebral oedema).

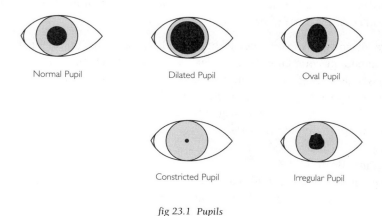

fig 23.1 Pupils

Trauma

Surgical instruments have been known to rest or even be dropped on the eye during surgery. If this occurs notify an ophthalmologist, even if the damage appears minimal. He will examine the fundus with an ophthalmoscope. There may be medico-legal consequences.

Pressure on the eye from an anaesthetic mask can cause retinal haemorrhages and detachment. Diabetic patients are especially at risk. Hypertensive anaesthesia has also caused vitreous haemorrhages.

Drugs

In susceptable patients atropine, glycopyrrolate, ketamine and trimetephan can precipitate acute closed-angle glaucoma. It presents with agonisingly painful red eye, corneal clouding and a dilated pupil. The vision goes fuzzy, and the patient may become nauseated and vomit. This event is an emergency, and if not treated promptly the patient will go blind. If you suspect acute glaucoma start acetazolamide 10mg/kg intravenously, and an infusion of 3ml/kg of 20% mannitol. Call an ophthalmologist for help.

Blindness

- Rarely, transient blindness occurs after transurethral resection of the prostate (see page 79);
- retinal haemorrhages caused by pressure from the mask can go on to blindness;
- epidural injection can cause blindness[6].

Cataracts (see page 61)

FINGERNAILS

If a patient has long fingernails and lies on her hands the pressure from the nails can ulcerate the skin. This can happen surprisingly quickly in comatose patients.

HAIR

Coagulated dry blood occasionally remains in the hair after head and neck surgery. Dried blood is hard to get out, and putrifies if it is left. Wash and comb the hair with aqueous cetrimide being careful not to get it in the eyes. Rinse with ample water.

HEADACHE

Headache occurs in 10 - 30 per cent of patients particularly after minor surgery. Those people who suffer from frequent tension headaches are more prone to get them postoperatively. Place a cool wet towel on the forehead. Start with simple analgesics, such as paracetamol 500 - 1000 mg. If the patient cannot take oral medication, use paracetamol supositories. Pethidine 0.5 - 1mg/kg is a stonger alternative, but avoid morphine which can aggravate headaches.

Other causes of headaches include:
- intraoperative tension on neck muscles or cervical spine joints;
- spinal headache, after epidural or spinal analgesia, especially after spinal tap;
- underventilation;
- hypoxia;
- caffeine withdrawal;
- severe hypertension;
- water intoxication (see page 126);

- opioids, especially morphine;
- intraoperative hypotension or hypoxia;
- bright fluorescent light.

HICCUPS

Hiccups frequently occur after laparoscopy, or more rarely after abdominal procedures when the operation has been close to the diaphragm. Usually they respond to gentle sucking out of the pharynx. If hiccups persist, metoclopromide 5 - 10 mg intravenously, or ephidrine 5 mg intravenously may help. Sometimes hiccups resist treatment. In the past chlorpromazine has been used but it is inappropriate, it doesn't work, and it causes prolonged sedation and hypotension.

HOARSE VOICE

A hoarse or croaky voice is more likely in patients who have been intubated for some hours. The endotracheal tube forcibly abducts the vocal cords and may actually dent them. The hoarse voice usually resolves in a few hours. Recurrent laryngeal nerve damage can occur during a thyroidectomy or operation on the neck. This will paralyse one or both of the vocal cords. Characteristcally the patient is unable to say "Eeeee" in a higher pitched voice. Inform the surgeon if you suspect this complication. Infants and children with a hoarse voice following intubation may go on to get airway obstruction some hours later. Children with stridor or a hoarse voice should be admitted and closely observed (see page 323 for management of stridor).

LATEX ALLERGY

Latex allergy has become a major occupational health problem among exposed individuals.[7] The disruptive consequences of this allergy are considerable. Sensitized workers develop symptoms which include urticaria, asthma, rhinoconjunctivitis, and anaphylaxis. This is probably mediated by the elevated level of latex allergen, carried by the glove powder in the rubber gloves, commonly used in operating theatre suites. Sensitized workers must have a safe environment. Low allergen powdered gloves are available, or better still use only powder free latex gloves or gloves made from non-latex material.

NUMBNESS AND TINGLING

Numbness (*anaesthesia*) or pins-and-needles (*paraesthesia*) occurs when a nerve is damaged. On the operating table, poor positioning of a patient can cause peripheral nerve damage. The nerve can be stretched, compressed, or made ischaemic (usually with a torniquet). The incidence is about 1:800 operations. Injury is more common in alcoholics and diabetics; possibly because these patients are already susceptible to peripheral neuropathies.

Apart from direct damage during surgery the commonest injuries are to the brachial plexus where the ulnar nerve is most frequently involved. Brachial plexus palsies also occur when an arm is hyper-extended from the shoulder on an arm board during the anaesthetic. This presents with wrist drop and weakness in the arm.

If the arm is not protected properly on the operating table, there is a risk of injuring the ulnar nerve as it passes through the groove on the medial epicondyle at the elbow. It can also be injured by a direct hit to the 'funny bone', usually on the frame of the trolley. Damage presents with numbness and tingling along the ulnar side of the hand to the little finger. The common peroneal nerve in the leg can be compressed while the patient's legs are in stirrups on the operating table. The patient develops foot drop, with numbness and tingling over the lower leg.

During attempts to maintain an airway the facial nerve can be compressed against the mandible. This will cause a facial palsy and drooping mouth, or eyelid, on the affected side.

Extravasation of irritating substances such as thiopentone, in the medial side of the anticubital fossa can damage the median nerve. This presents in recovery room as numbness over the palm and clumsiness of the fingers. The anticubital fossa will be painful and inflamed.

Regional neural blockade sometimes damages nerves, but the diagnosis is not normally made in recovery room. Patients who have had a brachial plexus block or other regional anaesthetic sometimes feel distressed with tingling and paraesthesia as the blockade wears off. Give analgesia.

PACEMAKERS

Patients with heart block have pacemakers to provide the heart with a rhythm that maintains an adequate cardiac output. Patients sometimes come to theatre with their pacemaker permanently implanted or temporarily inserted.

Assess pacemaker function when a patient arrives in the recovery room. Do a 12-lead ECG. Note the heart rate and rhythm, compare this with the patient's pulse. Check the ECG for the pacemaker spikes that precede the R-wave.

Normal serum potassium levels are necessary for a pacemaker to function well. If arrhythmias occur, or the pacemaker misbehaves; check the serum potassium. Diathermy or electrosurgery will not upset modern pacemakers, but older models can be damaged by current surges. Cardioversion can damage pacemakers. If possible consult a cardiologist before performing cardioversion on a patient with a pacemaker in place.

Do not insert central lines or pulmonary flotation (Swan Ganz®) catheters into patients with pacemakers, because you may dislodge the pacemaker wire from the right venticle.

PALLOR

If the patient appears abnormally pale and sweaty it may be due to one of the following drugs; pethidine, oxytocin,vasopressin (Por8®), desmopressin (DDAVP®).

Also consider:
- hypoxia;
- shock;
- bleeding;
- pain;
- hypoglycaemia;
- angina;
- nausea;
- anaemia.

INITIAL MANAGEMENT
- give high flow oxygen;
- ask the patient if he has chest pain;
- attach the pulse oximeter, ECG, and noninvasive blood pressure monitor;
- reassure the patient;
- take finger prick blood for glucose measurement.

FURTHER MANAGEMENT
This depends on the diagnosis, see appropriate sections in other parts of the book.

RIGIDITY

Muscle rigidity usually wears off after a few minutes. Persistant muscle rigidity is a sign of malignant hyperpyrexia (see page 263). It is often associated with shivering and shaking (see below) or hypothermia (see page 145). While the rigidity lasts the patient may clamp his jaws so tightly shut that they cannot be opened. This is called trismus. Trismus is dangerous because the tongue may be caught between the teeth and injured, or even partially severed, dental caps can be dislodged, or the patient may occlude his airway. Guedel airways have a metal phlange to prevent the lumen being crushed. To make the patient open his mouth pass a soft catheter through his nose until it touches the posterior pharyngeal wall. This will make him shake his head from side to side, grimace and gag and reflexly open his mouth.

> *Keep the patient's lips, and tongue out*
> *of the way of his teeth until he wakes up.*

Muscle rigidity can also be caused by some drugs including, promethazine, metoclopromide, fentanyl and droperidol. The *extrapyramidal syndrome* consists of muscle rigidity, and oculogyric crises with nystagmus. Patients can be very frightened by this side effect. To relieve anxiety give midazolam 0.1 - 0.2 mg/kg intraveously. Treat the rigidity with benztropine (Cogentin®) 0.015 mg/kg slowly intravenously.

SNORING

Never allow your patients to snore. Snoring is a sign of airway obstruction. Clear and support the airway (see page 325).

SHAKING AND SHIVERING[8]

Not all shaking or shivering is due to hypothermia. Many cold patients do not shiver, and furthermore some shaking patients are not cold. The term shivering is best reserved for the cold patient and shaking for the one who is not cold.

Between 20 and 50 per cent of all patients will shiver or shake after general anaesthesia. It also occurs after spinal and epidural anaesthesia. Sometimes the shaking is violent, especially in fit teenagers or young adults. Take care to prevent the patients from hurting themselves. Try to keep the airway in until the risk of shaking has passed, once it starts it is difficult to insert an airway.

Patients are more likely to shake if:
• they are teenage or young adult males;
• the operation is lengthy;

- they have been allowed to breath spontaneously for more than about 30 minutes on a volatile agent;
- an opioid or anticholinergic agent has been used for premedication;
- they have been hyperventilated during the procedure;
- analgesia is inadequate;
- after drainage of abscesses, when it may be a sign of a septic shower of bacteria entering the circulation. Take blood cultures, and consider commencing antibiotics, especially if this is accompanied by hypotension or poor oxygenation.

Shivers and shakes are characterized by:

- vasocontriction;
- pilo-erection (goose bumps);
- clonus;
- spike activity on an EEG;
- increased oxygen consumption;
- increased intraocular pressure.

Shivering and shaking raises the patient's metabolic rate enormously, with oxygen requirements rising to 5 and 8 times normal. This places extraordinary demands on the heart's ability to supply the tissues with enough oxygen to prevent hypoxia. In a patient with marginal myocardial reserves, the heart often cannot keep up; resulting in cardiac failure, myocardial ischemia, lactic acidosis and tissue hypoxia.

MANAGEMENT

Give oxygen by mask. Pethidine has a direct effect on hypothalmic temperature regulating centres to depress shivering and shaking. Use a small dose of pethidine of up to 0.33 mg/kg intravenously. It is even effective if naloxone has already been given, but you will need up to 1mg/kg or more[9]. About 75 per cent of patients respond to pethidine, but if this fails try doxapram 0.25 mg/kg intravenously.[10]

Morphine and fentanyl are not effective against shivering or shaking.

THEORIES ABOUT SHAKING

There are many theories about the causes of shaking seen after general anaesthesia. Suggested causes have been hyperventilation during the anaesthetic, adrenal suppression, pyrogen release, decreased sympathetic activity, and metabolic alkalosis. Electromyographic studies suggest unmodulated spinal cord activity returns before higher centres in the brain have recovered from the anaesthetic agent.[11] In other words the spinal cord wakes up before the brain does.

High flows of oxygen protect
shivering patients from hypoxia.

SORE THROAT

If asked postoperatively, almost half the patients complain of sore throats. The causes are:

- atropine, or dry gases that dessicate the mucosa;
- damage to the mucus membrane during intubation;
- pharyngeal packs;
- bronchcoscopy.

Reassure the patient that sore throats almost always resolve in 24 - 36 hours.

SWEATING

Sweating (*diaphoresis*) is a sign that something is seriously wrong.
It is associated with:

- nausea;
- hypotension;
- hypoglycaemia;
- hypoxia;
- malignant hyperpyrexia.

- cardiac failure;
- hypercarbia;
- opioids, especially pethidine given to a patient who is not in pain;

INITIAL MANAGEMENT
- Reassure the patient;
- give high flow oxygen by mask;
- ask the patient whether he has chest pain. If so treat as angina (see page 277);
- check for pneumothorax by asking the patient if he can take a deep breath;
- notify the anaesthetist;
- attach a pulse oximeter, blood pressure cuff and ECG monitor;
- perform a test for blood glucose;

Further management depends on the diagnosis.

TEETH

The anaesthetist sometimes damages teeth during intubation. Many patients' teeth are in poor repair with caries and gum disease. Teeth and gums break down suprisingly quickly when there is chronic illness. If the patient has been assessed fully preoperatively there should be a report of the condition of his teeth in the notes. Patients emerging from an inhalational anaesthetic often bite down very hard. This masseter spasm (trismus) is probably physiologically similar to that seen during shivering and shaking (see page 451). Do not let them bite their tongue. Teeth, and especially bridges and crowns can be damaged if the mouth is forced open. A nasopharyngeal airway is useful if the oral airway is obstructed. Choose a size one or two sizes smaller than the appropriate endotracheal tube. Lubricate the nasal airway liberally with 2% lignocaine gel, and pass it straight backwards along the floor of the nose. Do not push it upwards.

THIRST AND DRY MOUTH

Some patients will complain of a dry mouth and lips. There are commercial preparations that will help, or ask your pharmacy to make up a lemon flavoured ointment to smear on their lips. Avoid glycerine based ointments because they dry the lips even further. Dry mouths make some patients restless. Give them small sips of water, or let them suck on a wet gauze or ice. In many recovery rooms, after minor surgery it is possible for the patients to have a small drink. Check with the surgeon and anaesthetist before offering fluids.

WEAKNESS (SEE PAGE 441)

1. Smith T,(1998). *Anaesthesia and Intensive Care*, 26: 689.
2. Liu WH,Thorp TA, (1991). *Anaesthesia*, 46:435-7.
3. MacLeod AD, Maycock AE, (1993). *Anaesthesia and Intensive Care*, 21:653-4.
4. Oncel L,Hasgeli M, *et al.* (1998). *Journal of Laryngology and Oteology*, 106: 783-7.
5. Miller A, Olkkkola KT, *et al.* (1990). *British Journal of Anaesthesia*, 65: 826-8.
6. Victory RA, Hass P, *et al.* (1991). *Anaesthesia*, 46:940-1.
7. Arellano R, Bradley J, Sussman G. (1992). *Anaesthesiology*, 905-8.
8. Crossley AW, (1993). *British Journal of Hospital Medicine*, 49: 204-8.
9. Clayborn LE, Hirsch RA, (1983). *Anaesthesiology*, 59: (3A); S280.
10. Crossley AW, (1993). *British Journal of Hospital Medicine*, 49:204-8.
11. Sessler D. I., Israel D., *et al.* (1988). *Anesthesiology,* 68: 843–850.

24. Crisis Management

Be Prepared

Emergencies happen! Before the start of each day check all your trolleys and equipment, including your defibrillator, and make sure all new staff are shown where everything is kept.

A calamity is something which causes great harm.

When you are not sure about the cause of an emergency list the problems individually. Identify your differential diagnosis. It is best to do this on a white board near the patient so that everyone can immediately work out what is happening

JOHN SMITH 79 YRS

TURP under spinal anaesthetic at 15.15 hrs

Irrigation fluid glycine - 24 L

PHx. Hypertension → renal impairment

(Creatinine 15 mmol/l)

Mx   ß-blockers

Osteoarthritis Mx NSAID

IHD → AMI x 2   96,98

CCF   Mx Frusemide, K+ supplement

15.40 Admitted to recovery room
BP 140/90, P 88   35.8°C
O2 Sat 92% FiO$_2$ 28%
IV Normal saline 1000 mls - 8/24

16.20 Confused, and restless,
wheezy Mx 60% O$_2$, ECG Glucose 12

16.25 JVP + 10 cm, cyanosed BP 160/90 HR 116
Satn 89%

16.30 CXR and blood gases ordered.

16.33 Convulsion thiopentone 200 mg IV, IPPV
100% O$_2$

16.40 Blood gases, FBE, U+Es, glucose,
blood cultures.
Diff diagnosis: arrhythmia, water overload,
sepsis, hypoglycaemia,
glycine toxicity, previous epilepsy,
pulmonary oedema

fig 24.1 An example of a white board record used during the development of a crisis.

Crisis protocol

A crisis protocol is an organised approach to the management of the patient whose life is in danger. It is often difficult to diagnose what has happened to the patient but the fundamentals of basic life support are the same for all emergencies.

Prepare a set of flow charts (*algorithms*) on 12.5 x 20 cm filing cards for the diagnosis and management of emergencies. These cards will be your crisis protocols. Put them in a filing box on the desk where everyone can refer to them.

Many recovery rooms practise simulated disasters once a month so everyone knows what to do.

Successful management of emergencies depends on
practise, practise, practise.

As you practise these crisis protocols consider:
• What is the normal response?
• What is the worst that can happen?
• How do I assess the problem?
• What is the immediate management?
• How should the problem be followed up?

When your patient suddenly deteriorates, for instance his blood pressure falls, or he has a convulsion or can't breathe follow your crisis protocol. Because you will have to act quickly, the diagnosis and treatment must be performed concurrently, even when the cause of the problem is far from clear.

Analyze the crisis using the steps of: diagnosise, differential diagnosis and management. These are:
• What is the problem?
• What else can it be?
• What are we going to do about it?

Don't panic. Emergencies happen!

Managing emergencies

In an emergency your priorities are to keep your patient alive while you find out what is wrong; that is, you identify the problems.

Remember:
• keep your patient alive;
• then work out what is wrong.

Keep Your Patient Alive

Start with the THREE C's

Call for help, the emergency trolley and the defibrillator;

Check pulse, colour, oximeter and ECG;

Check the clock, and note the time on the white board.

MONITOR: ECG, blood pressure, pulse rate and rhythm, respiratory rate, oximetery.
GIVE: High flow oxygen.

GET HELP:
Help. It takes four people to manage a crisis:
Person 1. To look after the airway.

Person 2. To manage the cardiovascular system, and perform external cardiac massage if needed.

Person 3. To get drugs and equipment, and take blood tests.

Person 4. To supervise the resuscitation and write the problems and treatment on a white board where everyone can see it. This person is 'allowed' to help the others too.

Emergency trolley and other equipment as needed;

Look in history for clues eg. allergies, previous pneumothorax etc;

Prepare to take samples for laboratory analysis, blood gases, glucose, electrolytes, chest X-ray.

Check the carotid pulse
then follow the A B C D E F plan

Airway
Check the patency of the airway. Gently inspect the pharynx with a laryngoscope, suck out mucus, blood and other debris. Consider upper and lower airway obstruction from outside the airway, in the airway wall, and foreign body in the lumen.

Breathing
Check that air is moving in and out of the lungs. If you hold the chin up you can feel this in the palm of your hand. Insert an airway. Check the

oxygen saturation. Assist breathing with bag and mask, give supplemental oxygen.

Circulation

Feel for a carotid pulse. If it is absent call for help, and start *acute cardiac life support* (ACLS) protocol. Check the blood pressure and pulse, rate and rhythm, re-evaluate the perfusion status and attach the ECG.

Drugs

Review drugs for effects or side effects. If blood, drugs, or plasma expanders are being infused, then consider some form of reaction; turn off the drip.

Consider:
Wrong drug, Wrong rate, Wrong route.

Endocrine

Consider:
Hypoglycaemia. Check blood glucose with a glucose meter.
Hypothyroidism as a cause of delayed emergence.
Hypoadrenalism as a cause of refractory hypotension.

Fitting?

Consider:
Hypoxia.
Hypoglycaemia.
Hypocalcaemia.
Hyperpyrexia.
Hypocarbia.
Water intoxication.
Epilepsy, eclampsia.
Drugs: propofol, local anaesthetics, benzodiazepine withdrawal.

WORK OUT WHAT IS WRONG

What is it? What else could it be? What are we going to do about it?

Often the cause is obvious such as a cardiac arrhythmia, or laryngospasm, but you will still need to

LOOK, LISTEN and FEEL

The formula is 444. There are 4 things to look for, 4 to listen for, and 4 to feel.

LOOK
1. Wound sites and drains.
2. Appearance: Pallor? Cyanosis? Flushing? Sweating? Agitation?
3. Respiration: rates, depth, rhythm.
4. Neck: Jugular vein distension? Swelling of tissues? Tracheal deviation?

Blood loss is usually apparent, but it can be overlooked if it happens under the sheets. Blocked chest drains can cause respiratory difficulty. Difficulty in breathing can indicate airway obstruction, inadequate reversal of muscle relaxants, cardiac failure, or allergy. Bleeding into the neck can cause airway obstruction and cause the face to become suffused. Distended neck veins may indicate tension pneumothorax, cardiac tamponade, TURP syndrome, or gross fluid overload or pulmonary embolism by clot or air. A tension pneumothorax may push the trachea to the opposite side. Strip the patient to reveal abdominal swelling, and any other problems.

LISTEN TO
1. Patient's complaints.
2. Air entry: Wheezes with mouth open?
3. Stridor and other breathing noises.
4. Heart sounds (muffled, murmur, gallop).

If a patient says something is wrong, never pass it off as 'psychological'. If he says he can't breathe, then something is wrong. Listen to the breath sounds with a stethoscope. Assess their adequacy, pattern, and distribution. Possible problems include bronchospasm, pulmonary oedema, lobe collapse, pneumothorax, haemothorax, cardiac tamponade.

Stridor is a sign of impending total airway obstruction - it is an medical emergency - get help immediately. Wheeze suggests: aspiration, asthma, acute pulmonary oedema, allergy to drugs or infusions, or embolism. Heart sounds may be muffled if there is a pneumothorax or pericardial effusion - this is a difficult sign to interpret.

FEEL
1. Heart and pulse: rate? intensity? rhythm?
2. Head: sweaty? fever?
3. Hands: perfusion? grip strength, and leg movement on both sides?
4. Head lift to check residual muscle relaxation.

Take both wrists and feel the pulse. Check the carotid pulse and the femoral pulses. Look for differences in volume and rhythm. The ECG will assist in revealing arrhythmias. Cold hands are an excellent sign of sympathetic discharge, and warn of problems such as haemorrhage, hypoxia, hypoglycaemia, and pain. Warm hands and a bounding pulse suggest hypercarbia, thyrotoxicosis. Sweating or fever suggest a reaction to blood or drugs, malignant hyperthermia, serotinergic syndrome, thyrotoxic crisis, and neuroleptic malignant syndrome. Loss of grip strength or weakness in the legs on one side of the body alone suggests cerebral ischaemia, or on both sides the effects of residual muscle relaxants, neostigmine overdose, myasthenia or other neuropathies and myopathies.

A MINI INDEX OF COMMON PROBLEMS

Air embolism	see page 335	Hyperpyrexia	see page 263
Allergic reaction	see page 438	Hypertension	see page 261
Angina	see page 277	Hypoadrenalism	see page 432
Aspiration	see page 329	Hypoglycaemia	see page 416
Bleeding	see page 341	Hypotension	see page 257
Bradycardia	see page 267	Hypothyroidism	see page 434
Breathlessness	see page 301	Hypoxia	see page 295
Cardiac tamponade	see page 286	Malignant hypertension	see page 263
Confusion	see page 437	Nausea and vomiting	see page 231
Convulsions	see page 465	Pneumothorax	see page 333
Coughing	see page 318	Pulmonary embolism	see page 335
Crying	see page 440	Restlessness	see page 437
Cyanosis	see page 316	Sweating	see page 435
Death	see page 441	Tachycardia	see page 270
Delayed emergence	see page 441	Water intoxication	see page 81
Epilepsy	see page 422	Wheezing	see page 322

AIRWAY OBSTRUCTION

Unless this is recognised and relieved immediately the patient will die. Recovery rooms exist to prevent this emergency. Vigilance is the best prophylaxis. Read more on page 323.

Shock

Shock is a clinical syndrome that occurs when perfusion is inadequate to meet the metabolic needs of tissues. It involves both the failure to provide sufficient oxygen and nutrients, and the failure to remove the waste products of metabolism.

Characteristically shock causes a metabolic acidosis with a release of lactic acid into the circulation causing a falling pH (rising hydrogen ion concentration). It is always associated with tissue hypoxia.

There are two types of shock: *hypovolaemic shock* with reduced blood volume and extracellular fluid volume; and normovolaemic shock where the blood volume is normal but there is a failure of a sufficient head of blood pressure to perfuse the tissues.

Hypovolaemic shock

Hypovolaemic shock is caused by an inadequate left ventricular preload. If the blood volume is reduced by 15 - 20 per cent and cardiac output falls, and if untreated the clinical syndrome of shock will probably occur. The prognosis for haemorrhagic shock is good if it is treated quickly and vigorously.

Causes include:
- haemorrhage;
- bowel ileus;
- burns;
- polyuric renal failure;
- prolonged vomiting.

Typically arterial blood gas studies reveal hypoxaemia and hypoxia with PaO_2 below 60 mmHg, oxygen saturation less than 90 per cent, and a metabolic acidosis with pH less than 7.30 and low or very low bicarbonate levels. The patient will have a tachycardia, urine output of less than 30 ml/kg/hr, poor peripheral perfusion with cold extremities. If severe the patient may be pale, sweaty and exhibit air hunger with *Kussmaul's breathing*.

Normovolaemic shock

Causes include:
- anaphylaxis;
- cardiac failure;
- tension pneumothorax;
- hypothyroidism;
- Addisonian crisis.

Three special subgroups of normovolaemic shock are *cardiogenic shock*, *anaphylaxis*, and *septic shock*.

CARDIOGENIC SHOCK
Cardiogenic shock is a complex clinical syndrome characterized by ventricular failure, inadequate tissue perfusion, and impaired cellular metabolism. Even with the best treatment the mortality rate approaches 70 per cent. Causes include cardiomyopathy, cardiac arrhythmias, cardiac ischaemia or infarction.

ANAPHYLAXIS AND DRUG REACTIONS
Review the drugs the patient has recently received for possible side effects. If blood, drugs, or plasma expanders are being infused, then consider some form of reaction; turn off the drip.

Consider:
Wrong drug, Wrong rate, Wrong route.

Anaphylaxis is an acute life threatening allergic reaction following an injection of a specific antigen such as penicillin, other drugs, or blood within a few minutes. There is sudden cardiovascular collapse after this antigenic challenge. In the recovery room ninety per cent occur almost immediately after giving a drug.

Early signs include:
• sensation of warmth or itching especially in the groin or axilla;
• flushing over the upper part of the body;
• acute anxiety, restlesness, panic;
• nausea and vomiting;
• feelings of tightness in the chest.

Later:
• erythematous or urticarial rash similar to hives;
• developing oedema of face, eyelids and neck;
• crampy abdominal pain.

Progressing to:
• hypotension sometimes severe enough to cause coma;
• bronchospasm, cough, dyspnoea, wheeze;
• laryngeal oedema with dyspnoea, stridor, drooling and hoarse voice;
• tissue hypoxia with cyanosis; arrrhythmias and cardiac arrest.

Laryngeal oedema is life threatening. The onset of stridor warns that total airway obtruction is only moments away (for management see point 9 below). If the patient is conscious he becomes extremely frightened.

PRINCIPLES:

1. Suspect any unexpected reaction to a drug as an anaphylactic reaction.

2. The patient frequently deteriorates rapidly.

3. Use adrenaline at the first suspicion of anaphylaxis. It is rapid and effective.

4. Use adrenaline first, because steroids and antihistamines take some hours to work.

5. Additional vasopressors are rarely needed. The combination of adrenaline and plasma volume replacement will return the cardiac output to acceptable levels.

6. Do not use Haemaccel® or dextrans as plasma expanders in cases of suspected anaphylaxis.

ANAPHYLACTIC AND ANAPHYLACTOID REACTIONS

The reaction occurs when re-exposure to an agent triggers mast cells to degranulate and release pharmacologically active substances such as histamine, prostaglandins, leutkotrienes, and platelet activating factor.

ANAPHYLACTIC REACTIONS are immune mediated responses involving previous exposure to a foreign substance (usually, but not always, a protein) which provokes the production of an antibody called immunoglobulin E (IgE). On re-exposure to the same antigen it combines with the IgE on the surface of mast cells, or basophils. These immune cells guard the interface with the outside world (lung, gut, skin, eyes), and when challenged, release large amounts of histamine and other inflammatory mediators. Only a tiny amount of antigen is needed to evoke a huge reponse. The sudden vasodilation and catastrophic fall in blood pressure can cause cardiac arrest. If the patient survives the first insult, capillary beds all over the body, but especially in the lungs and gut, leak large amounts of fluid into the tissues. This causes airway, facial and pulmonary oedema.

ANAPHYLACTOID RESPONSES occur when some drug, or chemical causes histamine release either locally, or throughout the body. The reaction is not immune mediated, does not require previous exposure, does not involve IgE but is related to the dose and speed of injection.

MANAGEMENT:

Monitor: Pulse rate, automated blood pressure, oximeter, ECG.

Laboratory: blood gases may be needed.

IMMEDIATE MANAGEMENT:

1. Stop the administration of the agent suspected of causing the reaction.

2. Give high flow oxygen by mask.

3. Call for assistance; get the emergency trolley and prepare for rapid infusion of fluids.

4. Lay the patient down flat and raise the limbs. Do not tilt head down.

5. If unconscious clear the airway and assist ventilation as necessary.

6. First give adrenaline.

   For adults: Use adrenaline 1:1000 (1 mg/ml), and give it intramuscularly. If the patient weighs less than 50 kg give 0.25 ml, between 50 and 100 kg give 0.5 ml, and over 100 kg give 0.75 ml.

   For children: Dilute 1 ml of 1:1000 adrenaline, and make it up to 10 mls in saline. This gives you a solution of adrenaline 1:10 000. Use this diluted adrenaline to give 0.25 ml/year of age slowly intravenously over 5 minutes.

7. Now start a wide bore peripheral drip with normal saline. Do not use a colloid because this has been implicated in anaphylaxis.

8. Use intravenous adrenaline if either: there is no response to the intramuscular adrenaline, or there is no blood pressure or pulse recordable. For adults give adrenaline 5 ml of 1:10 000 slowly over 5 minutes. For children give adrenaline 0.1 ml/kg of adrenaline 1:10 000 slowly over 5 minutes.

9. Facial oedema is a grave sign of impending airway obstruction. An emergency airway will be needed. This will require skilled anaesthetic help, because the swelling caused by the oedema may obscure and then suddenly obstruct the laryngeal opening. If the anaesthetist is not trained in this emergency, then it is better to consider inserting a percutaneous mini-tracheostomy (Minitrak®) or perform a formal tracheostomy.

Once the patient's blood pressure is restored you can:

1. Give hydrocortisone 5 mg/kg intravenously.

2. Give promethazine (Phenergan®) 0.5 mg/kg intravenous slowly over 10 minutes

3. Treat bronchospasm with 2 ml salbutamol 0.5% through a nebulizer and face mask.

4. If bronchospasm remains unrelieved then give salbutamol 1.5 microgram/kg intravenously.

5. If wheeze still persists after 10 minutes, then repeat the dose of salbutamol.

6. If wheeze still persists, suspect aspirated foreign material.

SEPTIC SHOCK

Septic shock is caused by gram positive bacteria, gram negative bacteria, or fungi (most commonly Candida species). It can occur in the recovery room following drainage of abscesses or pus, following bowel resection, or after urological surgery.

Septic shock occurs when endotoxins and cytokines have been released into the circulation causing catastrophic cardiovascular collapse.

CONVULSIONS (ALSO FITTING AND DELIRIUM)

A fitting patient?
always exclude hypoxia and hypoglycaemia first.

Causes of convulsions include:
- hypoxia and hypoglycaemia - these are life threatening events;
- pyrexia (see also septic shock above);
- hypocalcaemia;
- an epileptic patient who has not taken his medication;
- water overload, TURP syndrome;
- eclampsia;
- malignant hypertension.

Drugs that can cause fitting are local anaesthetics, propofol, enflurane, methohexitone, pethidine and the anticholinergics; rarely benzodiazepine or antiparkinsonian drug withdrawal.

IMMEDIATE MANAGEMENT:

Check the carotid pulse, if it is not present then treat for cardiac arrest.
1. Call for help.
2. Clear the airway.
3. Support breathing.
4. Give high-flow oxygen by mask.
5. Lay the patient on to his side.
6. Attach ECG, pulse oximeter, and automated blood pressure machine.
7. Stay with the patient and ensure the airway is patent.

8. Bring the emergency trolley.
9. Check the blood sugar level.

FURTHER MANAGEMENT:

Fitting is usually controlled with:

1. Thiopentone (Pentothal®), 2 – 5 mg/kg intravenously.
2. Diazepam (Valium®), 0.15 mg/kg intravenously (up to 20 mg in an adult).
3. Phenytoin (Dilantin®, Epinutin®), 250 mg intravenously. And if patient has not already been receiving phenytoin, then up to 1 gram can be safely given over 30 minutes.

If the patient remains comatose, re-intubate to guard the airway against aspiration of gastric contents, pass a urinary catheter and a nasogastric tube. Prepare to transfer him to intensive care.

CHEST PAIN

Causes of chest pain include:
- angina (see page 277);
- pneumothorax (see page 333);
- air emboli (see page 335);
- pulmonary emboli (see page 336);
- trauma during surgery (in one case it was the assistant's elbow resting on the chest while holding a retractor).

ENDOCRINE EMERGENCIES

Consider:

Hypoglycaemia as a cause of agitation and sweating.

Hypothyroidism as a cause of delayed emergence.

Hypoadrenalism as a cause of refractory hypotension.

1. Lindner, KH, Burkhard D, Lancet (1997). 349: 535-7.
2. 'Guidelines for Cardiopulmonary Resuscitation'. (1992). *Journal of the American Medical Association*, 268: 2171-298.
3. 'Guidelines for Basic and Advance Life Support'. European Resuscitation Council (1992). *Resuscitation*, 24: 103-22.
4. 'The Australian Resuscitation Council Guidelines'. (1993). *Medical Journal of Australia*, 159; 616-21.

25. Equipment

Airways - Nasopharyngeal (see page 480)

Airways - Oropharyngeal

Guedal airways are normally disposible items. They have a reinforced mouth piece to stop the patient clenching his teeth and obstructing the airflow.

Size 4   for huge men.

Size 3   for adult men.

Size 2   for women, and men without teeth, and for children. down to the age of 18 months.

Size 1   for children under the age of 18 months.

Size 0   small for neonates.

Size 00   tiny.

In the elderly, especially if they have no teeth, try using a smaller rather than a larger size to maintain the airway.

Batteries

Laryngoscopes, torches, and clocks use disposable alkaline batteries. Alkaline 1.5 volt batteries come in four sizes AA, A, C, and D. Some apparatus uses 9 volt batteries. Have a ready supply of batteries on hand. They should be stored in a dry airtight container in a cool place.

RECHARGEABLE BATTERIES

Some apparatus such as a defibrillator uses rechargeable batteries. To make sure they are in good working order, charge them to the recommended levels, and for the recommended times. Do not overcharge these batteries.

To extend their life, some types of rechargeable batteries periodically need to be completely discharged, and then slightly overcharged. Properly maintained, they will give service for 3 to 5 years, or more than 1000 charges. Include this procedure on your regular maintenance program.

BLOOD PRESSURE MONITORS

Manual

Mercury sphygmomanometers with solid mountings are more reliable, robust and easier to repair than anaeroid devices. Choose ones with a bright (preferably yellow) scale, that is easier to read from a distance. Mount them at eye level to prevent parallax errors when reading the scale.

Anaeroid ones have a clock-face type dial. These are easier to read, but to remain accurate need recalibrating every 3 months. In humid areas the mechanism rusts quickly.

In addition to standard cuffs, you will need a broader cuff for obese adults, and a narrower cuff for children and thin adults. Wrap around cuffs are more durable than Velcro®, or hook ones and a local tailor can make you spares. In the tropics the rubber bladders perish quickly. Keep a supply of spares in an airtight container in cool dry place.

Non-invasive

Non-invasive blood pressure monitors (NBP) are popular because they release staff to attend to other matters while monitoring the blood pressure at regular intervals, and give warnings if the blood pressure rises or falls beyond set limits. The mean pressure is the most accurate. Well known makes are reliable and robust. They do not work well if the patient has an arrythmia. If the blood pressure is low they will keep starting again, looking for the pulse and if the blood pressure is high they can damage the patient's arm because they make the cuff very tight. If you suspect any of these problems, use a manual monitor.

Invasive

Invasive blood pressure measurement involves inserting a small cannula into an artery (usually the radial artery), and connecting it to a pressure transducer with plastic catheters. The signal is processed; and systolic, diastolic, and mean blood pressures along with the pulse wave form are displayed on a screen. Catheters can be either too soft or too hard; this interferes with the fluid dynamics of the system. With incorrectly matched catheters, fluid dynamic errors may be as much as 80 per cent. In other words the monitor may show a systolic blood pressure of 240 mmHg when the correct blood pressure is only 160 mmHg. Make sure that your lines and catheters conform to the manufacturer's recommendations. If you are unhappy with the readings check with a manual monitor.

BLOOD WARMERS

Blood warmers help prevent hypothermia.

WATER-BATH BLOOD WARMERS heat the blood by passing it through a coil immersed in water maintained at a constant temperature. The temperature of the water bath should never exceed 40°C. Their major disadvantages are that water slops out if the bath is knocked or tilted, and the coil slows the rate of transfusions,

DRY HEAT BLOOD WARMERS warm the blood by passing it close to a heated plate or cylinder. The Atom™ Blood Warmer (BW385L) is the first of a new generation of blood warmers that do not require dedicated disposables and, the makers claim, will accept any giving set.

It is difficult to run a rapid transfusion through a standard blood warmer. To overcome this problem there are two expensive systems available, the Level 1™ delivers 500 ml/min, and Rapid Infusion System™ 1500 ml/min.

Make sure your blood warmer has some means of indicating the temperature, a thermostat control, and preferably an alarm.

BRONCHOSCOPES

Have a sterile bronchoscopy tray with both adult and paediatric bronchoscopes available in the theatre suite. Make sure that the light source, cables, oxygen supply, suction devices and grasping forceps are all compatible, and in working order. Check this on your regular maintenance program.

FIBREOPTIC BRONCHOSCOPES are more appropriate for diagnostic work, they require special care and are not as useful for retrieving foreign objects from the lower airways as a rigid bronchoscope.

CENTRAL VENOUS LINES

Central venous lines should be radio-opaque. Do not buy the ones that are introduced through needles, because the needles can cut the cannula leaving the cut end in the vein. The best types are inserted using a vein dilator and a Seldinger wire. Manometers for central venous pressure measurement are disposable. The water column manometer (illustrated on page 36) is quite accurate and easy to use. An improvised manometer mounting board can be made with a half meter ruler.

CLOCKS

A clock with a clear-sweep second hand should be visible from all over the recovery room. These are cheap, readily available and run on batteries. Include battery replacement as part of your routine maintenance program. Use the 24-hour clock routinely for noting times on charts or records.

For example

midnight = 00.00 hr

10.20 am = 10.20 hr

Noon = 12.00 hr

8 pm = 20.00 hr

DEFIBRILLATOR

The defibrillator is an essential piece of equipment to treat cardiac arrest and some arrhythmias. In a small hospital share one defibrillator with the whole theatre block. Keep it with the resuscitation trolley in the recovery room. There are many types, but the most useful are portable and light weight, run on mains power or rechargeable batteries, and have their own internal ECG monitor. Include the care of the defibrillator on your regular maintenance program.

Since defibrillators put out as much as 7000 volts at 400 joules they are dangerous if not handled properly. Staff have been electrocuted while demonstrating its use on each other. Practice using the defibrillator but not while it is charged up. Defibrillators need special conductive jelly or conductive pads. Make sure they are available. In hot climates slightly moisten the pads with saline if they are dry. Do not allow the saline to leave the area of the pad or a short circuit may result. Do not use a non-conductive jelly (such as KY Jelly®) or water because it will cause deep burns during cardioversion.

As well as treating cardiac arrest, defibrillators are used to restore sinus rhythm in a patient with atrial fibrillation, and some supraventricular tachycardias. Reversion of these rhythms uses low-energy pulses. The shock pulse from the defibrillator needs to reach the heart at the peak of the R-wave on the ECG. Most defibrillators have the facility to detect the peak of the R-wave, and will deliver the shock pulse at the right time regardless of when the paddles are discharged. To use this facility switch the defibrillator to synchronised mode.

Defibrillators which give a truncated biphasic wave form of 130 joule pulse instead of the monopolar 200 joule damped sine wave are now available.[1] These are small light and inexpensive. They are also thought to be less damaging to the heart muscle.

ECG AND PHYSIOLOGICAL MONITORS

There are many ECG monitors on the market. It is wise to order them from the same manufacturer who supplies other monitoring apparatus to the hospital. This gives you greater bargaining power, and eases servicing and maintenance. Desirable features include a clear display, which can be read from 2 to 3 metres away, audible pulse monitoring, and pulse rate display, a cascade mechanism to view up to the last 30 seconds of trace, and a screen freeze function to allow analysis of a trace pattern. It is also helpful to have a paper trace readout to record arrhythmias for later analysis. This is an expensive option, and is not essential if your budget is tight.

Monitors are becoming increasingly sophisticated, and many have multiple functions enabling ECG, oximeters, non invasive blood pressure and various other parameters to be measured and displayed. Some have menu driven displays and colours to show different parameters on the screen.

Ordering electronic equipment for humid climates?
Make sure that the components are sealed against moisture and mould.

Keep spare cables and sensors in stock. Be careful not to bend the cables, particularly near their sockets. When they are not in use coil them loosely and store them carefully.

The ECG is not a good monitor for hypoxia, and it is not a substitute for a pulse oximeter. By the time hypoxic damage is evident on the ECG, much damage will have occurred.

MOBILE PHONES have been reported to interfere with monitoring equipment, and some hospitals have banned their use within the hospital precincts. This is excessively cautious, in fact, analogue phones are unlikely to cause any problems. The more powerful digital phones cause interference if used within 2 metres of a monitor.[1] Suitable mobile phones are available and if you have funds these are very convenient for each recovery nurse who can use them to communicate with the ward, and does not have to leave the patient to go to the main desk.

EMERGENCY TROLLEY

In the USA these are called *emergency carts* or *crash carts*. Recovery rooms must have a well designed and equipped emergency trolley ready for immediate use. They should carry all the drugs and equipment needed for the resuscitation of any collapsed patient. Keep a laminated plastic sheet, listing all the required items, tied to the trolley. Restock immediately after use (see page 563). Discourage lazy staff from using this trolley as a source of stock for routine procedures.

It is wise to leave drugs in their boxes until they are needed. Many mistakes have been made in selecting an emergency drug by inaccurate recognition of an ampoule's shape and colour. Drugs should be stored in alphabetical order of their generic names. Keep a list of their trade names and generic names with them.

ENDOTRACHEAL TUBES

Clear plastic tubes are preferable. You will need a range of sizes for different ages. Sizes are measured on their internal diameter. Children under the age of ten usually do not require cuffed tubes, however above this age cuffs are needed for a good gas seal, and to prevent fluid entering the lower airways.

ENDOTRACHEAL TUBE SIZES	
NEONATES	< 1 kg: 2. 5 mm 1–3. 5 kg: 3. 0 mm 3. 5– 6. 5 kg: 3. 5 mm
INFANTS	10 kg: 4. 0 mm 12 kg: 4. 5 mm
CHILDREN TO 16 YEARS OF AGE	$\dfrac{age}{4} + 4$ = size of tube
ADULTS	60 kg: 8. 0 mm 70 kg: 9. 0 mm

The distance from the teeth to the midpoint of the trachea[2]

$$= \frac{\text{height (cm)} + 2}{10}$$

add 3 cm to allow space to tie or fix the tube.

In the larger tubes a 'Murphy eye', which is a second hole near the distal end of the tube, prevents occlusion if the tip becomes obstructed.

Check the tubes you buy are non-irritant. They should have either 'IT' or 'Z 79' printed on the side of the tube. If you are still using rubber endotracheal tubes, periodically check them to see that they are not perished. Dispose of the old metal connectors and use well-made tight-fitting plastic 15 mm connectors.

FACE MASKS (SEE ALSO OXYGEN THERAPY DEVICES PAGE 482)

Keep a full range of anaesthetic face masks on the emergency trolley. Everyone working in the recovery room must be able to *bag and mask* a patient until help arrives (see fig 25.9, page 487).

GLUCOSE METERS

Glucose meters are small electronic devices that accurately measure blood glucose using a drop of blood from a finger or heel prick. Some machines are simpler to use than others. Keep the instructions on how to use the device with the meter. They use special reagent strips; store them in a cool dry place. Do not take blood from the toes or feet of diabetics, or patients with peripheral vascular disease because they are likely to get infected. Serious ulcers can cause the patient to lose a limb.

HAEMOGLOBINOMETERS

These compact, cheap and accurate electronic devices read the level of haemoglobin on a reagent strip. Most of them are easy to use. Microcuvettes used in some makes are damaged by humidity giving inaccuracte results.[3]

HUMIDIFIERS

Humidity is a measure of the amount of water vapour present in a gas. Humidifiers increase the amount of water vapour in the inhaled gases, helping prevent the tracheobroncheal mucosa from drying out, and preserving the action of surfactant in lowering surface tension within the alveolus. Humidification is especially important in those with acute or chronic respiratory disorders, especially smokers.

CONDENSER HUMIDIFIERS (such as the Humid Vent®)also known as a Heat and Moisture exchanger (HME) are disposable and weigh about 40 grams. They provide effective heat and moisture exchange, and help prevent the bronchial mucosa from drying out. They are attached to the upper end of an endotracheal tube and are often used during anaesthetics. As the patient breathes out, the expired water vapour collects in the baffles of the humidifier

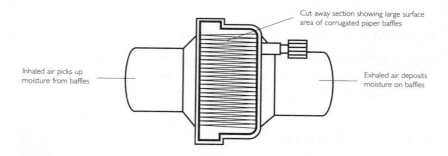

fig 25.1 Condenser humidifier

When the patient breathes in, the dry air rushes past the moisture-laden baffles and partially saturates with water vapour. These devices are only useful if the patient is receiving ventilatory support. Do not leave them on a patient who is spontaneously breathing through an endotracheal tube or laryngeal mask as they easily become blocked with sputum and may totally obstruct the patient's breathing. Another device known as a 'Hot Pot' is an alternative.[4]

Special condenser humidifiers are available for tracheostomies. If their baffles become clogged with sputum the end blows off so that the airway cannot obstruct.

HEATED HUMIDIFIERS are useful to warm hypothermic patients who are being ventilated. They deliver gas at 37°- 40°C at a relative humidity of 100 per cent. By humidifying gas in the trachea they prevent drying of the mucosa, preserve ciliary function, and keep the mucus fluid. The ones designed for ventilated patients are expensive. Fill them with sterile water rather than tap water because it may contain pathogens such as Legionella.

They have thermistor probes near the patient's airway that warn of overheating, because temperatures above 42°C will cause tracheal burns. Heated humidifiers require a lot of nursing attention. Make sure you have a service guarantee, proper instructions, and a service book with exploded diagrams showing all the parts, and how they fit together.

Cheap, compact heated humidifiers are available for the spontaneously breathing patient. Active airway heating and humidification is not an effective means of warming hypothermic patients. Infrared radiation is effective in controlling post operative shivering but is not useful for rewarming patients.

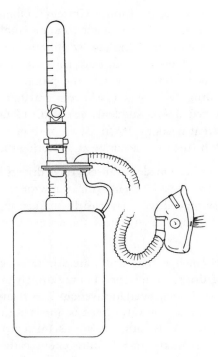

fig 25.2 Aquapack®

BUBBLE-THROUGH HUMIDIFIERS, where gas is passed through cold water, are barely effective. Use only sterile water. Tap water is a good source of aerosol infection especially in warmer climates.

INFUSION SETS

Special infusion sets are available for blood transfusions with 120 micron filters. There are several variations in the giving sets available. A useful one has a squeeze pump incorporated into the line for rapid transfusion. A Y-giving set for blood or platelet transfusion is available. These sets have an internal diameter of 3.2 mm. Large-bore trauma sets 5.72 mm internal diameter are available for rapid transfusion.

INFUSION PUMPS, SYRINGE DRIVERS, AND DRIP SET REGULATORS

SYRINGE DRIVERS (such as the Atom®, Graseby®, Ohmeda® and Terumo®) use the turn of a screw to deliver small accurate volumes of fluid from a syringe. They are useful for giving precise amounts of concentrated drug. At flow rates under 10 mls per hour most have a slow start up time, and it may be as long as 10 minutes before the pump is delivering a steady flow.Inadvertant drug delivery is a risk from gravitational syphoning and also if an obstructed line is suddenly released.[5] Obtain a sturdy pump, adaptable to different syringes. Try to use the syringe recommended by the makers. This will be the most accurate at delivering the prescribed dose

Fatal mistakes have been made because syringe drivers have been set at the wrong flow rate. The most frequent error is in wrongly setting the decimal point. A good syringe driver has clearly marked figures. Two trained personnel should independently check the drugs, dilutions and the pump settings.

INFUSION PUMPS (such as the Imed®) are drip rate regulators and deliver a set number of drips, or mls per hour, through an intravenous line. Infusion pumps need a dedicated intravenous line. If anything else is to run through that line, a one way valve must be inserted to prevent back flow. Multilumen central venous catheters are useful for running up to three separate infusions through a single intravenous catheter. Problems with infusion pumps include unintentional delivery if they are not set up correctly. A useful alternative to an infusion pump is a Dial-a-Flow®. These cheap, disposable, small drip set regulators are ideal for those recovery rooms who only occasionally need a precisely controlled infusions rates. Plug one into an intravenous infusion set, follow the instructions and you will find they are accurate enough for most infusions.

LARYNGEAL MASKS

Laryngeal masks were introduced into general anaesthetic practice in 1989 and are justifiably popular. It is far easier to maintain an airway with a laryngeal mask than with a normal rubber face mask. Laryngeal masks are made from a special grade silicone rubber. They are good for about 40 uses or 2 years, which ever comes first. Once damaged they cannot be repaired. They are inserted through the mouth and fit like a hood over the larynx. A cuff is then inflated to achieve a loose seal in the pharynx. There are modified laryngeal masks available for special use. One has an armoured and flexible tube, another is rigid and can be used for intubation.

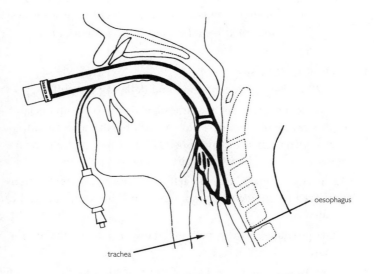

oesophagus

trachea

fig 25.3 Laryngeal mask in situ

Advantages[6] are that they:
• maintain a good airway;
• are easy to use;
• are atraumatic and do not irritate the upper airway;
• can be used with a CO_2 analyzer;
• can be used in patients who are difficult to intubate;
• do not require muscle relaxants to insert;
• are less likely to cause sore throats, coughing or bucking than an endotracheal tube;
• are reusable after sterilization.

Disadvantages are that they:
• difficult to use in babies;
• unsuitable for surgery of the face, or neck or in patients with degenerative cervical spine disease;

- do not protect the airway against vomiting or regurgitation of stomach contents;
- are expensive;
- attempted ventilation may fill the stomach with gas under tension;
- are unsuitable for fat patients who frequently have hiatus hernias, and may regurgitate gastric contents;

The laryngeal mask does not prevent regurgitation
and must only be used in fasted patients.

HINTS FOR THEIR USE[7]
- Use a 20 ml syringe for inflating and deflating the cuff.
- A patient emerging from anaesthesia is likely to clamp his jaws shut, bite the airway and obstruct it. Fold a piece of gauze and use it to prevent the patient biting down on the tube. There is not enough room for both a laryngeal mask and a Guedal airway in most patients.
- The laryngeal mask can be left in place while the patient is being transferred to the recovery room and until he wakes up and care for his own airway.
- Where possible recover patients lying on their side in the recovery position.
- To give oxygen attach a light T-piece made out of corrugated plastic tubing to the mask (see fig 25.7, page 484).

LARYNGEAL MASKS		
SIZES		**CUFF INFLATION**
size 1	neonate	2–4 ml
size 2	small child	10 ml
size 2.5	large child	15 ml
size 3	small adult	20 ml
size 4	large adult	30 ml

- Wait for the patient to take out his own laryngeal mask. If he coughs or gags on the mask remove it for him. There is no need to deflate the cuff as this brings the pharyngeal fluid out with it. Check to see no residual fluid remains in the pharynx or mouth that could be aspirated.

- Be careful not to rip the laryngeal mask past the teeth, or you may tear it.
- Laryngeal masks can be used to intubate patients who have difficult airways. Insert either a small endotracheal tube, or a fibre optic bronchoscope down the lumen of the mask and through the larynx. A specially modified laryngeal mask is available.

CLEANING AND STERILIZATION
- Put the dirty laryngeal mask straight into a bowl or jug of water. Dried secretions are difficult to wash off.
- Soak the mask thoroughly in soapy water and use a bottle brush to gently clean the lumen. Rinse it thoroughly in clean water.
- Do not use glutaraldehyde (Cidex®), formaldehyde or ethylene oxide. Laryngeal masks may be autoclaved at low pressures and temperatures. Do not use the high-pressure high-temperature autoclave. To prevent the cuff from bursting as it is heated, deflate the mask almost completely before autoclaving.

Don't throw the laryngeal mask away.
It is expensive and not disposable.

LARYNGOSCOPES

Many companies sell laryngoscopes, but unfortunately there is no standardization in design so that parts of one make of laryngoscope are not interchangeable with other models. There are dozens of shapes, sizes and designs, some are made of plastic, and others of metal. When you are buying laryngoscopes for your recovery room, buy the same make and model as the rest of the hospital. This means parts can be interchanged.

Choose a type with a detachable blade that can be easily washed and autoclaved if necessary. Do not autoclave blades if they have a fibreoptic light cable because it will be destroyed. Handles rust easily so do not autoclave them; just remove the batteries, wash the outside and dry it carefully. Sometimes the electrical contact between the blade and the contact on the handle becomes corroded. Clean it with a piece of steel wool until the brass just shines. The strike strip from a box of matches is another useful abrasive to clean the contacts.

Check each day that the light is bright and white. If the light is dim or yellow check that the contacts are clean and shiny and that the batteries are fresh. A dim light is not due to a faulty bulb; they either work or they do not. Keep a good supply of spare bulbs on hand because they blow out easily; especially if the laryngoscope is knocked or dropped.

Most useful of the blades are:

- The Mackintosh curved blade. It comes in three sizes child, standard, and large and is the most commonly used blade for adult use. The standard sized (medium) blade is satisfactory for most needs, but have at least one of each of the other blades available.
- Kessel blade for fat patients with short necks. Have at least one of these available.
- Paediatric blades for infants are straight. Choose one with the light near the tip such as the Warne or Weston blade.
- To complete the range it is useful to have a right handed blade available.

Keep these laryngoscopes on your difficult intubation trolley with other specialized equipment.

NASOPHARYNGEAL AIRWAYS[8]

It is worthwhile having a range of these available. They are useful in those adults whose airways are difficult to maintain. Size 5, 6 and 7 will cover most needs. Commercially available nasopharyngeal airways are made of soft plastic with a flange to prevent them slipping in too far. They can, however, be made by cutting a 15 cm length of old soft silastic endotracheal tube. Push a safety pin through the outer end so that the tube cannot disappear into the nose. Lubricate well and insert by pushing them gently straight back, parallel with the floor of the nose. Do not push them upwards.

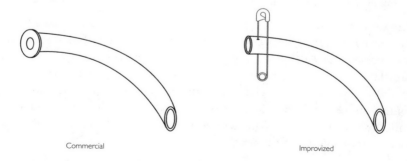

Commercial   Improvized

fig 25.4 Nasopharyngeal airways

NERVE STIMULATOR

Nerve stimulators are useful to assess the degree and type of neuromuscular block in patients who remain paralysed after the end of an anaesthetic (see page 442).

OXYGEN CONCENTRATORS[9]

In regions where bottled oxygen is expensive or difficult to obtain *oxygen concentrators* can provide an economical supply of nearly pure oxygen from air. If you are working in an isolated hospital, oxygen concentrators are a most worthwhile proposition. The purchase price of a concentrator is about half the cost of a year's supply of the same amount of oxygen from cylinders. The compressors in these units run on mains electric current but in emergencies they will run on the output from a small generator. The power consumption of a concentrator is only 350 watt, even a petrol generator or a truck battery fitted with an oscillator will give 600 watt.

Room air is basically a mixture of two gases: 21% oxygen and 79% nitrogen. This air is drawn into the machine through a series of filters and compressed to a pressure of 4 atmospheres. It is then passed into a canister of manufactured zeolite (a form of aluminium silicate) which acts as a molecular sieve. Nitrogen binds to the zeolite and oxygen passes on to a storage tank. After about 20 seconds the zeolite sieve becomes saturated with nitrogen, and the supply of compressed air is automatically diverted to a second canister where the process is repeated. This gives a constant output of oxygen. While the pressure in the second canister is at 20 PSI the pressure in the first is reduced to zero. Most of the nitrogen then comes off the zeolite, and is released to the atmosphere. A small back flow of oxygen from the alternative cylinder assists the process.

The life of the zeolite crystals is about 20 000 hours, or about 10 years. The gas emerging from the two cannisters and into the reservoir chamber is about 95% oxygen. This oxygen can be drawn off at about 4 litres/minute

WHO Performance Standard
The World Health Organisation has set down minimum standards of performance under extreme conditions of heat, humidity, vibration and atmospheric pollution. The Puritan Bennett 'Companion' (Model 492 A), the Healthdyne (Model BX 5000), and the DeVilbiss (Model DeVO/MC44) are the first three oxygen concentrators to successfully meet all these standards. These concentrators are easy to use; the controls are simply an on/off switch and a flow meter. There is a pressure alarm which sounds when the unit is first turned on. If it sounds during use it usually means the filters need changing. More on the approved machines can be obtained from the WHO office, 1211 Geneva 27, Switzerland.

without any loss in concentration. Higher flows result in lower percentages of oxygen. The concentrators are not suitable to drive ventilators or compressed gas anaesthesia machines such as a Boyles machine. Remember, if the power fails there is only 2 - 3 minutes oxygen stored in the machine.

Servicing is required about every 5000 hours, it is not difficult and can be carried out by the user. Make sure you are given all the instructions for this when you purchase the machine. You should also be given at least 2 years supply of spare parts.

If you are investing in oxygen concentrators you should buy two. Keep them clean and assign responsibility for them to one, named, person.

OXYGEN CYLINDERS

There are four sizes of oxygen cylinders normally available:

G cylinder contains 7000 litres = 7 cubic meters (200 - 260 cubic feet);
E cylinder contains 3500 litres = 3.5 cubic meters (100 - 130 cubic feet);
D cylinder contains 1400 litres = 1.4 cubic meters (40 - 50 cubic feet);
C cylinder contains 400 litres = 0.4 cubic metres (12 - 15 cubic feet);

The gas in the cylinders is at extremely high pressure (120 000 kPa or 2000 lb per square inch). Handle the cylinders carefully, Do not drop them, they have been known to explode with devastating effects similar to a bomb. Chain large cylinders upright so they cannot fall over. Store them in a cool place well away from direct sunlight. Do not accept delivery if they show signs of rust or the neck is damaged.

Make sure you have the right key to turn them on and off. Keep a supply of spare keys available. Cylinders need to be *cracked* before use. To *crack* a cylinder turn it on gently for an instant before connecting to the apparatus. This blows any dust or grit out of the neck of the cylinder that could otherwise damage the apparatus. Do not crack cylinders near inflammable or explosive gases. Oxygen is neither explosive nor flammable, but it vigorously supports combustion.

OXYGEN DELIVERY DEVICES

Fixed oxygen delivery masks (Hudson®, McGraw® Airlife®) deliver an oxygen air mixture. The masks are designed to give fixed percentages of oxygen. Oxygen flows through a small hole, called a venturi entraining air. The concentration remains roughly fixed.

The standard oxygen mask gives about:
- 35% oxygen at a flow rate of 4 litres a minute;
- 50% oxygen at a flow rate of 6 litres a minute;
- 60% oxygen at a flow rate of 10 litres per minute.

At flow rates less than 4.5 litres per minute some re-breathing occurs. The masks do not deliver the intended oxygen concentration if the patient is taking deep breaths. For over breathing patients increase the oxygen flow rate to 10 - 14 litres per minute. A tight fit is not necessary because the high flow rate constantly replenishes the oxygen supply.

Masks should be made of clear plastic so you can see the colour of the patient's lips and the fog which form when the patient breathes. Do not purchase coloured masks because these obscure cyanosis. Masks can be washed, thoroughly cleaned and used again. Do not autoclave them because they melt.

NASAL CATHETERS
Do not use these routinely in the recovery room. The oxygen delivery even at 10 l/min, flow is inadequate.

TRACHEOSTOMY MASKS fit over a tracheostomy tube. They raise the oxygen content of the inspired air by a variable amount depending on how deeply the patient is breathing.

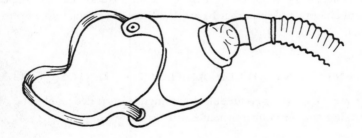

Fig 25.5 Tracheostomy mask

T-PIECES are attached directly to an endotracheal tube, laryngeal mask, or tracheostomy tube. Usually made of wide-bore plastic corrugated tube, their advantage is that they are non-rebreathing with low resistance to gas flow, and do not increase the effort of breathing. Humidified gas is delivered at 6 - 8 litres per minute through one limb of the T, while expired air is washed out of the system by the fresh gas flow. The expiratory limb should not have a volume exceeding 2 ml/kg ml in an adult. The volume of the expiratory limb in children should not exceed 0.5 ml/kg body weight. Never attach the fresh gas flow to a high-pressure gas source, and preferably attach it to a heated *blow over humidifier*.

T pieces are simply made and effective. They are ideal for weaning patients before extubation, and for giving oxygen to patients in the recovery room who have, either a tracheostomy, or laryngeal mask in place.

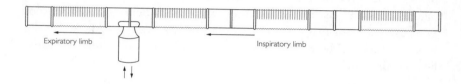

Expiratory limb   Inspiratory limb

fig 25.6 T-piece

Head Boxes and Incubators

These are only useful for infants. Head boxes require high flow rates, and it is necessary to monitor the oxygen concentration close to the child's face. Incubators and humidicribs at 3 - 8 litres per minute give up to 40% oxygen.

PATIENT CONTROLLED ANALGESIA DEVICES (PCA)[10]

There are many pumps suitable for patient controlled analgesia. When purchasing one for your unit make sure:

- it has battery backup;
- disposable items are readily available;
- it is easy to use;
- it is tamper proof;
- it indicates the number of times the patient has pressed the button;
- it has internal safeguards that shut the machine down if any malfunction is detected;
- maintenance and servicing is readily available.

Pressure Infusion Bags

Pressure infusion bags are used to squeeze plastic bags containing intravenous fluids. Many are poorly designed and made. Check the one you buy has a clearly marked pressure gauge, and is constructed of strong woven material that will not burst or tear. The bulb used to inflate them should be large enough to rapidly and easily inflate the device.

AN INSTANT PRESSURE INFLATOR BAG

A temporary device can easily be made. Carefully cut open the ends of a tough outer plastic bag in which many litre bags of intravenous fluid are delivered. Reinforce this with non-stretchable cloth surgical adhesive dressing (such as sticky zinc oxide tape) or Sleek® so that it can withstand pressure. Then attach a blood pressure cuff inflation bulb to an empty plastic litre bag. Slip the litre bag inside the reinforced outer bag to act as a bladder. A bag of blood attached to its giving set can then be compressed between the reinforced outer case and the inflatable inner bladder.

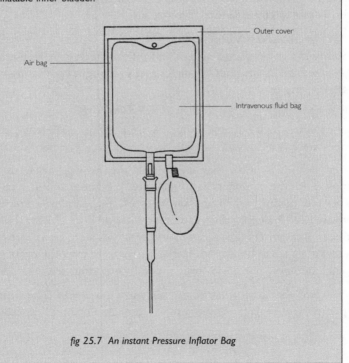

fig 25.7 An instant Pressure Inflator Bag

PULSE OXIMETERS[11]

Pulse oximeters measure the differential absorption of red, and infrared light, by oxygenated and deoxygenated haemoglobin. A light emitting diode located in a finger tip, or ear lobe probe sends light waves through the test site, and monitors the reflected wavelengths coming back as the blood passes through the capillaries. During systole, the extra surge of arterial blood absorbs additional light, and the reflected intensity falls. In this way the pulse can be detected. The difference in intensities is sensed by a photodetector in the probe, and the signal is fed into a microprocessor, that calculates the saturation, and pulse rate, and displays the reading on a screen.

Pulse oximeters give an early warning of hypoxia. They are the single most useful electronic device for monitoring in the recovery room. Every recovery room should have a pulse oximeter for each bay. Well known makes are accurate if the patient is warm. They measure the oxygen saturation of haemoglobin as blood passes through the capillaries of the skin. Points to check before purchase are:

• size, weight and portability;
• ability to run on mains current and internal rechargeable batteries;
• display easily seen from all angles and in all light conditions;
• alarms easy to set;
• probes robust, easy to repair or cheap to replace.

Probes come in a suitable range of sizes to suit different patients. Ear probes are useful for patients who have cold hands or poor circulation.

When testing a pulse oximeter check the display when the probe is exposed to the ambient light. Do not purchase a unit that shows a saturation reading when the probe is off the patient. Some makes are confused by flickering fluorescent or incandescent electric bulbs, where ambient light enters the sensor causing interference. This can be overcome by making a small light proof bag or sleeve to fit over the probe and finger to exclude light. The cover from a blood gas syringe makes a good sleeve.

Probes are the items that cause the most problems. They can be very expensive to replace. Some probes can be repaired especially if the electrical connections have worked loose from repeated bending of the wire running to the sensor. An unmatched probe, that is not designed for your particular oximeter, can burn the patient's finger.

RESPIROMETERS

THE WRIGHT'S RESPIROMETER® is a fragile instrument. It has delicate vanes that rotate to turn a series of fine cogs. These move a needle on a dial to register the volume of gas passing through the instrument. Respirometers are easily damaged if dropped. If someone blows into them hard it will tear the vanes and shred the cogs.

Don't blow hard into a Wright's respirometer,
they are easy to damage, and expensive to replace.

THE DRAGER VOLUMETER® is bulky and more robust. It has a useful timing device which stops the measurement after one minute, making it easy to standardize measurements. This device may be autoclaved and is a better choice for a remote hospital.

RESUSCITATION BAGS

The two commonly used self inflating types are the Ambu bag® and the Laerdal bag®. These bags are useful for transporting a patient when you are away from a compressed gas supply, because their shape automatically restores itself after it has been squeezed. The bags have a volume of about

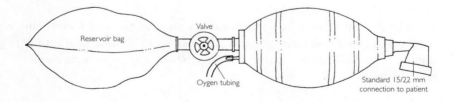

fig 25.8 Self-inflating resuscitation bag

1600 ml. Air is entrained through a one-way valve, and oxygen can be added if necessary. To enrich the inspired oxygen a reservoir bag must be attached to the Laerdal bag to act as an oxygen store. Turn the oxygen on to full flow which should be 10 - 15 litres per minute. Less flow than this is no better than room air. Resuscitation bags are not easy to use. They require practice under supervision until you feel competent.

A Mapleson C circuit, sometimes known as the Magill circuit, is useful in recovery room.

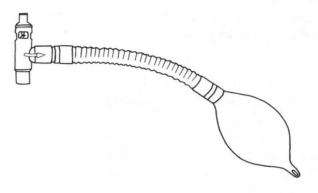

fig 25.9 Mapleson C circuit

It is easy to use in the resuscitation of a non-breathing patient. It has a major disadvantage; if it is attached to a spontaneously breathing patient he will rapidly become hypercarbic.

> *Do not use a Mapleson C circuit*
> *on a spontaneously breathing patient.*

To make this circuit safe for a spontaneously breathing patient remove the bag from the end and turn the fresh gas flow up to at least 10 litres per minute. This will convert it into a T-piece where carbon dioxide cannot accumulate.

SPACE BLANKETS

Space blankets are thin shiny metallic-like sheets made from Mylar®. This is an exceptionally strong plastic material which has a layer of silver, a few molecules thick, adsorbed on to it. Mylar sheets are hard to break, but tear easily. Put the silver side next to the patient. They are excellent for minimizing radiant heat loss, however as they conduct heat readily they need to be separated from the patient's skin by a sheet or blankets which will seal a layer of insulation around them. They also conduct electricity so keep them away from electrical apparatus. They are highly inflammable, and quickly burn with intense heat to form a shrunken, molten ball of red hot plastic.

A cheap and probably better alternative is *bubble* plastic used for packing fragile items for posting. This can be wrapped around the patient, cut to size and stapled with an ordinary office stapling machine. It is especially useful for keeping infants or neonates warm.

Spirit level

Spirit levels are used for levelling transducers or central venous measuring lines with the isophlebotic line on the body. One can easily be made from a six foot (1.8 metre) length of plastic tubing that has its ends joined to make a loop. Half fill the tubing with coloured water (stained with methylene blue or ink). Join the ends together, seal the join with water proof tape, and label it so it is not discarded (see page 36).

Stethoscopes

People borrow stethescopes and do not return them. Buy easily identifiable coloured ones. Most disposable stethoscopes are not suitable for recovery room use.

Suckers

Y-CATHETERS are used for either tracheal suction where they are passed down an endotracheal tube, or for pharyngeal suction where they are passed through the nose or mouth, to remove fluids collecting in the pharynx. Use only sterile catheters for tracheal suction.

Y-catheters are soft and flexible; they should be transparent, with a single hole at the tip. They must be long enough to pass beyond the end of an unshortened endotracheal tube. Their outer diameter (OD) should clearly labelled in millimetres. Since 1993, Charriere size (known as French gauge) has been dropped as the international standard.

Do not buy one with an additional side hole or eye near the tip of the catheter. If the end hole becomes blocked by secretions the side hole will suck on to the mucosa and damage it. Argyle Aeroflo® catheters are cleverly designed to prevent this sort of damage. For endotracheal tubes, size 5 or less, select an appropriate sucker for every tube. The sucker must never be more than half the width of the internal diameter of the endotracheal tube.

RIGID SUCKERS are made out of metal or plastic. They are sometimes called Yankeur, or dental suckers. Make sure their tips are firmly in place because they might come loose and be either swallowed or inhaled. If buying reusable suckers, check they are easily cleaned and sterilized.

SUCTION

The most important piece of equipment in the recovery room is a high-capacity, high-flow suction. This may come from a wall-outlet or an electrical pump. Foot pumps, and other devices are occasionally used. Whatever suction unit you use must run perfectly, and be strong enough to suck up the most viscid mucus or vomit. Each suction point must be capable of permitting a free flow of air of not less than 80 litres a minute and achieve an occluded suction of not less than 460 mmHg (60 kPa).

To prevent the suction inlet becoming blocked, have a fluid trap (usually a three litre glass or plastic container) between the sucker and the pump. This trap collects the secretions, blood and other fluids and prevents the pump becoming clogged with muck. Most suction pumps have a sintered brass filter at the wall inlet. These frequently become clogged which lowers the suction pressure. Establish a maintenance routine to clean, and replace these filters every few days. Change the tubing between patients, replace the collection bottles every shift, and get the hospital engineers to check the pressures and flows at the start of every day.

TEMPERATURE

Every recovery room needs a device for measuring low temperatures, because many patients will be hypothermic when they arrive in the recovery room. Normal clinical thermometers do not register below 35.5°C. Recently developed infra-red tympanic thermometers[12] accurately measure the patient's temperature. Devices such as The Genius™ (Model 3000A) and the The Cyclops 33™ are accurate, respond rapidly and are easy to use. The hypothalamus, where the thermoregulatory control centre is located, and the tympanic membrane share the same blood supply. They give the best estimate of temperature. Be very careful when you place them in the ear.

Cheap but less accurate thermistor tipped catheters can be placed in the rectum or oesophagus. Do not put these devices in the ear, because you risk damaging the delicate tympanic membrane and auditory canal. Swan-Ganz® catheters, too can give an accurate core temperature because they measure the temperature of the blood in the pulmonary artery.

TORCHES

Keep torches where they can easily be found in the dark if the lights fail. Have one torch available for every two beds. Each needs spare bulbs and batteries. Torches are also used for testing pupillary reflexes. A better way to do this is to use the standard 100 W incandescent bulb from a radial arm lamp held 60 cm (2 feet) from the patient's face.

TROLLEYS

Tables and sets of drawers on wheels are known as carts in the USA and Canada, and trolleys in the UK and elsewhere. These are designed to be taken to the patient's bedside for various procedures, for example, arrest trolleys (crash carts). The best ones have strong, large sprung castor wheels, and are made of stainless steel. Painted, or coated trolleys tend to chip and this makes them difficult to clean. Make sure the drawers cannot fall out and have stout runners to withstand heavy use.

Decide how many trolleys your recovery room needs. Depending on how busy you are you may need dedicated trolleys for paediatrics, difficult intubations and bronchoscopies. See appendix VII for examples of trolley set ups.

PATIENT TROLLEYS suitable for the recovery room have a specific standard dedicated to their design. Purchase those that conform to your local standard.

- Quickly tilted head or foot down at least 25° from the horizontal;
- the patient should be able to sit up with support;
- an adjustable foot rest or bed-end to stop the patient sliding down;
- a firm base and mattress;
- trolley sides or rails are necessary to prevent the patient rolling off. They must be easily retracted or removable;

- removable poles to carry intravenous fluids;
- holders for drainage bottles and bags and urine bags;
- large castor wheels for easy manoeuvrable;
- easily applied brakes;
- portable oxygen and suction easily available. This will require a cylinder, regulator, a flow device and a suction device on each trolley. This can be provided with a Twin-O-Vac® or similar device;
- a tray for carrying small articles such as the patient's history, false teeth and belongings.

VENTILATORS

Ventilators that have been inappropriately purchased or donated often become an embarrassing and expensive mistake. There are many makes and models and one is sure to fit your requirements. Seek expert advice. Make sure that the one you get will work in your recovery room. If you have a restricted supply of compressed gas, do not purchase a gas driven ventilator that is going to use many litres a minute to run; the Bird® ventilator and the Campbell® ventilator require between 11 litres and 25 litres of compressed gas a minute to power them.

If you have an unreliable electrical supply make sure that your auxiliary generators can cope with the load. Your ventilator should have an alarm to warn you if the patient has become disconnected. In case of ventilator malfunction, have a self-inflating bag near by so that you can use to ventilate the patient. Make sure all the connections can be attached to an endotracheal tube. Always have a clean ventilator ready. You may need it in a hurry.

If the patient is difficult to ventilate check the following:
- blocked tube, blood, foreign body, tissue or secretion;
- kinked tube, or patient biting on tube;
- cuff herniation;
- blocked breathing circuit;
- pneumothorax;
- bronchospasm.

THE MANLEY MULTIVENT® is a simple, reliable ventilator developed for the geographically isolated hospital. It can be powered either by compressed gas from a standard cylinder or electricity. It cannot, however, be triggered by the patient which limits its use to the paralysed or deeply sedated patient.

WARMING BLANKETS

SPACE BLANKETS (see page 488)

FORCED AIR WARMING DEVICES blow warm air into a light plastic envelope which is laid around the patient. They are highly effective in preventing further heat loss, and help rewarm the patient in the recovery room. One of the most widely used is the 'Bair Hugger™'; which when set on high, can increase body temperature by about 1.5°C/hr.[13]

1. Australian and New Zealand Intensive Care Society, Circular Sept 1994. ANZICS, *College of Surgeons*, Melbourne, Australia.
2. Eagle CC. (1992). *Anaesthesia and Intensive Care*, 20: 156 - 160.
3. Henderon MA, Irwin MG (1995). *Anaesthesia and Intensive Care*, 23: 407.
4. Hyson JM, Sessler DI, J. (1992). *Clinical Anaesthesia*, 4: 194-9.
5. Rooke GA, Bowdle TA, (1994). *Anaesthesia and Analgesia*, 78: 150-6.
6. John RE, Hill S. (1991). *Anaesthesia*, 46: 366-7.
7. Brimacombe J, Berry A. (1993). *Anaesthesia*, 48:670-1.
8. Stoneham HD. (1993). *Anaesthesia*, 48: 575 -580.
9. Dobson MB, (1992). *Tropical Doctor*, 22: 56-8.
10. Rowbotham J, (1992). editorial, *British Journal of Anaesthesia*, 68: 331-2.
11. Clayton RK, Webb AC. (1991). *Anaesthesia*, 46: 3 - 10.
12. Edge G, Morgan M. (1993). *Anaesthesia*, 48: 604 -7.
13. Sessler AI, Moayeri A. (1990). *Anesthesiology*, 70:424-7.

26. EQUIPMENT –
PURCHASING AND SAFETY

When setting up a recovery room one of the most challenging tasks is to decide what equipment is needed, what is available, reliable and good value for money. Make sure any electrical equipment you buy conforms to the international safety standard for electromedical equipment (IEC 601-1). Do not approach supply companies until everyone agrees on the decisions.

When buying equipment keep in mind the KISS criteria. KISS stands for Keep It Simple and Safe. Equipment must be easy to operate, preferably so easy that just by looking at it you can work out what it does, and how to use it, without referring to an instruction book. Important functions such as alarm settings, should be obvious. Remember many staff will use it and some may not have been trained in its use. Simplicity is important. Do not buy complicated equipment. Try to use the same equipment as the rest of the hospital; this means bits and pieces can be borrowed from, or shared with, other departments. It also helps the purchasing officer to buy and stock spare parts, and to negotiate on cheaper bulk purchases of disposables. Check with other nearby recovery units about the reliability, and ease of servicing of the equipment you intend to buy.

SPECIAL PROBLEMS FOR THE ISOLATED HOSPITAL

Nominate one member of your department to be in charge of the purchase, care, and maintenance of equipment. This is an important and time consuming job.

How to find out what is available

In the UK, the Department of Health periodically publishes evaluations of available equipment in *Health Equipment Information*. In Australasia there is a master reference manual published annually by MIMS (Medical International Statistics) called *Hospital Equipment and Supplies*. This thick book gives comprehensive details on almost everything that is commercially available in the region. Included are such data as catalogue numbers, addresses and telephone numbers of suppliers. Unfortunately there is no attempt to evaluate the equipment. These catalogues are expensive, but if you write to MIMS Publishing in your official capacity they may send your hospital a free copy. In Australasia the address is MIMS, 49 Albany Street, Crows Nest, New South Wales, 2065, Australia. The World Health Organisation is collecting data on reliable, robust and economical equipment for use in the isolated hospital.

Work out why you need the equipment in the first place:

• Will it improve patient safety. Such as a pulse oximeter?

• Will it help staff work more efficiently by doing a routine chore better; such as a non-invasive blood pressure machine?

• Can it do something that was impossible before; such as an oxygen concentrator?

• Does it need a special power source? A gas powered ventilator is useless unless there is a reliable and cheap source of compressed gas to run it. Many isolated hospitals have to work with an erratic and unreliable power supply.

Equipment must be robust and reliable. Robustness is important, and reliability, essential. Fragile equipment is useless if it constantly needs maintenance, or has to be sent a long distance for repairs. Reliability is essential. Before purchasing any piece of equipment, find out how often it breaks down. In engineering terms this is known as the MTBF (*mean time between failures*). For instance, for the best of the oxygen concentrators, this is about 6000 hours of operating time. Find out what happens when it does break down. Does it break down in a safe way? If in doubt about the reliability of the equipment, or its suitability for the task, telephone your nearest university teaching hospital and consult either the Biomedical Engineering Department or the Department of Anaesthesia. They should be able to give you helpful and unbiased advice.

When buying expensive equipment, such as electronic monitors or ventilators; involve the engineering staff in the planning phase. Consider their advice on technical matters about the choice of equipment, and what sort of training they need; and particularly, the manufacturer's ability to provide support such as manuals, maintenance contracts, spare parts, and training films or familiarity courses.

Do not buy equipment unless the company is willing to release circuit diagrams, and detailed workshop manuals of the equipment. Servicing is almost impossible if these diagrams are not available. Get at least two copies of the operator's manual and the maintenance manual; one for the hospital's biomedical engineers, and one to keep in the department. Check that they are complete and relevant to your piece of equipment. These manuals are an essential part of the equipment. They must be easy to understand, and have clear diagrams so that you can teach others. Poorly written, poorly translated, or incomplete manuals make equipment difficult to use, maintain and repair. Poor instruction manuals may also indicate that the equipment has not been carefully designed in the first place and may be unreliable. Sending equipment away for repairs or servicing can take many months and is very expensive. Often a local technician can do the work if he has access to the workshop manuals

Where do spare parts come from? Getting spare parts from another country can take months. Make sure there is an *after sales' service*, with a reliable supply of spare parts. It is a good idea to order spare parts when the equipment is purchased. Even with normal wear and tear some pieces will begin to break down almost immediately; for example the rubber suction bulbs, or rubber straps of an electrocardiograph, and blood pressure cuff bladders. This is especially true in tropical climates where rubber perishes quickly.

SERVICING (WITH SPECIAL REFERENCE TO THE ISOLATED HOSPITAL)

Of all the areas in which the isolated hospital has problems servicing causes the most difficulty. Lying around departments of most isolated hospitals is broken down or unusable equipment. Thoughtful planning avoids such waste.

Most equipment requires simple servicing by the people who use it. Establish a regular program of checking the equipment with clear orders on what to is to be done, and enforce them or else it may not happen! Every time a service is carried out, enter it in a book kept with the equipment.

This includes:
• daily, or pre-use checks;
• routine calibration;
• daily or pre-use cleaning and the reporting of faults;
• ensuring accessories are serviceable and complete;
• consumerable items are available.

Regular checks should be done by the biomedical engineers. To make things proceed smoothly the following questions need to be considered:
• what is to be maintained?
• how it is to be maintained?
• when is it to be maintained?
• is the maintenance effective?

To answer the first question draw up an inventory or register of equipment that needs maintenance. Before putting equipment into use it needs to be commissioned. This involves setting up a maintenance program and training staff to use and care for the equipment. The regular maintenance schedule must balance the manufacturer's recommendations with how often the equipment is used. Obviously the more often the equipment is used, the more frequently it should be checked.

Documentation is crucial, and card index systems are best in a smaller hospital. We hesitate to recommend computer based systems in an isolated hospital because they require expert staff run them. If the computer breaks down (and proper back-ups have not been made) all your data can be lost.

Some items of biomedical equipment such as blood gas machines require periodic calibration by an outside agency. Try as far as possible to calibrate the apparatus on the spot to avoid long periods without the equipment, and the risk of damage during transport. Bring the technician to the machine, try not to send the machine to the technician.

If servicing and maintenance is beyond the resources of your biomedical engineers it is possible for regions, or even countries, to co-operate to share a technician at regular intervals. This reduces costs, and increases efficiency.

If it cannot be repaired, condemn broken biomedical equipment. Do not leave it in your department. Ask the Supply Department to organize its disposal, and attend to the proper inventory and accounting procedures. Consider modifying the equipment to extend its useful life, or using parts of it for other things.

If a non disposable piece of equipment causes trouble shortly after purchase, ring the supplying company and inform them immediately. If they are unhelpful you can always find an alternative supplier.

DISPOSABLES

It is tempting to buy disposable items, because they release staff from the chores of cleaning and sterilization. Disposables save wages, and time, and reduce the chance of cross infection. However they are expensive, and need lots of storage space. If you are working in a isolated hospital think carefully before you discard, or stop using reusable items such stainless steel dishes, glass syringes, metal suckers and linen drapes. Circumstances can make disposables unobtainable. Once the routines for cleaning and sterilising reusable items is abandoned, it is hard to start again.

An inventory system is needed to automatically re-order disposables. Delegate this clerical function to, either the pharmacy, or the supply office.

Re-using disposable items is a controversial issue. Many disposable items, which have not been exposed to blood, or body fluids, can be washed, and then sterilised and safely reused. In many countries medicolegal problems make re-use impracticable.

Budgets

Most hospitals require every service area, such as the recovery room to have their own budget with the freedom, within set limits, to purchase and maintain their equipment. Until you are familiar with budgets it is worthwhile sitting down with a hospital administrator to check through the figures to see how the department is managing financially.

Safety in the Recovery Room

Electrical safety

Make sure that all equipment has been checked by an accredited technician before it is put into service, such as an electrician, an or electrical engineer from your hospitals biophysics department.

Report anything you suspect is faulty, such as:
• kinks in wires;
• plugs not fitting their sockets properly;
• worn or frayed electric leads;
• damaged outer coats on power cables;
• instances where someone has felt tingling, or has received a minor shock;
• spillage of liquid into electrical equipment.

Disconnect the suspect equipment, put a large 'Unsafe -Do not use' label on it, and report it.

Other points include:
• keep electric leads as short as practicable;
• keep electrical leads off hot surface, pipes or taps;
• do not use extension cords, because of the danger of fluid entering the junction;
• do not stand on a wet floor when operating or plugging in electrical equipment;
• do not stand on electric leads, or run trolleys over them.

(Electrical safety in the design of the recovery room - see page 506.)

Fire safety

All staff should have lectures about what to do in the case of a fire. and attend a *fire drill* at least twice a year.

Put up notices in conspicuous places giving clear, simple instructions about what to do in the case of fire. You will need to **RACE** to prevent tragedy.

Rescue	Remove patients to a safe place.
Alarm	Sound alarm.
Contain	Close windows and doors to isolate the fire.
Extinguish	Only attempt to put out the fire if you are certain of what you are doing.

Put Anglia® or similar evacuation sheets under each mattress on the trolleys. These tough sheets have handles, straps and buckles and use the mattress to wrap the patient in a protective shell. It is easy to drag this shell along the floor, and even down stairs, if necessary.

The best type of fire extinguish for recovery room is one that uses carbon dioxide. This copes with fires involving wood and paper, flammable liquids, live electrical equipment, and oil. Ensure fire extinguishers, fire hoses and fire blankets are installed in prominent places. Get the advice of your local fire department on this matter. Be sure to include maintenance of your fire equipment on your routine maintenance program.

27. Design of the Recovery Room

Ideal Requirements:

- public and private access;
- mini laboratory and access to blood gas machine;
- blood bank nearby and large blood fridge;
- pharmacy, checked and stocked every day;
- overhead radiographic imaging;
- administration area with computer connection to hospital computer;
- step down area with small kitchen for day patients and their relatives;
- staff call room.

Site of the Recovery Room

Shortly after the first anaesthetic was given in 1846, Florence Nightingale recognized the need for a special area, and special nursing care of patients recovering from ether anaesthesia. She wrote in her book 'Notes on Hospitals 'that the patient should be placed in a small room near to the ward, with clean fresh sand on the floor, clean bedclothes, and windows to admit the sunlight and fresh air.[1]

The recovery room is normally part of the operating suite, located close to where the anaesthetic was given, but readily accessible to medical staff who are in their street clothes. Staff tea rooms should be nearby so that the doctors, having a break at the end of a case can have quick access to the patients if needed. It is also useful if there is a communicating window between the holding bay, where patients arrive for theatre, with their escorting nurses, and the recovery room. Patients who are ready to leave can then be sent back with these escorts. Preferably, have the intensive care unit on the same level, and close to the recovery room. In hospitals with fewer than 200 beds it may be useful to have the intensive care unit next to the operating theatre. The recovery room can then be a functional part of the intensive care unit, but remain a separate area, away from the normal intensive care beds.

Make sure doctors in their street clothes
still have access to your recovery room.

Such an arrangement means that staff, facilities, and equipment can be shared between the two areas. A further advantage is that after hours, when there are less staff on the wards, patients can be recovered over night in the intensive care unit. The big disadvantage is the risk of transferring infection from the intensive care patients to the surgical patient. Staff will need education, and discipline to prevent this nosocomial infection. Hand washing, and the wearing of protective gowns are crucial parts of this program.

STANDARDS

There are many things to consider when planning, and building a recovery room. Fortunately architects, and engineers have access to help in the form of standards. Standards are sets of specifications that cover almost everything to do with the construction, design, safety, purchase, and applications of buildings, and equipment used in hospitals. Many countries including Australia, United Kingdom, and the European community, and USA have their own standards that specify such things as the design of buildings, the supply of piped gases, the quality of lighting, the fittings for anaesthetic apparatus, the formulation of drugs, electrical safety, hospital signs, medical records, and so on.

The International Organization of Standardization (ISO) based in Switzerland is struggling to get agreement between the various national standardization bodies, and is slowly bringing them into line. This means that apparatus designed, and used in one country, can be used equally safely in another; and the various fittings, pipes and colour codes, are uniform. In the European Community the Comité Européen de Normalisation has made rapid progress towards standardization, and their determinations were made mandatory in 1992.

Make sure that anything you design, builds, or buy complies with the accepted standards in your area. We have drawn freely on various standards to list ideas that may help you to design, and manage your recovery room. Our emphasis is on the needs of geographically isolated hospital.

PLAN FOR THE RECOVERY ROOM

The following section is an overview of the major features of a well-designed recovery room.

Square recovery rooms are more efficient than rectangular ones. Arrange the trolley bays around three walls, with a nurses' station, and open storage space on the fourth wall. The number of bed or trolley spaces should be sufficient for expected peak loads. You will need about 3 recovery room trolley bays for each operating theatre. Make sure there is easy access to the patient's head, and an adequate working area around the patient. Two metres on either side of the trolley is ideal. Allow about 12 square metres of space for support utilities. Modular cupboards can be expanded to meet the future requirements. Each trolley bay needs at least 1 cubic metre (9 cubic feet) of storage space within the room, and at least 3 square metres (28 square feet) of shelving and storage nearby.

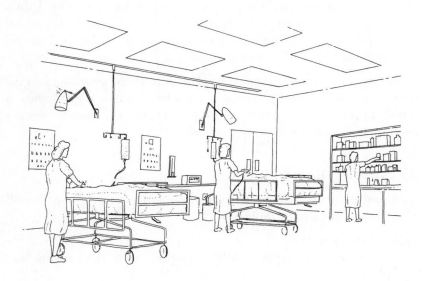

fig 27.1 Recovery room

*Too much storage space is better
than too little.*

Plan an open, and uncluttered recovery room, with no structures obstructing your view. If there is an unavoidable structure arrange mirrors to overcome your blind spot. Every trolley bay should be visible from anywhere within the room. If you design a central island for your nurse station be careful with heights. The bench top should still be low enough for staff, who are sitting, to see over.

If the recovery room is designed as part of the intensive care unit, consider building an *isolation room* for managing patients with infections, contaminated wounds, and those who are immunosupressed. This room should have both negative, and positive air conditioning.

> *Make sure nothing obstructs*
> *your view of the patients.*

Make sure the patient trolleys can move easily around the room, with a minimum number of corners to negotiate. Have two wide doors for access; one from the operating theatre, and one to the wards. Ideally these should be at opposite ends of the recovery room.

All the recovery room bays should be identical with the same things in the same place. Do not design bays that are mirror images of each other, a confusing technique favoured by many architects. Consistancy ensures easy access to equipment and safe practice.

RECOVERY ROOM BAYS

Each patient trolley bay needs its own *service utilities* mounted on the wall at the head of the patient trolley.

Ideally there should be:
- two high-pressure oxygen outlets equipped with flow meters and nipples;
- two high-vacuum, high-flow suction outlets, including receiver, tubing, rigid hand piece, and a range of suction catheters;
- two high pressure medical air outlets;
- six electric (general) power outlets;
- one mobile examination lamp, that can be swung to provide light to any point on the patient;
- at least two shelves with slightly raised edges to prevent things falling on the floor;
- appropriate facilities for mounting monitoring equipment;
- somewhere to keep the patient's chart;
- storage space or bins for the day patient's belongings.

Equipment

Provide each recovery room bay with:

- a sphygmomanometer attached to the wall at eye height;
- a good stethoscope;
- over head runners similar to curtain rails are preferable to drip stands;
- a place to keep the patient's chart;
- suction equipment, sterile suction catheters;
- oropharyngeal airways, and nasopharyngeal airways;
- sterile disposable gloves; (preferably powder free)
- unsterile disposable protective gloves in small, medium and large sizes;
- a pressure infusion bag for giving intravenous fluids rapidly;
- clear plastic masks so you can see the patient's mouth and lips;
- oxygen tubing with connectors;
- T-pieces for delivering oxygen to intubated patients, or those returning with a laryngeal mask still in place;
- self inflating bag, Laerdal® or Ambu®;
- a pulse oximeter;
- bowls, and kidney dishes;
- small hand towels;
- paper tissues;
- scissors;
- tape, gauze, mouth swabs;
- sealable plastic bags for transport of potentially infected fluids;
- containers for haematology, and pathology specimens;
- blood gas syringes;
- a range of needles, syringes, and skin cleaning preparation.

These last three groups of items can be stored in a separate trolley for the use of all the bays. This reduces the amount of stocking for all the bays.

If any of this non-disposible equipment is faulty, complain immediately to the manufacturer or supplying company. Ask for a replacement or your money back.

RECOVERY ROOM FACILITIES

AIR-CONDITIONING should maintain the temperature of the recovery room at between 21°C and 24°C with the capability of increasing it to 26°C, and with a relative humidity of between 40 and 60 per cent under all conditions with at least 6 air changes each hour. Anaesthetic gas pollution can be high in the recovery room, because patients continue to exhale the gases for some time after leaving the operating theatre.

EMERGENCY POWER is essential in case the mains supply fails. This should automatically switch on if there is mains power failure. To avoid the recovery room being plunged into total darkness have one or more emergency battery powered lights, that automatically switch on when the mains power supply fails.

ELECTRICAL SAFETY. *Macroshock* causes electrocution, with the heart going into ventricular fibrillation. *Microshock* occurs when a tiny current of a few millivolts passes through an electrolyte infusion or pacemaker wire to cause ventricular fibrillation. *Isolation transformers* or *core balance earth leakage devices* protect against macroshock.

ELECTRICAL PROTECTION DEVICES

Ordinary wiring used in domestic houses has its electrical protection (*Class A*) limited to fuses, and an earth wire in the cord. The recovery room should be a *Body Protected Area (Class B)* giving protection from macroshock in event of an accident. Macroshock protection is provided by either *isolation transformers* or *core balance earth leakage devices*. Isolation transformers may be fitted to the main electricity supply. These prevent a person being electrocuted if they touch the electrically live (or active) wire of the power supply while in contact with an earth. They are designed so that current cannot flow through a person or other electrical conductor to the earth. They are expensive, and need regular maintenance. A far cheaper alternative is a core balance earth leakage device. It detects a current flowing to earth, and automatically cuts off the power supply before it causes harm. For most recovery rooms this device is sufficient to minimise the risk of electrocution. To ensure they work properly all earth points in the ward need a common heavy copper grounding cable. The engineering specifications for these areas are set out in special safety standards. Cardiac-protected areas (*Class Z*) are similar to Class B areas but include special wiring to ensure no exposed surfaces of the plumbing, electrical equipment monitors etc, in the vicinity of the patient can create, and electrical gradient sufficient to cause microelectrocution.

EMERGENCY STATION. Establish an emergency station where the defibrillator, and trolleys (*crash carts*) for managing a cardiac arrest, and other emergencies are kept. Keep this easily accessible. The emergency station needs its own power outlets to keep the portable equipment's batteries charged.

FLOORING. Lay a non-slip floor, with a non-absorbent surface of uniform colour that can be easily cleaned. Patterned or speckled flooring hides dirt, and makes it difficult to find small objects that have fallen on the floor.

HAND WASHING. Ideally, there should be one hand basin with hot and cold running water, a liquid-soap dispenser, paper towels, and a waste bin to every two trolley bays. To prevent cross contamination linen towels should not be used. Avoid installing hot air hand dryers because they are noisy, and spray germs, and skin squames all over the room.

IMPREST SYSTEM. A drug and disposables *Imprest system* makes restocking easy. This is a system for holding commonly used items in the recovery room. It is the duty of the pharmacist, and supply officer to check, and restock them as they are used. Recovery rooms use a wide range of drugs. Store them lockable drug cupboard. A set of recessed shelves with a door that is rolled down at the end of the day is ideal. Organize the drug cupboard in such a way that drugs can be quickly found. Post an alphabetical list of available drugs under both their generic and trade names. It is a good idea to have a third list with the drugs classified under their pharmacological actions, for example a list of antibiotics, cardiac drugs, etc.

LIBRARY. Have an unlocked bookcase built to house a small library of reference books.

LIGHTING. Consider the advantages of windows and natural light for both the patients and the staff. If natural daylight is not available, light the room with special colour-corrected fluorescent tubes. Do not use blue-light fluorescent tubes, or incandescent light bulbs, because they make it difficult to judge the patient's colour, and delay the recognition of cyanosis. The lights should provide 100 candela for every 10 square metres of floor space. Effectively, this is enough light to read the printing on a drug ampoule at arm's length with one eye covered. For most purposes two 25 watt fluorescent tubes are enough to cover 10 square metres.

LINEN AND LAUNDRY. Make provision for the collection of soiled linen, and other contaminated waste. Plan for the orderly disposal of paper, and clean plastic. Have a meeting to decide what can be safely be recycled, then make the process easy with clearly labelled containers.

NOTICE BOARD and a white board with erasable pens for teaching, and planning patient management. This can also be used to display daily staff rosters.

PAINTING. Paint walls, and ceilings light, neutral colours. Avoid colours such as blues, reds, greens or yellows, because they reflect misleadingly on the patient's skin.

PATIENT TROLLEYS. A minimum of three patient transport trolleys will be needed for each working theatre; one for attending to the patient in theatre, one for the patient in recovery room, and one for transporting the patient back to the ward. There are special international standards for the design of these trolleys.

If your hospital is suitably designed, patients having major surgery can have their own beds brought to recovery room.

PIPED GASES. Fit all piped gases with failure alarms that are easily identified by both a sound and a light. Install these in a conspicuous place. Frame a set of instructions on what to do if the alarm sounds, and screw them to the wall next to the warning light. Supplies of oxygen, and suction for emergencies are best kept under every trolley bay.

PLUMBING. Share toilets, and space for equipment cleaning with the operating theatres.

TELEPHONES. Noisy telephones disturb patients, and demand to be answered. Install a phone with an audible but non irritating ring. Use this phone for paging and answering paging calls. Trivial in-coming and outgoing calls are a nuisance, discourage them. They are best handled by the theatre receptionist or secretary. Consider personal mobile phones for individual staff members. These mean the ward can be contacted or a doctor paged from the trolley bay and the patient not left unattended.

UTILITY CABLES. The desk, and nurses' station will need power points. Install a utility cable duct to carry cables for telephones, intercoms, computers, and paging systems. Make these ducts easily accessible to allow you to lay more cables in the future.

VOICE PAGING. this useful for summoning help in emergencies.

X-RAY MACHINES. Install a suitable power outlet for the portable X-ray machine used in your hospital. An overhead radiograph fixture is ideal. Use X-rays in recovery room as infrequently as possible. Patients should be sent to the X-ray department on the way to the ward unless it is an emerency.

X-RAY VIEWING SCREENS. Attach X-ray viewing screens, and a bright light for examining films on the wall near the nurses' desk.

EQUIPMENT FOR THE RECOVERY ROOM

BLOOD WARMERS. In-line blood warmers to reduce transfusion pain, help prevent hypothermia, reduce the viscosity of blood, and prevent damage from cold agglutinins.

EMERGENCY ALARM. Site a large red panic button on the wall above each trolley bay to call for help. The best buzzer is one with an urgent repeating sequence that can be heard throughout the operating theatres, rest rooms, and changing rooms. To prevent these being accidentally activated, design them to pull on rather than push on. Identify them with large clear signs. Test them daily.

EMERGENCY TROLLEYS (CRASH CARTS). Keep trays or trolleys (carts) set up, and ready to use for the management of anaphylaxis, malignant hyperthermia, emergency airway care, emergency bronchoscopy, insertion of thoracic drains, minor surgical procedures, and vascular access. Each needs its own set of protocols attached to it. It helps to have a large, clear colour photograph of each setup so that the trays can be checked quickly, and are always put together the same way. Photos enable you to tell quickly what is missing. Trolleys used infrequently for malignant hyperthermia and bronchoscopy can be shared with the anaesthetic department. For set ups of typical trolleys (see appendix VII).

FIRE CONTROL EQUIPMENT. Fit fire control equipment, and smoke detection devices in the recovery room (see page 500). Appoint staff as fire monitors, and take their photographs. Display their names, photographs, and duties, in case of emergency, at the entrance to the recovery room. These people will be in charge if a fire breaks out. Remember to train new personnel. Every one working in the recovery room should have a written instruction on the back of their identification labels about to what to do in the case of fire, or other emergencies requiring evacuation. Hold evacuation practices twice a year, and ask random questions, for example "Where is the nearest fire extinguisher?".

MONITORS. At least one patient physiology monitor is needed for every bay. This should be mounted at eye level and have a large screen. Most have a number of features such as ECG, pulse oximetry, end expired carbon dioxide, inspired oxygen concentration, blood, and other pressure modules, parameter trending, and non-invasive blood pressure monitoring (see page 468). For the district hospital physiology monitoring you will need, at least, a pulse oximeter for each patient. ECG, non-invasive blood pressure monitors can be shared between two, or three bays as necessary.

REFRIGERATORS
You will need two refrigerators:
1. A refrigerator for storing heat labile drugs, and other items such as ice used for testing the efficacy of local blocks.

2. A special thermostatically controlled refrigerator for storing blood products and vaccines. It should have a clock-chart, and an alarm to warn if its temperature has risen or fallen outside set limits; even when the recovery room is unattended. If this alarm go off, check with the blood bank, because you may need to discard the biological products. This fridge can be shared with the whole operating suite. It should have ready access to the haemotology department. A delivery hoist and dedicated phone are ideal.

RESPIROMETERS (anemometers) measure the volume of air moving in or out of the lungs (see page 487).

SCREENS OR CURTAINS. Some means of screening each patient for privacy, or if problems arise.

SHARPS DISPOSAL is a major issue; especially with the increasing risk of HIV, Hepatitis B, and C transmission due to needle stick injuries. Immediately after use sharps, such as needles and empty ampoules, must be put into rigid sharp puncture proof containers. Have one container at each trolley bay. Do not over fill these containers. When they are full, seal them, and send them to be incinerated. Before handling the containers check that no needle points are sticking through the walls of the container. Most hospitals now have formal programs for safely dealing with, and disposing of sharps.

VENTILATOR. A mechanical ventilator with a humidifier, and all the necessary sterile tubing and connections. This should be checked and primed every day. This can be attached to an available anaesthetic machine.

WARMING CUPBOARD. A warming cupboard for warming blankets, towels, and fluids.

1. Nightingale F. (1863). Notes on Hospitals page 89, Publishers: Longman, Roberts and Green.

28. STAFFING AND MANAGEMENT

MANAGEMENT'S RESPONSIBILITY TO RECOVERY ROOM

It is the hospital management's responsibility to ensure that adequate nursing personnel, support staff and the appropriate drugs and equipment are available. Support staff include administrators, clerical staff, engineering staff, pharmacists and technicians. Before taking responsibility for the care of patients, the staff must be assessed as competent to carry out their duties. It is negligent to leave unstable postoperative patients in unskilled hands. Many countries such as the UK, USA and Australasia have special *standards* drawn up by professional bodies to lay down an acceptable standard of care for the patient in recovery room. It may help to consult the nursing or medical professional associations in your area.

Sir Robert Macintosh, the first Professor of Anaesthetics at Oxford University, said in 1970 that he regarded recovery rooms as one of the greatest advances in anaesthesia. Coroners, throughout world, affirm the recovery room as the most important room in the hospital, for it is here the patient is at the greatest risk of coming to harm.

During normal office hours most work is with patients having elective operations. Work in the recovery room starts at the beginning of the operating lists, and finishes an hour or two after the last operation. Emergencies are usually dealt with at the end of day's routine operating and at night. Most recovery rooms are properly staffed during the day, but it is important to maintain proper staffing after hours too. The hospital's management needs to be reminded that emergency patients operated on after hours are often those most in need of highly specialized care.

Nursing staff

Maintain a flexible ratio of experienced nurses to patients. The American Society of Post Anaesthetic Nurses (ASPAN) suggests sensible criteria for the allocation of nurses in the recovery room.

CLASS I. Uncomplicated patients who are conscious and stable require one trained nurse for three patients.

CLASS II. Uncomplicated paediatric patients who are stable and conscious, or patients who have undergone major surgery, or adult patients who are stable and unconscious, require one trained nurse for two patients.

CLASS III. Patients requiring life support care need one trained nurse for each patient.

There should always be two nurses in the recovery room, even if there is only one patient. One of these should be an experienced recovery room nurse. Nurses without sufficient recovery room experience need direct supervision, and should not be left on their own.

High dependency patients, such as those following neurosurgery, thoracic, vascular, or emergency trauma surgery need more nursing care than those undergoing more minor surgery. Lists with large numbers of short cases will require extra nurses.

NURSING BANKS

Nursing banks are organized by many hospitals to provide relief personnel to cover illness, holidays and times of peak activity. Many nurses prefer part time work. Sometimes it may be necessary to employ temporary staff from nursing agencies. These nurses may not have adequate experience in recovery room and will require extra supervision.

ORDERLIES OR TECHNICIANS

Orderlies or technicians are needed to lift, transport and position patients, and help with equipment. Have at least one strong, competent orderly always available.

TRAINING

Staff who know what they are doing are impressive, and it is training and experience that make them competent. Recovery room nursing is a skilled and demanding task. Training requires a structured post-graduate course, assimilating both operating theatre techniques, and intensive care nursing. It can be reinforced by rotating the recovery room staff through areas such as intensive care, high dependency units, and coronary care units. Establish a structured continuous education program to keep staff up to date.

For safety and efficient management
there must be enough trained staff.

Medical staff

In most operating theatres the anaesthetist responsible for the anaesthetic is also responsible for the recovery room care of the same patient.

Administration

The recovery room is usually supervized by, either the Medical Director of Anaesthesia, or the Nursing Director of the Operating Theatre Suite. An experienced recovery room nurse should manage the area. Clerical staff are needed to answer phones, keep track of supplies, run errands and so on.

PLANNING is often delegated to an *operating theatre committee* composed of nurses, medical staff, and administrators. Some tips to make this committee run smoothly are that it should:
• be small, with no more than six members;
• hold regular meetings;
• have defined written responsibilities;
• have an agenda circulated some days before the meeting.

When confronted with a task to plan the committee should:
• define the task to be accomplished;
• provide appropriate resources to accomplish the task;
• establish people to be responsible for each phase;
• appoint someone to co-ordinate, and follow-up the task;
• set deadlines;
• keep good records.

ROSTERS are best made up at least a fortnight in advance.

POLICY MANUALS help standardize protocols, procedures, and lines of communication. Write them in collaboration with all the staff in the operating theatres. It is the job of the operating theatre committee to organise this task.

PROTOCOLS AND GUIDELINES. *Protocols* are designed to be followed precisely, while *guidelines* allow latitude for common sense. *Policies* lay out a course of action for the future. Protocols ensure everyone does things the same way. Most administrative and clinical situations recur, and every hospital has its own routine and ways of coping with these situations. It is not easy to transplant routines from one hospital to another, so develop your own protocols, and guidelines about to what to do in given circumstances. Develop routines so that everyone approaches these recurring problems in the same way. Protocols and guidelines make audits easy.

Develop and keep nursing and medical protocols together, because it needs an informed and willing team to provide good holistic patient management. Nursing care has five elements: assessment, nursing diagnosis, development of a care plan, its implementation, and evaluation of the plan. This takes into account relevant preoperative emotional, psychosocial, and safety needs. Medical care includes the recognition of ordered, and the diagnosis of disordered, physiology and biochemistry of the patient, and their therapeutic management. The doctor is responsible for the overall physical, and mental welfare of his patient. This includes the duty of informing the patient of the risks of therapeutic intervention.

Review the guidelines and protocols regularly at unit meetings. You will need protocols for:

- checking of equipment and drugs;
- transfer of patient from operating theatre to the recovery room;
- handover of the patient from theatre staff to recovery room staff;
- observation and documentation of details about the patient;
- emergency procedures;
- discharge criteria and procedures;
- responsibilities of categories of staff.

Once routines are established errors are less likely to occur. Written guidelines help ward staff manage the more complex postoperative problems such as, management of epidural catheters, or airway problems after thyroidectomy.

Protocols need to be concise, clearly written and helpful. Keep them in the unit where they can be consulted. Do not make them too wordy or no one will read them. A successful policy, protocol and guideline book will soon look well thumbed and dog-eared.

A LIBRARY for reference is particularly useful after hours. Do not lock the books away. You never know when you may have to look up something urgently. References could include books on topics such as nursing, practical pharmacology, a synopsis of anaesthesia, and techniques of local anaesthesia. Collect useful articles from journals.

A MESSAGE BOOK is useful to pass on messages to staff on later shifts. Use it to keep track of equipment lent to other parts of the hospital, and to follow up ideas, new techniques, staff with special roster requests and so on.

MAINTENANCE BOOKS ensure the weekly check of the defibrillator, and regular servicing of equipment have been done properly.

WEEKLY MEETINGS are a part of the quality assurance program. Establish regular meetings to discuss cases, and problems and to keep staff up-to-date with recent advances. Involve all staff in educational and peer review meetings.

AUDITS are part of a quality control process. They help you find potential problems, as well as revealing occasionally surprising information to help you improve patient care, and justify the resources needed in the recovery room. Once you think you have corrected a problem, repeat your audit to make sure it really has been solved. This check is called *closing the audit*. Audits are sometimes a tedious chore, but do make a huge difference in the quality of care.

Do not attempt to review every patient at every audit. For example, take a homogeneous sample of ENT patients. Prepare a simple list of problems that arise in day-to-day routines, such as, restlessness after nasal surgery, sore eyes, or vomiting. These problems delay the discharge of patients. Survey the incidence of these problems for a month, and then use the results to find trends that will help improve efficiency and patient care. Perhaps you may find a high incidence of sore eyes and trace the cause back to the skin preparation used by one particular surgeon. There may be a delay in getting the patients back to the ward at the end of the morning. Staggered lunch breaks for the orderlies might solve this problem.

ERRORS, INCIDENTS, AND ACCIDENTS[1] are bound to occur. Some errors are trivial and others disastrous, but error is unfortunately a part of every human activity. Accidents do happen, and not all errors are blame worthy. Normal people, under normal circumstances do not make mistakes on purpose. It is easy to be wise in hindsight.

Document them accurately including written reports from all the staff involved. The statements must contain facts only - do not try to interpret what happened. If there are likely to be medicolegal consequences ask the administrators in your hospital to help you prepare these statements.

Understanding why incidents occur is the first step in crisis management, and their analysis is useful to prevent them occurring again. The staff, the patients, their diseases, and the technology used in recovery room is a complex dynamic system, and those familiar with *Chaos theory* will know that a minor incident can set up a chain reaction of a series of subtle, and possibly undetected events coming together to explode as a catastrophe. Collect a record of incidents with sufficient detail to allow you to identify events and their contributing factors. Note what went wrong, and who, what, when, why and how it occurred. Include contributing factors such as fatigue, rostering problems, power failures and so on.

1 Runciman WB, Sellen A, *et al.* (1993). *Anaesthesia and Intensive Care*, 21: 506-19.

APPENDIX I.
DRUG INFUSIONS

Some drugs need to be administered at a constant rate for a number of hours or days. This is best achieved by an infusion. A solution is prepared with a known concentration of drug. This is delivered at a rate calculated to keep the blood concentration of the drug at a fairly constant level. A loading dose is needed for most drugs. The advantages of an infusion are that the effect of the drug is smoother, a lower overall dose is required and the need for repeated injections is eliminated.

There are three ways of administering an infusion.
1. Syringe drivers give small volumes of concentrated drug through a catheter placed in one of the large central veins such as the superior vena cava. The drugs are usually so concentrated that they will injure smaller peripheral veins and may cause severe tissue damage if extravasation occurs.

Never infuse concentrated drugs
through peripheral veins.

2. Infusion pumps (see page 475) give larger volumes of fluid. Generally the drugs are less concentrated and often it is possible to safely infuse them into smaller peripheral veins.

3. Convert ml/hr to drops/min:
$$\text{ml/hr} \times \text{drops/ml} \times 1/60 \text{ drops/min} = \text{drops/min}.$$

For example, if 30 ml/hr are to be given through an ordinary drip set which delivers 15 drops/ml, how many drops a minute would this require?
$$30 \times 15 \times 1/60 = 7.5 \text{ drops/min}.$$

The best way to regulate this would be to measure it over 2 minutes so that $2 \times 7.5 = 15$ drops would come every 2 minutes.

Prepare written protocols for each drug used. In them, set down the dose of the drug and the required pump or syringe drive settings. Include details of the expected effects, complications, and management of these complications. Staff should be familiar with all the effects and expected problems before the infusion starts. Establish clear written instructions about limits of the parameters of blood pressure, pulse rate, respiratory rate and other variables. These are best set out on a whiteboard mounted on the wall near the head of the patient so that all staff can easily see them.

Each potent drug needs its own dedicated separate intravenous line. It is unwise to use one catheter for the infusion of a number of drugs. Do not 'piggy back' lines by using multi-entry ports or plug infusions into intravenous lines carrying other intravenous infusions. For safety, potent drugs should be infused through a multilumen central venous catheter, with each lumen carrying only one drug.

For safety infuse only one drug
through each intravenous line.

Be careful of the 'dead space' in lines and catheters. Unfamiliarity with the concept of dead space can cause dangerous problems. Prime (that means 'fill') the lines with the solution containing the drug. This prevents a delay in the drug reaching the patient. Unless properly primed it will take time for the drug solution to fill the volume of the tubing. This volume is called the 'dead space'. Beware of inadvertently flushing this dead space because the patient may get a large dose of unwanted drug. For this reason, never inject anything into a line through which concentrated drug is being infused.

Patient's name _____	Unit record number _____
Ward _____ Date _____	Time prepared _____
Prepared by _____	Checked by _____
Drug and dose added _____
_____
_____
Concentration _____
Duration of infusion _____	Time to finish _____

To prevent errors, the drug concentration, and the rate of infusion, must always be checked independently, by two separate trained staff who understand the equipment and how to use it.

In the doses recommended below, the concentration of drug has been chosen so that the pump settings, in mls per hr, represent some simple numerical function of the drug dose in units per hr. For example if morphine is to be given then a setting of 4 ml/hr will give a dose of 4 mg/hr.

Attach an intravenous additive label to bags, flasks, or syringes containing drugs.

Patients receiving infusions need constant monitoring and careful nursing care. Patients must never be left unattended. Everyone needs to be familiar with the pharmacology of the drugs, their actions, and side effects. Written protocols are needed and the patient's cardiovascular and other parameters need to be carefully specified.

IMPORTANT NOTICE

Most of the following drugs are highly concentrated and cause severe thrombophlebitis and tissue necrosis if infused into peripheral veins. So infuse them into central veins only through a central venous catheter.

When infusing vasoactive or cardiac drugs always monitor cardiac rate and rhythm with an ECG and continuous record blood pressure using an intra-arterial cannula.

DRUG INFUSIONS AND DILUTIONS

DRUG	DILUTION	DOSE
ADRENALINE* Epinephrine in USA 1 ml of 1/1000 = 1 mg 10 ml of 1/10 000 = 1 mg	Adrenaline 3 mg Make up to 50 ml in 5% dextrose	1 ml/hr = 1 microgram/min 1–30 microgram/min Increase dose by 1 microgram/min until desired effect
AMIODARONE*	Amiodarone 300 mg in 50 ml of 5% dextrose. (Not stable in saline). No need to use glass syringes	Loading dose: 25 microgram/kg/min for 4 hr May be given at 5 mg/kg over 20 min if urgent Maintenance: 5–15 microgram/kg/min

* Infuse these drugs only through a central venous catheter.

DRUG	DILUTION	DOSE
DOPAMINE*	Dopamine 300 mg Make up to 50 ml in 5% dextrose	1 ml/hr = 100 microgram/min Increase dose by 1 microgram/kg/min until desired effect Low (renal) dose: 3–5 microgram/kg/min Beta effect: 5–25 microgram/kg/min Alpha effect: > 25 microgram/kg/min
DOBUTAMINE*	Dobutamine 250 mg Make up to 41.5 ml in 5% dextrose	1 ml/hr=100µg/min 2.5–15 microgram/kg/min
DOPEXAMINE*	Dopexamine 10 mg Make up to 41.5 ml in 5% dextrose	1 ml/hr = 4 µg/hr 0.1–1 mg/kg/hr
FRUSEMIDE Furosemide in USA	Frusemide 100 mg Make up to 50 ml in normal (0.9%) saline	1 ml/hr = 2 mg/hr Loading dose: 0.5 mg/kg Maintenance dose: 0.1–1 mg/kg/hr Protect from light
GLYCERL TRINITRATE* 'GTN' 'Nitroglycerine'	Glyceryl trinitrate 100 mg Make up to 41.5 ml in 5% dextrose	1 ml/hr = 40 microgram/min Maintenance dose: 1–5 microgram/kg/min Increase dose by 2–40 microgram/min
HEPARIN 1 mg = 100 units	Heparin 25 000 units make up to 25 ml in 5% dextrose	1 ml/hr = 1000 units/hr Low dose: 75 units/kg stat then 10 – 15 units/kg/hr Full heparinization: 200 units/kg stat then 15 – 30 units/kg/hr
INSULIN	Insulin (act rapid) 50 units Make up to 50 ml in 5% dextrose or haemacel®	1 ml/hr = 1 unit/hr sugar 6-8 give 2mls/hr sugar 8-10 3mls/hr sugar 10-14 4mls/hr
ISOPRENALINE*	Isoprenaline 3 mg Make up to 50 ml in 5% dextrose	1 ml/hr = 1 microgram/min 1–20 microgram/min

* Infuse these drugs only through a central venous catheter.

DRUG	DILUTION	DOSE
LIGNOCAINE Lidocaine in USA 'Xylocard'	Lignocaine 1000 mg Make up to 41.5 ml in 5% dextrose	1 ml/hr = 0.5 mg/min Run at: 8 ml/hr for 1st hr 6 ml/hr for 2nd hr 4 ml/hr for next 24 hrs
MILRINONE*	Milrinone 30 mg Make up to 50 ml in 5% dextrose	1 ml/hr = 10 microgram/min Min. 0.37 microgram/kg/min Av. 0.5 microgram/kg/min Max. 0.75 microgram/kg/min
MORPHINE	Morphine 50 mg Make up to 50 ml in 5% dextrose	1 ml/hr = 1 mg/hr Loading dose: 0.1 – 0.5 mg/kg Normal requirements 0.02 – 0.1 mg/kg/hr
NIMODOPINE		Initial dose: 15 microgram/kg/hr for 2 hr If BP remains stable, then increase to 30 microgram/kg/hr
NITROGLYCERINE *	see Glyceryl trinitrate	
NITROPRUSSIDE* 'Nipride'	Nitroprusside 50 mg Make up to 41.5 ml in 5% dextrose Do not exceed dose of 10 µg/kg/minute	1 ml/hr = 20 microgram/min 0.5 – 10 microgram/kg/min The average dose is 1.5 microgram/kg/min Max effect seen in 3 minutes. Dose increments: 0.5 microgram/kg
NORADRENALINE* Norepinephrine in USA	Noradrenaline 3 mg Make up to 50 ml in 5% dextrose	1 ml/hr = 1 microgram/min 1–30 microgram/min Increase dose by 1 microgram/min until desired effect.
PETHIDINE	Pethidine 500 mg Make up to 50 ml in 5% dextrose	1 ml/hr = 10 mg/hr Loading dose: 0.75–1.5 mg/kg Maintenance dose: 0.1–0.4 mg/kg/hr

* Infuse these drugs only through a central venous catheter.

DRUG	DILUTION	DOSE
PROCAINAMIDE	Procainamide 1000 mg Make up to 41.5 ml in 5% dextrose	1 ml/hr = 0.5 mg/min Run at: 8 ml/hr for 1st hr 6 ml/hr for 2nd hr 4 ml/hr for next 24 hrs
PROTAMINE	Use undiluted 500 mg in 50 ml	1 ml/hr = 10 mg/hr Dose: Take previously administered heparin dose (units/hr) and divide it by 100
VERAPAMIL 'Cordilox'	Verapamil 50 mg Make up to 50 ml in 5% dextrose	1 ml/hr = 1 mg/hr Loading dose: 1 mg/min up to 10 mg (10 ml of 10% calcium gluconate may be needed to control hypotension) **or** 0.1 – 0.15 mg/kg IV over 10 minutes

CATECHOLAMINES USED IN TREATMENT OF SHOCK

ADRENALINE (EPINEPHRINE) is a hormone of exercise. It is a useful drug in the treatment of systolic dysfunction. Adrenaline is both an alpha and beta stimulator. At low doses the effects are predominantly beta but as the dose increases the alpha effects take over. In small doses of 0.1 microgram/kg β_1, and particularly β_2 effects prevail. The result is an increases in cardiac rate and force of contraction (β_1 effect) which raises the cardiac output, and vasodilation in skeletal muscle beds. As a result the systolic blood pressure rises, and as muscle blood flow increases, the diastolic blood pressure falls. The overall effect is an increase in pulse pressure. If the dose of adrenaline is increased, then alpha effects predominate with vasoconstriction, particularly in skin, gut, and kidney.

It is best to use a syringe pump. Dilute 3 mg of adrenaline in 5% dextrose and make it up to 50 ml, (1 ml/hour = 1 microgram/min). Infuse it into a central vein through its own dedicated line, because in this concentrated form it will necrose peripheral veins. In adults start with a dose of 1 microgram/min and increase the dose by 0.5 microgram (0.5 ml/hour) every 3 - 5 minutes until the desired effect is achieved. The effective dose range is 1-20 microgram/min. On stopping the infusion the effects wear off in 6 - 8 minutes.

DOPAMINE[1] is a biochemical precursor of noradrenaline synthesized in adrenergic nerve endings and the adrenal medulla. Dopamine stimulates two types of dopamine receptors (DA_1 and DA_2) as well as $alpha_1$ and $alpha_2$ and $ß_1$ adrenergic receptors. DA_1 receptors are found in great number in mesenteric and renal vascular beds. Their stimulation causes smooth muscle relaxation and vasodilation. Dopamine is widely used for the treatment of acute cardiac failure and normovolaemic shock.

Dopamine has different effects depending on the dose given. At doses of 3 microgram/kg/min its effects are mainly dopaminergic, improving cardiac output and renal blood flow, but with little effect on blood pressure or pulse rate. This dose is called renal dose dopamine. At doses of 5 -15 microgram/kg/min it increases the rate and force of cardiac contraction to improve cardiac output. This is the beta range of dopamine. At doses greater than 15 - 20 microgram/kg/min dopamine cause vasoconstriction and increases cardiac work disproportionately. This is called the alpha range of dopamine.

Use a syringe pump. Dilute 300 mg of dopamine in 5% dextrose and make it up to 50 ml, (1 ml/hour = 100 microgram/min). Infuse it into a central vein through its own dedicated line., because in this concentrated form it will necrose peripheral veins. In adults start with a dose of 2 microgram/kg/min and increase the dose by 1 microgram/kg/min (1 ml/hour) every 3 - 5 minutes until the desired effect is achieved. The effective dose range is 200 - 1500 microgram/min. There is little to be gained by pushing the dose into the alpha range, instead combine it with adrenaline or even noradrenaline. On stopping the infusion the effects wear off in 2 - 4 minutes.

DOBUTAMINE is a good stimulator of cardiac contractility. In low doses dobutamine increases cardiac output, and decreases systemic and pulmonary vascular resistance. It does not maintain the blood pressure as effectively as dopamine, but has the advantage of increasing cardiac output without a parallel increase in heart rate. Since the heart rate is slower, and the blood pressure is slightly higher, then myocardial perfusion is better maintained than with drugs that increase the heart rate. This is a valuable asset for the ischaemic, failing heart. Dobutamine does not dilate the renal vasculature. At doses greater than 10 microgram/kg/min the pulse rate starts to rise.

Use a syringe pump. Dilute 250 mg of dopamine in 5% dextrose and make it up to 41.5 ml (1 ml/hour = 100 microgram/min). In this concentrated form it will necrose peripheral veins, so infuse it into a central vein through its own dedicated line. In adults start with a dose of 2 microgram/kg/min and increase the dose by 1 microgram/kg/min (1 ml/hr) every 3 - 5 minutes until the desired effect is achieved. The effective dose range is 2.5 - 15 microgram/kg/min. There is little to be gained by pushing the dose into the alpha range, instead combine it with adrenaline or even noradrenaline. On stopping the infusion the effects wear off in 4 - 6 minutes.

DOPEXAMINE is a synthetic catecholamine dilation blood vessels in muscle and splanchnic beds by stimulating stimulating $ß_2$ receptors. It causes renal vasodilation and improves renal blood flow by stimulating dopaminergic DA_1 receptors. It inhibits the neural reuptake of catecholamines an so increases the effects of endogenous adrenaline and noradrenaline. It increases the force of cardiac contraction and decreases peripheral resistance, this improves tissue blood flow.

Use a syringe pump. Dilute 50 mg of dopexamine in 5% dextrose and make it up to 41.5 ml (1 ml/hour = 20 microgram/min). In this concentrated form it will necrose peripheral veins, so infuse it into a central vein through its own dedicated line. In adults start with a dose of 20 microgram/min and increase the dose by 10 - 20 microgram/minute (1 ml/hour) every 3 - 5 minutes until the desired effect is achieved. The effective dose range is 0.5 - 60 microgram/kg/min. On stopping the infusion the effects wear off in 20 - 30 minutes.

NORDARENALINE (NOREPINEPHRINE) is a neurotransmitter for the immediate response to threatening situations. It is useful for the treatment of conditions where peripheral resistance failure causes a falling blood pressure. It is predominantly an alpha stimulator. It causes generalized vasoconstriction in most vascular beds and greatly increases peripheral vascular resistance so both the systolic and diastolic blood pressure rises. It increases blood pressure much more than cardiac output and if the patient has systolic dysfunction will make the cardiac failure worse.

Use a syringe pump. Dilute 3 mg of noradrenaline in 5% dextrose and make it up to 50 ml, (1 ml/hour = 1 microgram/min). Infuse it into a central vein through its own dedicated line., because in this concentrated form it will necrose peripheral veins. In adults start with a dose of 1 microgram/min and increase the dose by 0.5 microgram (0.5 ml/hr) every 3 - 5 minutes until the desired effect is achieved. The effective dose range is 1 - 30 microgram/min. On stopping the infusion the effects wear off in 2 - 4 minutes.

1. Murphy MB, Elliot WJ. (1990). *Critical Care Medicine*, 8(1):S14-8.

APPENDIX II.
BLOOD CROSS MATCH REQUIREMENTS

TYPICAL BLOOD LOSS ASSOCIATED WITH FRACTURES	
Radius and ulna	500
Humerus	800-1000
Rib	250+
Pelvis	3000 ++++
Femur	1000 - 3000
Tibia and fibula	750 - 1500

TYPICAL TRANSFUSION REQUIREMENTS FOR COMMON OPERATIONS	
OPERATION	**NUMBER OF UNITS**
Abdomino perineal resection	3
Abdominal lipectomy	2
Adrenalectomy	2
Amputation - below knee	G+H
Amputation - above knee	G+H
Anterior resection	2
Aortic aneurysm - elective	4
Aorto-femoral bypass	4
Aorto-iliac bypass	4
Appendicetomy	Nil
Apronectomy	2
Arthroscopy	Nil
Bowel resection	2
Burns debridement	lots, discuss with haematologist
Caesarean section	G+H
Carotid endarterectomy	G+H
Cholecystectomy - laparoscopic	G+H

(G+H = group and hold)

Cholecystectomy - open	G+H
Colectomy	2
Colostomy - formation or closure	G+H
Colposuspension	G+H
Cystectomy	4
Cystoscopy	Nil
Dilation & curette	Nil
Ecotopic - simple	G+H
Ectopic - ruptured	4
Femoro-popliteal bypass	2
Gastrectomy	2
Gastric stapling	G+H
Haemorroidectomy	Nil
Harrington's rods	4
Hepatectomy	6
Hiatus hernia repair - abdominal	G+H
Hiatus hernia repair - transthoracic	2
Hip replacement	3
Hysterectomy - abdominal	G+H
Hysterectomy - vaginal	G+H
Hysterectomy - Wertheims	2
Ilio-femoral bypass	2
Incisional hernia	Nil
Knee replacement	2
Laminectomy	G+H
Laparoscopy	Nil
Lumbar fusion - no graft	G+H
Lumbar fusion - with graft	2
Lumbar sympathectomy	G+H
Lung - lobectomy	2
Mammoplasty - reduction	G+H
Mastectomy - simple	G+H
Mastectomy - radical	2
Mastectomy + axillary clearance	2
Menisectomy	Nil
Myomectomy	G+H
Nephrectomy - Ca	4

(G+H = group and hold)

Nephrectomy - simple	2
Nephrolithotomy - open	4
Oesophagectomy	4
Ovarian cystectomy	G+H
Pancreatectomy - partial	4
Pancreatectomy - total	6
Pancreatic cyst	2
Parotidectomy	G+H
Pleurectomy	2
Pneumonectomy	4
Porto-caval shunt	4
Prostatectomy - open	2
Putti-Platt	Nil
Renal artery repair	3
Salphingoplasty	G+H
Spinal fusion	2
Splenectomy	2
Synovectomy - knee	G+H
Termination of pregnancy	G+H
Thymectomy	2
Thyroidectomy - simple	G+H
Thyroidectomy for Ca	G+H
Transcutaneous nephrolithotomy	G+H
Tubal ligation	G+H
TURP	G+H
Uretolithtomy	G+H
Vaginal repair	G+H
Varicose veins	Nil
Vulvectomy - radical	4
Vulvectomy - simple	2

(G+H = group and hold)

APPENDIX III.
USEFUL DATA

Standardization

Over the years countries have developed their own units of measurement; for instance the Europeans measured liquid volume in litres, the UK in imperial gallons, and the US in a different gallon. The Systeme Internationale d'Unites (SI system) was developed to overcome these difficulties. It has become standard to measure length in metres, mass in kilograms, and time in seconds, pressure in pascals, work in joules, volume in cubic metres and so on. Non-standard units are still widely used and include millimetres of mercury, litres, and degrees Fahrenheit. It will be many years before one drinks 0.180 3 10 - 3 cubic metres instead of a tumbler (or glass) of water, or say today's temperature is 300°K.

Factors

FACTOR	PREFIX	SYMBOL
10^6	mega	M
10^3	kilo	k
10^{-1}	deci	d
10^{-2}	centi	c
10^{-3}	milli	m
10^{-6}	micro	μ
10^{-9}	nano	n
10^{-12}	pico	p

Temperature

SI unit is the degree Kelvin, but Celsius is the usual notation.
Centigrade means the same as Celsius.

$$C° = (F° - 32) \times {}^5/_9$$
$$F° = (C° \times {}^9/_5) + 32$$

C°	F°	C°	F°	C°	F°
30	86.0	35	95.0	38	100.4
32	87.8	36	96.8	39	102.2
34	93.2	37	98.6	40	104.0

Length
SI unit is the metre
1 metre = 100 centimetres = 1000 millimetres
1 foot = 30.48 cm = 304.8 mm
1 inch = 2.54 cm =25.4 mm

Volume
SI unit is the cubic metre
1000 millilitres = 10 decilitres = 1 litre
1 teaspoon = 4.5 ml
1 tablespoon = 15 ml
1 teacup = 120 ml
1 tumbler = 240 ml
1 pint= 568 ml
1 fluid ounce = 28.42 ml

Conversion table for solution strengths
By definition a 1 per cent solution contains 1 gram of substance in every 100 ml of solution. This can also be written as 1:100 or 10 mg/ml.

DILUTION	SOLUTION	MG/ML
1:200 000	0.0002%	0.002 mg/ml
1:100 000	0.001%	0.01 mg/ml
1:10 000	0.01%	0.1 mg/ml
1:5000	0.02%	0.2 mg/ml
1:1000	0.1%	1.0 mg/ml
1:500	0.2%	2.0 mg/ml
1:200	0.5%	5.0 mg/ml
1:100	1.0%	10.0 mg/ml
1:50	2.0%	20.0 mg/ml
1:10	10.%	100.0 mg/ml

Pressure
SI unit is the pascal. A kilopascal is 1000 pascals. Some places measure pressures in kilopascals (kPa), whereas others measure it in millimetres of mercury (mmHg).

7.6 mmHg = 1 kPa
1 mmHg ≈ 13 Pa
Occasionally pressure is measured in centimetres of water
10 cmH2O = 1.36 mmHg

	SI UNIT	OLD UNIT	OLD TO SI	SI TO OLD
	kPa	mmHg	× 0.133	× 7.60
		cm H$_2$O	× 0.098	× 10.20
		lb per inch^2	× 6.894	× 0.145

mmHg	kPa	mmHg	kPa	mmHg	kPa	mmHg	kPa	mmHg	kPa
1	0.13	21	2.76	41	5.39	61	8.03	81	10.66
2	0.26	22	2.89	42	5.52	62	8.16	82	10.79
3	0.39	23	3.03	43	5.65	63	8.29	83	10.92
4	0.53	24	3.16	44	5.79	64	8.42	84	11.05
5	0.66	25	3.29	45	5.92	65	8.55	85	11.18
6	0.79	26	3.42	46	6.05	66	8.68	86	11.32
7	0.92	27	3.55	47	6.18	67	8.82	87	11.45
8	1.05	28	3.68	48	6.32	68	8.95	88	11.58
9	1.08	29	3.82	49	6.45	69	9.08	89	11.71
10	1.32	30	3.95	50	6.58	70	9.21	90	11.84
11	1.45	31	4.08	51	6.71	71	9.34	91	11.97
12	1.58	32	4.21	52	6.84	72	9.47	92	12.11
13	1.71	33	4.34	53	6.97	73	9.60	93	12.24
14	1.84	34	4.47	54	7.11	74	9.73	94	12.37
15	1.97	35	4.60	55	7.24	75	9.87	95	12.50
16	2.11	36	4.73	56	7.37	76	10.00	96	12.63
17	2.24	37	4.87	57	7.50	77	10.13	97	12.76
18	2.37	38	5.00	58	7.63	78	10.26	98	12.89
19	2.50	39	5.13	59	7.76	79	10.39	99	13.03
20	2.63	40	5.26	60	7.89	80	10.53	100	13.16

Weight

1 000 000 microgram = 1000 milligram = 1 gram = 0.001 kg

1 ounce (oz) = 28.35 g

1 pound (lb) = 0.4536 kg

1 stone = 14 lb = 6.35 kg

APPENDIX IV.
AUTONOMIC NERVOUS SYSTEM

Surgery and anaesthesia imposes a *physiological stress* on the body. The autonomic nervous system plays an important role in adapting the body to stress. At rest the body is running at a *basal metabolic rate*, producing just enough energy to keep it going. The internal environment of the body is kept in balance, a process called *homeostasis*, by a great number of co-ordinated processes. Once the body takes part in any activity a stress occurs, then homeostatic mechanisms adjust the body's response to restore equilibrium. Cardiovascular stresses may be as ordinary as getting out of a warm bed in the morning, where the blood tends to pool in your legs; or life threatening catastrophic haemorrhage.

Homoeostasis involves *feedback phenomena*. When a stress occurs a sensor mechanism detects the change, and a message is then sent to a *processor* that analyses and coordinates a *response*. The processor then sends a message to an *effector* that adjusts things so that the equilibrium is restored.

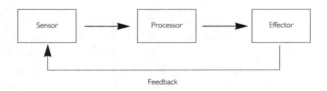

fig IV.1 Feedback

Feedback is part of most physiological processes in the body. Consider: you get hot, you sweat and cool down again. Temperature receptors (sensors) in the skin send messages to the thermoregulatory centre in your brain (processor) which sends messages down nerves to cause you to sweat (effector). You cool down, and the temperature receptors in the skin then stop sending messages to the brain.

The physiological *response* is usually proportional to the stress causing it. This response involves two sets of homeostatic mechanisms. The first is the autonomic nervous system (or *neural*) response, and the second is a hormonal (or *humoral*) response. The neural response works instantly; but the various hormonal responses take time to achieve their effect.

There are two components of the autonomic nervous system; the *sympathetic* (adrenergic) system, and the *parasympathetic* (cholinergic) system.

SYMPATHETIC NERVOUS SYSTEM

The sympathetic nervous system (SNS) is part of the body's *fight and flight response*.

In response to a stress the body uses the nervous system to get an instant effect with shorter duration. In contrast, hormones act more slowly but for a longer period.

The neurotransmitter of the sympathetic (adrenergic) system is *noradrenaline*. The humoral component is mediated through the hormone *adrenaline*, which is synthesized in the adrenal medulla. Noradrenaline and adrenaline are members of a group of chemical compounds called *catecholamines*.

Noradrenaline prepares the body for brief intense effort (to fight); and adrenaline dilates muscle vasculature, preparing the body for a sustained effort to run away (flight). In other words noradrenaline is the neurotransmitter for unavoidable life threatening situations: such as haemorrhage, heart failure, and the pain of surgery; while adrenaline is a hormone secreted predominantly for exercise. Following surgery the effects of these two catecholamines overlap.

Another hormone, *cortisol*, enables the body to maintain a sustained adrenergic response to a prolonged stress. Cortisol is a *steroid* synthesized in the adrenal cortex. Yet another steroid, called *aldosterone*, slows the excretion of sodium ion by the kidney in a patient who is bleeding or has lost some of their extracellular fluid volume.

In the USA noradrenaline is called norepinephrine; adrenaline is called *epinephrine*, and cortisone is called *cortisol*.

Catecholamines administered to stimulate the sympathetic nervous system are called *adrenergic drugs*. *Sympatheticomimetic* drugs mimic the effects of noradrenaline or adrenaline; and include ephedrine, metaraminol, phenylephrine, dopamine, and dobutamine.

There are two principal groups of adrenergic drugs; beta (ß) agonists and alpha (α) agonists. Agonists are drugs that stimulate receptors. Beta agonist drug increase the heart rate, and its force of contraction, they behave like small doses of adrenaline. Alpha agonists drug cause vasoconstriction in skin, muscle, kidney and gut, and behave like small doses of noradrenaline. Most of the synthetic adrenergic drugs, such as metarminol, ephedrine and dopamine, have varying degrees of both alpha and beta effects.

SUBTYPES OF ADRENERGIC RECEPTORS				
RECEPTOR	HEART	ARTERIOLES	LUNGS	OTHER
α_1	-	constricts	-	reduces gut mobility.
β_1	increases rate increases strength	dilates coronary arteries	-	glycogenolysis
β_2	increases rate increases strength	dilates most arteries	bronchodilation	tremor, tocolysis, hypokalaemia.
β_3	-	-	-	lipolysis.

Noradrenaline causes peripheral vasoconstriction raising the blood pressure. Very small doses of adrenaline cause tachycardia and peripheral vasodilation. The higher doses of adrenaline used in resuscitation have mixed alpha and beta effects increasing the heart rate and its force of contraction; but also causing vasoconstriction in the kidney, skin and gut, and vasodilation in muscle.

PARASYMPATHETIC NERVOUS SYSTEM

Parasympathetic nerve fibres arise in the cranial nerves (CN III, VII, IX and X); however the vagus nerve (CN X) is the most prominent. The neurotransmitter parasympathetic (cholinergic) nervous system is acetylcholine When stimulated the parasympathetic nervous system slows the heart rate, increases peristaltic activity of the gut, and constricts the pupils.

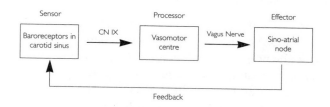

PARASYMPATHETIC FEEDBACK
A the blood pressure rises the pulse rate falls.

fig IV.2 Parasympathetic feedback

The parasympathetic nervous system's action on the heart is to slow down the rate of discharge of the sinoatrial node which slows the heart rate. Drugs that prevent enzymes breaking down acetylcholine cause a bradycardia; they include neostigmine, and physostigmine. In contrast, atropine blocks the braking effects of acetylcholine on the sino-atrial node, and causes tachycardia.

The paraympathetic system is often said to oppose the action of the sympathetic system. Although this is partly true, it is misleading to think this way. The parasympthetic nervous system is the homeostatic mechanism responsible for the hour to hour to housekeeping activity in the body such as digestion, slowing the heart rate, temperature regulation, emptying bladder and bowels.

APPENDIX V.
ARRHYTHMIAS

Medical and nursing staff who have direct responsibility for patient care in the recovery room should be able to recognize on the ECG trace, and treat the following arrhythmias.

1. Sinus tachycardia.
2. Sinus bradycardia.
3. Premature atrial contractions (PAC) and multifocal atrial tachycardia (MAT).
4. Paroxysmal supraventricular tachycardia (PSVT).
5. Atrial flutter.
6. Atrial fibrillation (AF).
7. Junctional rhythms.
8. Atrioventricular blocks of all degrees.
9. Premature ventricular contractions (PVC).
10. Ventricular tachycardias (VT) including Torsade de pointes.
11. Ventricular fibrillation (VF).
12. Asystole (cardiac standstill).

If arrhythmias occur they will cause the pulse to slow, or speed up, or become irregular.

NORMAL RHYTHMS
Sinus arrhythmia
This is a normal variant in young people. The heart speeds up during inspiration and slows down during expiration.

RHYTHM	irregular, rate faster on inspiration, slower on expiration
P-WAVE	normal
P:QRS	1:1
P–R INTERVAL	0.12 – 0.2 sec
ATRIAL RATE	bradycardia or normal sinus rhythm
QRS SHAPE	normal
QRS WIDTH	less than 0.12 sec
VENTRICULAR RATE	bradycardia up to 100 per minute

Sinus bradycardia
It is normal in fit young athletes who may have pulse rates as low as 45 beats per minute.

Abnormal Rhythms

1. Sinus tachycardia

A tachycardia is a pulse rate greater than 100 per minute. Never ignore tachycardia, it is warning sign that all may not be well. Find and treat the cause, do not just treat it symptomatically. Drugs such as atropine, adrenaline, pethidine, ephedrine and ketamine cause tachycardia.

Children's heart rates vary with age. A tachycardia in a child is a rate of more than 20 per cent above his baseline heart rate

Other causes include:
- pain;
- hypercarbia;
- agitation, restlessness;
- hypovolaemia, bleeding;
- heart failure;
- hypoglycaemia;
- drugs;
- hypoxia;
- airway obstruction
- shivering, shaking;
- following thyroid surgery;
- hyperthermia;
- cardiac arrhythmias;
- pneumothorax.

Lead II

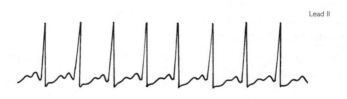

fig V.1 Sinus tachycardia

RHYTHM	regular
P-WAVE	normal position, but can be merged with previous T-wave
P:QRS	1:1
P-R INTERVAL	0.12 - 0.2 sec
ATRIAL RATE	100 - 150/min
QRS	normal shape
QRS WIDTH	less than 0.12 sec.
VENTRICULAR RATE	10 - 150/min

Treatment involves finding the cause.

2. Sinus bradycardia

A bradycardia is a pulse rate of less than 60 beats per minute. It is a common arrythmia in recovery room

Causes of bradycardia include:
- athletes;
- hypoxia, this is a grave sign;
- intraoperative fentanyl; especially if propofol has also been given;
- nausea;
- residual neostigmine;
- beta blockers, calcium channel blockade;
- painless urinary retention causing a distended bladder;
- hypothermia;
- reflex secondary to hypertension;
- myocardial ischaemia, and especially after antero-inferior infarction;
- raised intracranial pressure;
- spinal cord injury;
- airway suctioning;
- after carotid artery surgery;
- myxoedema.

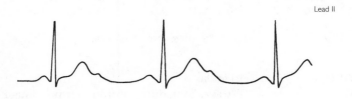

Lead II

fig V.2 Sinus bradycardia

RHYTHM	regular, or slightly irregular
P-WAVE	normal position and shape
P:QRS	1:1
P-R INTERVAL	0.12 - 20 sec
ATRIAL RATE	less than 60/min
QRS	normal shape
QRS WIDTH	less than 0.12 sec.
VENTRICULAR RATE	less than 60/min

Do not treat a sinus bradycardia if the pulse rate is above 45 per minutes, and the patient has warm hands, a good urine output, and is comfortable. If the pulse rate is less than 60 per minute, monitor the patient with a pulse oximeter until you are sure the cardiovascular state is stable. If the pulse rate is below 45 per minute, attach a pulse oximeter, and an ECG and check the rhythm. Myocardial ischaemia, hypotension, an escape rhythm or poor perfusion requires treatment. A sinus bradycardia will respond to a small dose of atropine 0.01 mg/kg intravenously, the effects last about 10 minutes. If it does not work immediately repeat it after 2 minutes. If the bradycardia persists, then consider the possibility of heart block. This may require an adrenaline infusion, at a rate of 1 - 10 microgram per minute, or a pacemaker.

3. Premature atrial contractions (PAC)

PACs arise from an ectopic atrial focus, and consequently shows an abnormally shaped P-wave. Sometimes they occur with right or left bundle branch blocks. Causes include sympathetic stimulation (pain, agitation, hypoxia), myocardial ischaemia and digoxin toxicity.

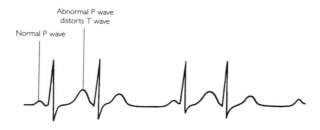

fig V.3 Premature atrial contractions

RHYTHM	irregular
P-WAVE	P-waves look different from normal sinus P-wave
P:QRS	1:1
P-R INTERVAL	0.12 - 0.2 sec
ATRIAL RATE	varies depending on underlying rhythm
QRS	normal shape
QRS WIDTH	less than 0.12 sec.
VENTRICULAR RATE	varies depending on underlying rhythm

Treat the cause and they usually resolve.

Digoxin toxicity may require supplemental potassium or occasionally digoxin antibodies.

MULTIFOCAL ATRIAL TACHYCARDIA (MAT)

Multifocal atrial tachycardia is characterized by irregular and different forms of P-waves (chaotic P-waves) with a ventricular rate of greater than 100 beats per minute. It is an arrhythmia usually seen in elderly patients who have severe ischaemic heart disease.

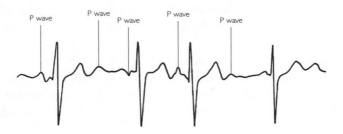

P wave P wave P wave P wave P wave

fig V.4 Multifocal atrial tachycardia

RHYTHM	irregular
P-WAVE	forms differ, chaotic P-waves may be on top of T waves
P:QRS	P-waves may arrive faster than QRS.
P-R INTERVAL	variable
ATRIAL RATE	150 - 200/min.
QRS	usually normal in shape unless altered by P-wave
QRS WIDTH	usually less than 0.12 sec.
VENTRICULAR RATE	depends on AV conduction

MAGNESIUM

Magnesium is an essential co-factor for the production of ATP used as an energy source in many biochemical reactions in the cell. It also counters the effects of calcium. Magnesium deficiency is associated with cardiac arrhythmias, cardiac failure and sudden cardiac death. It can precipitate refractory ventricular fibrillation. Magnesium supplementation is used to decrease the incidence of post-ischaemic arrhythmias. Suspect magnesium deficiency in patients who have been on diuretics, have had large intestinal fluid losses, or who are hypokalaemic. It also commonly occurs in diabetics and alcoholics. Because magnesium spreads evenly through out the extracellular fluid, you will need to give a loading dose. Magnesium is rapidly excreted by the kidney, therefore to maintain blood levels, follow the loading dose with a constant intravenous infusion.

It causes:
- presynaptic inhibition of neurotransmitter release in peripheral nerves;
- directly inhibits cardiac muscle contraction;
- vascular smooth muscle relaxation.
- tachycardia, because it blocks the action of the vagus nerve.

It is a useful:
- antiarrhythmic;
- bronchodilator;
- tocolytic reducing uterine contraction during labour;
- renal vasodilator increasing the renal blood flow;
- antihypertensive and anticonvulscent in eclampsia and pre-eclampsia.

Calcium antagonizes the cardiac and vascular effects of magnesium.

Treat MAT with magnesium sulphate 10 mmol (5 ml of 49.3% solution) intravenously over 5 minutes. Repeat if necessary.

4. Supraventricular tachycardias

In a fit young person the maximum rate the ventricles can respond to the SA node is about 220 - 240 per minute. This ability decreases with age. As a rule of thumb, treat tachycardias when the perfusion status is inadequate, or the rate rises too high.

The maximum acceptable heart rate = (200 - patient's age)

Supraventricular tachycardias usually have a rate of 150 - 250 per minute. The QRS look normal or occasionally the QRS is wide. Any cardiac failure is aggravated by a decrease in coronary blood flow that occurs with tachycardias. More than half the patients will have hypotension, with associated oliguria and deteriorating oxygenation.

Supraventricular tachycardias are the most common arrhythmias causing cardiovascular instability in infancy and childhood. SVT may produce heart rates near 240 beats per minute, but it may be as high as 300 beats per minute. Any SVT with wide QRS complexes (>120 milliseconds) should be assumed to be ventricular in origin.

Paroxysmal supraventricular tachycardia (PSVT)

PSVT is the most common of the supraventricular tachycardias. It usually begins and ends abruptly. Patients often describe sensations of fluttering (palpitations) in the chest. If the paroxysm is prolonged cardiac perfusion becomes impaired resulting in ischaemia, angina, a fall in cardiac output, hypotension, poor peripheral perfusion and oliguria. Immediate cardioversion is seldom needed if the pulse rate is less than 150 beats per minute.

Causes include:
• usually occurs in otherwise fit young people;
• Wolff-Parkinson-White syndrome. (WPW);
• ischaemic heart disease;
• rheumatic heart disease.

RHYTHM	regular
P-WAVE	within the QRS or on T-wave.
P:QRS	1:1
P-R INTERVAL	not visible
ATRIAL RATE	170 - 250/min.
QRS	normal

QRS WIDTH	less than 0.12 sec.
VENTRICULAR RATE	170 - 250/min.

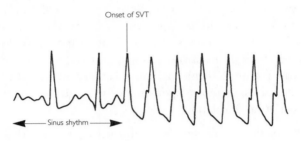

Onset of SVT

Sinus shythm

fig V.5 Paroxysmal supraventricular tachycardia

VAGAL MANOEUVRES

Supraventricular tachycardias can often be abruptly terminated with vagal stimulation. Attach an ECG, pulse oximeter and non-invasive blood pressure cuff. To start with, try putting an ice-cold sloppy wet towel on the patient's face. If this fails try gentle carotid sinus massage. The carotid sinus is close to the bifurcation of the common carotid artery, adjacent to the angle of the jaw. With the head turned to one side put your thumb over the point of maximum pulsation and firmly massage up and down along the length of the carotid artery by pressing it against the spine for no longer than 10 seconds. Try the right side first, and then the left side, but never both sides together. Keep your other hand on the radial pulse, and listen with a stethoscope over the apex of the heart. Carotid sinus massage may convert the rhythm to sinus rhythm, or slow the pulse rate down. If carotid sinus massage fails, treat the patient as a narrow complex tachycardia. It is unwise to do carotid sinus massage in patients with cerebrovascular or carotid artery disease.

If the vagal manoeuvres are unsuccessful, the patient's blood pressure is within normal limits, and he is not on ß-blockers; then try verapamil 5 mg intravenously over 2 minutes. Wait 15 minutes and repeat verapamil 10 mg intravenously.

If the patient is unstable, or has a low blood pressure, use synchronised cardioversion 75 - 100 joules. Increase this to 200 joules and then 300 joules. If the rhythm fails to revert do not use further cardioversion; in this case a pacemaker may be needed. Meanwhile try amiodarone or digoxin.

Restrict the use of verapamil to patients with narrow complex PSVT who have normal blood pressures. Do not use verapamil in patient's with wide QRS complexes, because it may be lethal.

WOLFF-PARKINSON-WHITE SYNDROME

Wolff-Parkinson-White (WPW) syndrome is caused by an abnormal conduction pathway (called the bundle of Kent) between the atria and the ventricles, through which impulses take a shortcut to the ventricles, bypassing the AV node. The ECG shows a characteristically short PR interval that often fuses with the QRS complex. This is called a fusion beat Sometimes the impulse re-enters the atria through another pathway setting up a rapid feed back on itself stimulating a fast ventricular response. The pulse rate can rise to 200/min or more. Patients with Wolff-Parkinson-White syndrome sometimes spontaneously go into supraventricular tachycardia or atrial fibrillation.

Atrial fibrillation in these patients is life threatening because the rapid atrial rate is not delayed at the AV node, and it may stimulate the ventricles up to 400 times per minute. The QRS complexes are widened (>120 msec), and can trigger ventricular fibrillation. Do not use digoxin, verapamil, or adenosine. These drugs slow transmission through the AV node, so then more impulses will take the short cut, and paradoxically increase the ventricular rate. Procainamide will sometimes slow the conduction through the aberrant pathway.

Do not use digoxin, verapamil or adenosine in patients with WPW syndrome

P wave with short PR interval

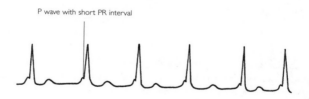

fig V.6 Wolff–Parkinson–White (WPW) syndrome

RHYTHM	regular
P-WAVE	may merge with QRS
P:QRS	1:1
P–R INTERVAL	less than 0.12 sec
ATRIAL RATE	bradycardia or normal sinus rhythm
QRS SHAPE	normal
QRS WIDTH	less than 0.12 sec
VENTRICULAR RATE	60–100/min

5. Atrial flutter

Atrial flutter is easily recognized because of the saw-toothed pattern of the P-waves on the ECG. The causes are similar to atrial fibrillation.

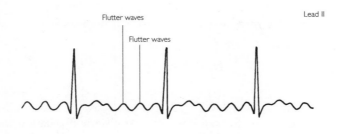

Flutter waves

Flutter waves

Lead II

fig V.7 Atrial flutter

RHYTHM	regular or irregular
P-WAVE	saw-toothed pattern
P:QRS	more P-waves than QRS complexes. The complexes may come in a fixed ratio in which case the ventricular rate will be regular.
P-R INTERVAL	difficult to measure
ATRIAL RATE	250-350/min
QRS	normal complex
QRS WIDTH	less than 0.12 sec
VENTRICULAR RATE	depends on AV conduction ratio.

Treat it as a narrow complex irregular rhythm

6. Atrial fibrillation (AF)

Atrial fibrillation is a common arrhythmia, and is usually a result of long standing ischaemic heart disease. It may arise for the first time following:

- thoracotomy, especially if the pericardium has been damaged;
- oesophagectomy;
- following thyroid surgery;
- pulmonary embolism.

Since atrial contraction contributes up to 25 per cent of the cardiac output the onset of atrial fibrillation can cause the cardiac output to fall enough to precipitate heart failure in patients with poor cardiac reserves.

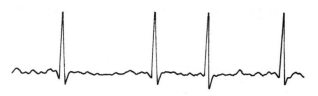

fig V.7 Atrial fibrillation

RHYTHM   irregular
P-WAVE   no formed P-waves, just chaotic fibrillation waves
P:QRS   more fibrillation waves than QRS complexes
P-R INTERVAL   none
ATRIAL RATE   greater than 350/min
QRS   normal
QRS WIDTH   less than 0.12 sec
VENTRICULAR RATE   varies, but in uncontrolled fibrillation is greater than
                        100/minute.

Treat atrial fibrillation as a narrow complex irregular arrhythmia. Aim to,
either revert the fibrillation to sinus rhythm, or failing that, to bring the
ventricular rate to under 100 beats per minute. If the rhythm starts in
operating theatre or recovery room, and the patient's perfusion is falling,
then consider cardioversion. Start with 1.0 joule/kg. Only attempt
3 countershocks. If this fails to convert the heart to sinus rhythm, then
control the ventricular rate with verapamil and digoxin.

7. Nodal or junctional escape rhythms
If the sinus node fails, the AV node usually takes over as the pacemaker for
the heart. This takeover mechanism protects the patient from asystole.

Causes:
• hypoxia;
• myocardial ischaemia;
• pain, especially visceral pain from the abdomen travelling via the vagus nerve;

RHYTHM   regular
P-WAVE   before, during, or after the QRS complex, inverted
P:QRS   P-waves less than, or equal to the number of QRS complexes
P-R INTERVAL   if present, less than 0.12 sec.
ATRIAL RATE   cannot always see the P-waves

QRS	normal
QRS WIDTH	less than 0.12 sec.
VENTRICULAR RATE	40 - 60/min.

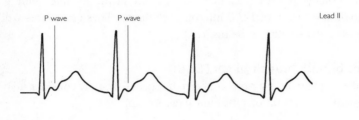

fig V.8 Nodal rhythm

Eliminate hypoxia and myocardial ischaemia as a cause.

If the patient is not hypoxic, and has a good perfusion status, no treatment is necessary. If the patient has cold hands, is cyanosed, or has a blood pressure less than 80 mmHg, then treat it with atropine 0.01 mg/kg intravenously. Repeat the atropine at 2 minute intervals if needed.

8. Atrioventricular blocks

Heart blocks occur when transmission of the cardiac impulse, is either blocked, or delayed on its normal journey through the heart. In recovery room always suspect myocardial ischaemia as the cause.

Causes include:
• right bundle branch block (RBBB);
• left bundle branch block (LBBB);
• first-degree heart block;
• second-degree heart block;
• complete heart block.

Exclude hypoxia or myocardial ischaemia if heart block occurs.

Causes include
• myocardial ischaemia and infarction;
• valvular disease;
• myocarditis;
• heart surgery;
• sometimes congenital.

MANAGEMENT
Aim to reduce cardiac work, and improve cardiac oxygenation. Give
oxygen, control hypertension, and pain. If the cardiac output falls, causing
hypotension, shortness of breath, or changes in mental state then treat the
block. Drugs that temporarily increase cardiac output are atropine 0.6 mg
intravenously, repeated as necessary; or if atropine fails then give an
adrenaline infusion of 1- 10 microgram/minute. These measures will allow
time for a pacemaker to be inserted.

Right bundle branch block (RBBB)
RBBB is not usually a serious concern. If it occurs acutely consider myocardial
ischaemia, infarction or pulmonary embolism.

Lead V₁

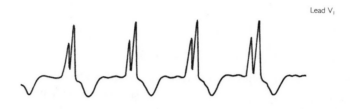

fig V.9 Right bundle branch block

RHYTHM	Can occur with any rhythm
P-WAVE	before QRS complex if the rhythm is sinus
P:QRS	1:1 if sinus rhythm, otherwise depends on underlying rhythm
P-R INTERVAL	depends on underlying rhythm
ATRIAL RATE	depends on underlying rhythm
QRS	often notched
QRS WIDTH	greater than 0.12 sec in right chest leads, and aVR and III
VENTRICULAR RATE	depends on underlying rhythm

Left bundle branch block (LBBB)
LBBB is usually a sign of severe heart disease. If it occurs acutely the patient
has probably had a myocardial infarction.

RHYTHM	can occur with any rhythm
P-WAVE	before QRS complex if the rhythm is sinus
P:QRS	1:1 if sinus rhythm, otherwise depends on underlying rhythm
P-R INTERVAL	depends on underlying rhythm
ATRIAL RATE	depends on underlying rhythm

QRS	may be notched
QRS WIDTH	greater than 0.12 sec in left chest leads, and I and II
VENTRICULAR RATE	depends on underlying rhythm

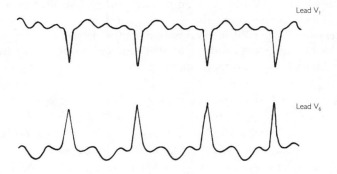

fig V.9 Left bundle branch block

First-degree AV block

First-degree AV block occurs if the PR interval is longer than 0.2 seconds, which is one large box on normal ECG paper. It means the impulse is delayed, usually at the AV node, and is a sign of myocardial ischaemia. It may progress to second- or third- degree heart block.

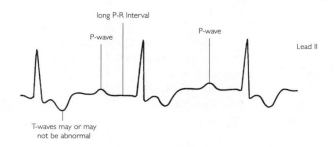

fig V.10 First-degree AV block

RHYTHM	regular
P-WAVE	uniform shape
P:QRS	1:1
P-R INTERVAL	prolonged more than 0.2 sec.
ATRIAL RATE	any sinus rate

QRS	normal complex
QRS WIDTH	less than 0.12 sec.
VENTRICULAR RATE	any sinus rate

Second-degree AV block, Wenckebach block (Möbitz type I)

This block occurs where the SA node fires at a regular rate, with a progressively longer PR interval until a ventricular beat is dropped. It is a sign of AV node ischaemia, and will respond to atropine. It is often transient, and may stop spontaneously.

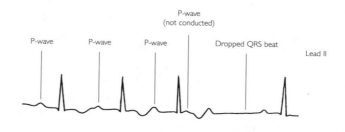

fig V.11   Second-degree AV block, Wenckebach block (Möbitz type I)

RHYTHM	irregular
P-WAVE	each QRS complex preceded by P-wave, but some P-waves do not trigger a QRS complex.
P:QRS	more P-waves than QRS complexes
P-R INTERVAL	prolonged more than 0.2 sec.
ATRIAL RATE	any sinus rate
QRS	normal complex
QRS WIDTH	less than 0.12 sec.
VENTRICULAR RATE	any sinus rate

Second-degree AV block, Möbitz type II block

This block occurs when there are missed atrial beats. The PR interval is normal, but the sick SA node is firing at irregular intervals. It may progress without warning to complete heart block. It is a sign of severe myocardial ischaemia, or anteroseptal myocardial infarction. Avoid atropine, because the SA node is already malfunctioning, and may it stop and make the block worse.

RHYTHM	irregular.
P-WAVE	each QRS complex preceded by P-wave, but some P-waves do not trigger a QRS complex.
P:QRS	more P-waves than QRS complexes
P-R INTERVAL	varies.
ATRIAL RATE	greater than the ventricular rate
QRS	less than 0.12 sec.
QRS WIDTH	normal.
VENTRICULAR RATE	any sinus rate.

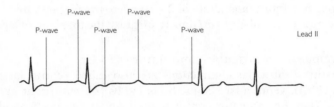

fig V.12 Second-degree AV block (Möbitz type II)

Third degree heart block (complete heart block)

Otherwise known as complete heart block occurs where the ventricles are not triggered by the SA node, and the atria and ventricles are contracting independently of each other. This results in poor perfusion, and a fixed cardiac output. Often it is accompanied by transient junctional escape rhythms.

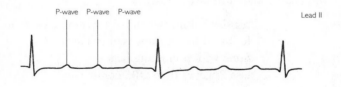

fig V.13 Third-degree AV block (complete heart block)

RHYTHM	regular atrial and ventricular rhythm.
P-WAVE	uniform shape.
P:QRS	more P-waves than QRS complexes.

P-R INTERVAL	varies.
ATRIAL RATE	greater than ventricular rate.
QRS	normal or widened.
QRS WIDTH	less than 0.12 sec if pacemaker cell is in the AV junction greater than 0.12 sec if pacemaker cell is in the ventricles.
VENTRICULAR RATE	40 - 60/min if escape pacemaker is in the AV junction. 20 - 40/min if the escape pacemaker is in the ventricles.

If the complexes are wide, avoid atropine. If the complexes are narrow then, in order try:
- atropine 0.5-1.0 mg (repeat in 3 - 5 minutes to a total dose of 0.04 mg/kg;
- transcutaneous pacemaker (TCP) is a stop gap measure;
- isoprenaline infusion of 0.5 - 20 microgram per minute;
- adrenaline infusion at a rate of 2 - 10 microgram/kg/minute.

These measures will give you time to organize the insertion of a pacemaker.

9. Premature ventricular contractions (PVC)

Premature ventricular contractions are also called ventricular premature beats (PVB), ventricular ectopic beats (VPBs) or ventricular extrasystoles (VEs). They are premature contractions arising from some irritable, ectopic focus in the ventricles that come earlier than expected in the cardiac cycle.

Causes include:
- caffeine, alcohol, and tobacco consumption, they occur in 50 per cent of the healthy population;
- hypertension;
- neurohumoral response to pain, anxiety or fear;
- drugs, such as digoxin, adrenoceptor agonists; tricyclic antidepressants and aminophylline;
- diuretics causing hypokalaemia, and hypomagnesaemia increase myocardial irritability;
- underlying cardiac disease, such as ischaemia, mitral valve prolapse, cardiomyopathy and aortic valve disease.

RHYTHM	regular, until interrupted by ectopic beat, and then followed by a compensatory pause.
P-WAVE	none with premature beat.
P:QRS	less P-waves than QRS complexes.
P-R INTERVAL	none for premature beat.
ATRIAL RATE	normal for sinus beats.
QRS	abnormal complex is wide and frequently in opposite direction to ST segment and T-wave.
QRS WIDTH	abnormal beat is wide, others less than 0.12 sec
VENTRICULAR RATE	depends on underlying rhythm.

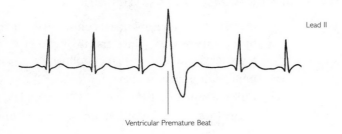

fig V.14 Ventricular premature beats

Eliminate hypoxia, or myocardial ischaemia as a cause. If the blood pressure, and pulse rate is within normal limits, the patient's perfusion is normal, and there are less than 5 ectopics per minute, no treatment is necessary. If there are 5, or more abnormal beats per minute, make sure that the patient is not hypoxic. More than 5 abnormal beats per minute are a minor predictor of serious sequela, such as, postoperative myocardial infarction, pulmonary oedema or ventricular tachycardia.[1]

BIGEMINY

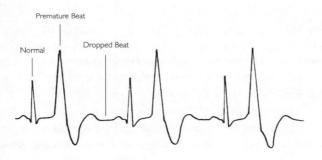

fig V.15 Bigeminy

Bigeminy occurs when a normal beat is followed by a ventricular ectopic beat, to be followed by a compensatory pause before the next cycle is started. Bigeminy signals more severe damage than the occasional ectopic beat. It is a sign of irritable myocardial muscle, due to one or more of: myocardial hypoxia, hypertension, digoxin toxicity, high catecholamine levels, hypokalaemia or hypomagnesaemia. Bigeminy usually either resolves spontaneously, or progresses to a ventricular tachycardia.

RHYTHM	irregularly regular, two beats close together followed by a compensatory pause and then two beats close together. Sometimes called coupling.
P-WAVE	none with premature beat.
P:QRS	Half the number of P-waves as QRS complexes.
P-R INTERVAL	normal for normal beats, absent for premature beats.
ATRIAL RATE	60-100/min.
QRS	normal beat followed by premature ventricular beat which is opposite in direction to ST segment and T wave.
QRS WIDTH	normal for normal beat, greater than 0.12 sec for premature contraction.
VENTRICULAR RATE	60-100/min.

The arrhythmia may resolve with treatment of any hypoxia, or hypertension. Otherwise try lignocaine 1.5 mg/kg intravenously, or if the patient has a tachycardia use a ß-blocker, such as esmolol or metoprolol. Treating the arrhythmia does not prevent it from progressing to a ventricular tachycardia. Using lignocaine is like covering a wound with a bandage, it only hides the underlying problem.

CARDIAC FAILURE AND VPBS
A patient with ventricular ectopic activity in the presence of myocardial ischaemia, and poor left ventricular function, is at high risk of sudden death. Following myocardial infarction, a ß-blocker reduces ectopic activity, and may improve prognosis. Hypertension causes myocardial ischaemia, and you may see ventricular ectopic beats. If you suspect myocardial ischaemia, then aim to improve myocardial oxygen supply, and to decrease myocardial work. Give oxygen, treat pain, reduce blood pressure if it is elevated, improve cardiac perfusion with nitroglycerine, or calcium channel blockers, and consider cautiously slowing the heart rate with a ß-blocker.

10. Ventricular tachycardia (VT)
Ventricular tachycardia is a life threatening arrhythmia, generally occurring in patients with poor left ventricular function. If it is sustained the patient rapidly becomes hypotensive, with poor peripheral perfusion. Ventricular tachycardia is defined as three, or more ventricular premature beats in succession.

Causes include:
- myocardial ischaemia and infarction;
- hypotension;
- inflammation;
- drug toxicity.

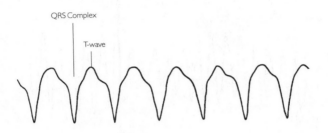

fig V.16 Ventricular tachycardia

RHYTHM	regular.
P-WAVE	absent.
P:QRS	absent.
P-R INTERVAL	none.
ATRIAL RATE	cannot be determined.
QRS	often notched or bizarre, and opposite in direction to ST segment and T-wave.
QRS WIDTH	greater than 0.12 sec.
VENTRICULAR RATE	100 - 250+/min.

A precordial thump may convert ventricular tachycardia to sinus rhythm. If the patient has a poor or absent perfusion status, do not delay, immediately use DC synchronized cardioversion. Treat pulseless VT as ventricular fibrillation. The patient who is alert with a good perfusion status, may revert with lignocaine 0.75 - 1.5 mg/kg intravenously given as a bolus. Because of the sluggish circulation, you need to allow up to 3 minutes for the drug to reach the heart. If you have given the drug into an arm vein, then elevate the arm to hasten venous return. This dose may be repeated at 5 - 10 minute intervals to a total of lignocaine 3 mg/kg. Follow this with a lignocaine infusion if needed. If this fails try procainamide 20 - 30 mg per minute.

Patients with severe left ventricular dysfunction sometimes get a paradoxical response to antiarrhythmic drugs. The drug makes the rhythm, or its rate, worse. If this happens stop the drugs, and use cardioversion.

TORSADE DE POINTES (POLYMORPHIC VT)

Torsade de pointe means twisting about a point. This is a type of rapid ventricular tachycardia with rapidly changing QRS morphology. It looks as though the QRS complexes are revolving, as a spiral, around a baseline axis. It may occur in patients on quinidine, and is often fatal.

Note "Spiral Pattern"

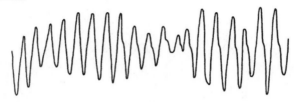

fig V.17 Torsade de pointes

RHYTHM	regular or irregular
P-WAVE	none
P:QRS	absent
P-R INTERVAL	absent
ATRIAL RATE	cannot be determined
QRS	alternating positive and negative deflection
QRS WIDTH	greater than 0.12/sec.
VENTRICULAR RATE	cannot be determined

First use DC countershock, and then give magnesium sulphate 2 gm intravenously over 2 minutes. Other antiarrhythmics are ineffective, and if the patient is hypotensive he usually will not survive long. Isoprenaline may be useful.

11. Ventricular Fibrillation (VF)

Ventricular fibrillation is chaotic quivering of the ventricles. There is no cardiac output, and it is lethal.

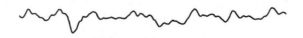

fig V.18 Ventricular fibrillation

RHYTHM	none
P-WAVE	none
P:QRS	absent
P-R INTERVAL	none
ATRIAL RATE	cannot be determined
QRS	irregular chaotic electrical activity with bizarre shapes
QRS WIDTH	coarse or fine waves
VENTRICULAR RATE	cannot be determined

Immediately defibrillate and manage as for a cardiac arrest according to your protocol.

12. Asystole (cardiac standstill)

This is usually fatal, and responds poorly to resuscitation efforts. The ECG shows a flat line with no carotid pulse detectable.

Line may wave slightly

fig V.19 Asystole

RATE	none
RHYTHM	none
P-WAVE	none
P:QRS	none
P-R INTERVAL	none
ATRIAL RATE	none
QRS	slowly fluctuating base line
QRS WIDTH	none
VENTRICULAR RATE	none

Immediately commence CPR, and ensure adequate oxygenation, and ventilation. Try to find out the reason. Exclude hypoxia, hypovolaemia, tension pneumothorax, and cardiac tamponade. Give 1 mg (1 ml of 1:1000) adrenaline intravenously. Follow the adrenaline with 20 ml of saline and lift the arm to hasten the drug to the central circulation. If there is no response within 3 - 5 minutes then double the dose of adrenaline. If there is still no response consider a small dose of sodium bicarbonate 0.25 mmol/kg given over 2 minutes. This is a lethal arrhythmia, with a poor prognosis.

Appendix VI.
Day Surgery Information

How does a general anaesthetic affect me?

When you are under an anaesthetic you are *not* asleep. The drugs used during the anaesthetic turn off the brain so that you cannot feel pain. Once you are unconscious, your brain cannot control your body's vital functions. This means that the anaesthetist has to take over the control of things like breathing and blood pressure for you.

How long does it take to wake up?

When the operation is finished you will be taken from the Operating Theatre to the Recovery Room. Here the nurse and the anaesthetist will look after you until you have recovered from the anaesthetic. It takes a few minutes to wake up, but you may remain drowsy for some time. You will stay in the Recovery Room for at least one hour until most of the effects of the anaesthetic have worn off.

How will I feel when I wake up?

At first ordinary sounds will seem louder than normal. To start with you may wonder where you are, and possibly have some pain at the operation site.

Why do I need the oxygen mask?

The oxygen helps flush out the anaesthetic gases from your body.

Do not take off your oxygen mask.

If you remove it too soon you may get a headache, or may even become confused. Usually oxygen is necessary only for a few minutes. But if you have had major hip or knee surgery, or have been receiving treatment for heart or lung problems, you may need oxygen for some time. Do not take off the oxygen mask until a doctor or nurse says it is safe for you to do so.

Why is the nurse asking me to take deep breaths?

As you are waking up nurse will call you by name and say "Your operation has finished, take some nice big deep breaths and move your legs". These deep breaths help the lungs start working normally again. This deep breaths are especially important if you are a smoker.

- Take a deep breath to gently fill your lungs.
- Hold the air in while you count slowly to three, and then let the air out.
- Repeat these 3 times and the have a rest.
- Then have a big cough.

It is a good idea to practice these exercises several times before you come into hospital.

Why should I move my legs around?

After an operation you may not move your legs around as much as normal. If blood clots form in the big sponge muscles of your calves or thighs these can cause very serious complications that may delay your discharge from hospital. To help prevent these clots, the nurses will show you how to do special exercises to speed up the blood flow through your legs. The nurses will remind you how to pump your feet and legs up and down as would if you were pressing the brake pedals in a car. You should do this at least 20 times every half hour until you are up and walking around. Of course you do not need to do this while you are asleep.

How much pain should I expect?

Tell the nurse if you have pain.

Severe pain is largely unnecessary and can be harmful. It is important to tell nurse if you have pain. The anaesthetist has many ways of controlling pain to keep you comfortable. Usually, the anaesthetist will give you something to help relive the pain before you wake up.

Will I feel sick or vomit?

Because the anaesthetic drugs are much better than they were even a few years ago, only a few patients vomit after their anaesthetic. If you do feel sick, tell nurse. Vomiting is still sometimes unavoidable.

What is the intravenous drip for?
You will have an intravenous drip running into a vein in your arm. Anaesthetists give these special fluids to help your kidneys flush the anaesthetic drugs from the body.

Can I catch a disease such as HIV/AIDS or hepatitis?
Each patient has brand new sterile drugs, needles, and syringes; so there is no chance that you will catch HIV or AIDS from this new anaesthetic equipment.

When can I drive a car?
Many of the effects of the anaesthetic wear off after a few hours, but it can take much longer in some cases. You may not react as quickly as normal to any emergency for up to 48 hours after an anaesthetic.

*You are warned that you must not drive a car
or use dangerous machinery
for at least 48 hours (two full days) after your anaesthetic*

If you do drive there is a high risk that you may have an accident. Avoid using any machinery which may injure you such as lawn mowers, chain saws, or any electrical or mechanical tools. Similarly you should not make any financial or legal decisions because you may not be able to think clearly. You should not cook because of the danger of tipping hot fluids over yourself.

*Please ask questions
if there is anything you do not understand.*

What about my teeth, dentures, caps, crowns and bridges?
When waking up from anaesthesia some patients grind their teeth and bite their lips. It is not possible to stop you doing this. We use a special rubber mouth guard device to help stop this happening, but sometimes teeth still get chipped and crowns become detached, and lips are bruised. We trust you understand that despite all care, this is a problem we cannot always prevent.

Appendix VII.
Trolley Setups

Emergency trolleys are best prepared in advance and stored for easy access. Those that are rarely required like malignant hyperthermia and bronchoscopy can be shared with the operating theatre. Photograph the layout and tie the photograph, encased in plastic, to the trolley. This makes it easy to check the setup each day. Discourage people from borrowing from these trolleys. Keep the trolleys as near as possible to the fridge and the defibrillator. If you are a small hospital without piped oxygen you will need to keep a full cylinder and regulator close too.

Trolleys include:
- IV access;
- reintubation, these two, which are most frequently required, can be combined into a general emergency trolley;
- cardiac arrest;
- paediatric this can be a tray on the bottom shelf of the main trolley which can be lifted up when required;
- anaphylaxis;
- thoracic aspiration (instructions for carrying out this procedure are on page 96);
- malignant hyperthermia;
- bronchoscopy;
- local anaesthetic trolley.

General Emergency Trolley

If you have a small recovery room you may wish to combine your main trolley. A typical set up for a general emergency trolley would include:
- an intravenous tray with all sizes of cannulas, spirit wipes and gauze;
- tubes for taking blood studies and a key to their coding;
- tubes for blood gas studies;
- boxes of non-sterile gloves, all sizes;
- two laryngoscope handles with batteries;
- extra batteries;
- laryngoscope blades (all sizes);
- stylettes and guide wires (malleable metal or plastic);
- water soluable lubricant;

- oropharyngeal airways, all sizes;
- nasophyngeal airways, all sizes;
- laryngeal masks (including an intubating laryngeal mask);
- cricothyroidotomy kit;
- retrograde intubation kit;
- self-inflating manual resuscitation bag, such as Ambu® or Laerdal®;
- face masks to fit this bag;
- oxygen tubing to connect the bag to the oxygen source;
- bronchoscopes with their light source: small, medium and large;
- cuffed endotracheal tubes, all sizes;
- catheter mounts and tight connections;
- 20 ml syringe for inflating tracheal cuffs;
- Magill forceps;
- wooden mouth-gags.

Drugs should be kept on the trolley and in the fridge, as appropriate. Leave a list of the fridge drugs on the trolley. The following drugs are suitable for the trolley, you will probably add others:
- two ampoules of thiopentone, with water to dilute them;
- ketamine;
- propofol;
- suxamethonium, put out two ampoules each day and keep the main suppply in the fridge;
- diazepam or diazemuls;
- midazolam;
- atropine 0.6mg;
- lignocaine 1% and 2%;
- dextrose 50%;
- adrenaline 1:1000 and 1:10 000;
- hydrocortisone 100mg;
- intravenous fluids and drip tubing.

LOCAL ANAESTHETIC TROLLEY

A local anaesthetic trolley should be ready at all times for the urgent insertion of a spinal or epidural. This should include;
- gown and sterile gloves, all sizes;
- four sterile drapes;
- sterile gauze;
- sponge holders;
- preparation solution such as cetrimide;

- local anaesthetic drugs;
- commercial packs for spinal and epidural procedures;
- spare needles and other individually packed sterile items if available;
- needles and syringes of various sizes;
- lignocaine 1% for skin analgesia.

THORACIC DRAIN TROLLEY

This trolley should hold the following:
- One medium stainless steel tray, or similar commercial packed tray;
- one small kidney dish;
- two small gallipots;
- one scalpel handle size 3;
- one toothed dissecting forcep;
- two pair of artery forceps;
- one suture scissors;
- one needle holder;
- one 1/0 atraumatic silk suture;
- one scapel blade size 10;
- sterile packs of cotton wool swabs;
- sterile packs of gauze;
- three sterile drapes.

Add to this:
- lignocaine 1%;
- disposable syringes and needles;
- povidone (Betadine®) skin preparation;
- drain tubes of various sizes including children's sizes;
- trochars, Argyle® or similar.

MALIGNANT HYPERTHERMIA TROLLEY

This trolley should be kept right beside the fridge and a supply of Ringer's lactate and normal saline should be set aside in the fridge for use in this crisis, if it should occur. Also in the fridge, dedicated to this emergency keep:
- nasogastric tubes;
- dantrolene sodium, at least 20 ampoules (shelf life is 3 years);
- regular insulin.

On the trolley keep the following:
- urinary catheter and insertion tray;

- a urinometer;
- fresh breathing circuit;
- temperature probe and recorder;
- cooling blanket (or note where this is stored);
- rectal tube;
- intravenous, CVP and Swan-Ganz catheters;
- tubes for blood gas and haematological studies;
- equipment for administering high flow oxygen;
- sterile distilled water, at least 2 litres;
- a sterile bowl for mixing dantrolene and this water;
- mannitol;
- frusemide;
- sodium bicarbonate 8.4% 100ml;
- dextrose 50%;
- procainamide hydrochloride.

REQUIREMENTS FOR RESCUSCITATION OF THE NEWBORN

These include;
- a high sloping trolley;
- a radient heater;
- oxygen, a flow meter, limited to a flow of 4l/min, and tubing;
- a suction which is set at 40 cm water pressure;
- suction catheters, sizes 5 - 10F;
- a bulb syringe;
- a meconium aspirator;
- sterile gloves, all sizes;
- a stethescope;
- a laryngoscope with straight blades;
- extra bulbs and batteries;
- airways, sizes 000, 00 and 0;
- small masks;
- endotracheal tubes, sizes 2.5 to 3.5. Check that the tube has an end on it which will fit into the mask mount if you need to intubate;
- laryngeal mask, size one;
- a neonatal Ambu® or Laedal® rescucitation bag;
- pulse oximeter with appropriate sensor for a baby;
- ECG;
- umbilical catheter, 3 - 5F;
- sterile umbilical vessel catheterization tray;

- needles and syringes, all sizes;
- 3 way taps;
- IV giving set with a burette;
- saline, 1/5N saline;
- albumen 5%;
- dextrose 10%;
- adrenaline 1:10 000;
- naloxone 0.4mg/ml;
- NaHCO$_3$ 0.5mEq/ml 4.2% 10cc ampoules;
- sterile water and saline 10cc ampoules;
- adhesive tape;
- scissors.

APPENDIX VIII.
ABBREVIATIONS

Abbreviations are frequently used by medical and nursing staff. They are sometimes specific to a particular area, and are a mystery to outsiders, but many are in common use. To avoid errors and mishaps use only abbreviations approved by your hospital. Even approved abbreviations can be misunderstood if they are not written clearly, and clear script is not a virtue of many doctors. Always explain abbreviations if there is the possibility they have more than one meaning, for example, DOA could mean dead on arrival, or date of admission; ARF could mean acute respiratory failure or acute renal failure; and Cx could mean cervical spine or cervix. This is a list of common abbreviations used in many hospitals.

Never act on an abbreviation
unless you are absolutely sure what it means.

a.c.	before food is given; it applies to medication.	ASAP	as soon as possible
		Assist	assistants
AC	alternating current	ATLS	advanced trauma life support
ABG	arterial blood gases	AUC	area under curve
ACE	angiotensin converting enzyme	AV shunt	arteriovenous shunt
ACLS	advanced cardiac life support	AV node	atrioventricular node
ADT	any damn thing	AXR	abdominal x-ray
AED	automatic external defibrillator	BA	bowel action
AF	atrial fibrillation	BCC	basal cell carcinoma
AIDS	acquired immune deficiency syndrome	BCLS	basic cardiac life support
		b.d.	twice daily
a.m.	before noon	BF	breast fed
AMI	acute myocardial infarction	BIP	bisthmus iodine paste
ANS	autonomic nervous system	BKA	below knee amputation
APACHE	acute physiology and chronic health evaluation	BP	blood pressure
APS	acute pain service	B.S.	blood sugar
APTT	activated partial thromboplastin time	BUN	bound urinary nitrogen
		BVM	bab valve mask unit
ARDS	adult respiratory distress syndrome	Bx	biopsy
		Ca	carcinoma
ARF	acute renal failure	Ca^{2+}	calcium ion

CaO₂	arterial oxygen content
CABG	coronary artery bypass graft
CAN	cardiac autonomic neuropathy
CAD	coronary artery disease
CAPD	ambulatory peritoneal dialysis
CAVDH	continuous arterio-venous haemodialysis
CCF	congestive cardiac failure
CDH	congenital dislocationof the hip
CE	continuing education
CETT	cuffed endotracheal tube
CK	creatinine kinase
CKMB	creatinine kinase isoenzyme—muscle band
Cl-	chloride ion
cm	centimetre
CMV	cytomegalovirus
CNS	central nervous system
CO₂	carbon dioxide
COAD	chronic obstructive airway disease
COPD	chronic obstructive pulmonary disease
CPAP	continuous positive airway pressure
CRF	chronic renal failure
CRI	cardiac risk index
CSF	cerebrospinal fluid
CT	computographic scan
CVA	cerebrovascular accident
CVC	central venous catheter
CVP	central venous pressure
CvO₂	mixed venus oxygen content
CWMS	colour,warmth, movement, sensation
Cx	cervix
Cx	cervical spine
C5	fifth cervical vertebra
CXR	chest X-ray
DDAVP®	desmopressin,
DB&C	deep breath and cough
DC	direct current

DPG	diphosphoglycerate
DOA	dead on arrival
DO₂	oxygen supply
DOB	date of birth
dTC	tubocurare
DUT	diabetic urine tests
Dx	diathermy
D5W	dextrose 5% in water
EACA	epsilon amino caproic acid
ECF	extracellular fluid
ECG	electrocardiograph
ED	emergency department
EKG	electrocardiograph
ELISA	enzyme-linked immunosorbent assay
EMB	early morning breakfast
EMLA	eutectic mixture of local anaesthetics
ENT	ear, nose and throat surgery
E/o	excision of
ER	emergency room
ERSF	end stage renal failure
ESWL	extracorporeal shock wave lithotripsy
ESU	electrosurgical unit (diathermy in the UK)
ETA	estimated time of arrival
ETT	endotracheal tube
EUA	examination under anaesthesia
FB	foreign body
FBC	fluid balance chart
FBE	full blood examination
FDA	Federal Drug Authority—an USA agency
FDP	fibrin degredation products
FEV₁	forced expiratory volume in one second
FF	free fluids
FHx	family history
FI	for investigation
FIO₂	fractional concentration of inspired oxygen
FNAB	fine-needle aspiration biopsy

FNH	febrile non-haemolytic reactions	ICF	intracellular fluid
FRC	functional residual capacity	IDDM	insulin dependent diabetes mellitus
FS	frozen section	IgA	immunoglobin A, (others are M, E.and G).
FSH	follicle stimulating hormone		
FVC	forced vital capacity	IHD	ischaemic heart disease
FWD	full ward diet	IMV	intermittent manditory ventilation
FWT	full ward test of urine		
G	gauge	INR	International normalized ratio (see PTT)
GA	general anaesthesia	IPPV	intermittent positive pressure ventilation
GABA	gamma aminobutyric acid		
GAMP	general anaesthetic, manipulation and plaster	ISQ	in status quo (meaning 'unchanged')
GCS	Glasgow Coma Scale	I.U.	International units
GGT	gamma-glutamyltransferase	IUD	intrauterine device
GFR	glomerular filtration rate	IV	intravenous
GTN	glyceryl trinitrate	IVI	intravenous injection
Gyn	gynaecology	JVP	jugular venous pressure
Hb	haemoglobin	K^+	potassium ion
HCO_3	bicarbonate ion	KCl	potassium chloride
HFV	high frequency ventilation	kg	kilogram
HIC	head injury chart	kPa	kilopasacal
HITs	heparin induced thrombocytopaenia	LA	local anaesthesia
		Lac	laceration
HIV	human immunodeficiency virus	LBBB	left bundle branch block
		LDH	lactic dehydrogenase
HNPU	has not passed urine	LIF	left iliac fossa
HOCUM	hypertrophic obstructive cardiomyopathy	LMA	laryngeal mask airway
		LOC	loss of consciousness
HPV	hypoxic pulmonary vasoconstriction	LP	lumbar puncture
		LUQ	left upper quadrant
hrly	hourly	LVF	left ventricular failure
HSV	herpes simplex virus	L3-4	interspace between 3rd and 4th lumbar vertebrae
Htn	hypertension		
HT	hypertension	m^2	square metre
HTR	haemolytic transfusion reactions	mane	in the morning
		MAC	minimum anaesthetic concentration
HTLV	human T cell lymphotrophic virus		
		MAC	monitored anaesthetic care
Hx	history	MAHA	micro-angiopathic haemolytic anaemia
i.d.	internal diameter		
I/M	intramuscular	MAO	mono-amine oxidase
ICC	intercostal catheter		

MAOI	mono-amine oxidase inhibitor	nocte	at night
MAP	mean arterial pressure	NO	nitric oxide
MAR	medicine administration record	NOF	neck of femur
MAT	multifocal atrial tachycardia	NPA	nasopharyngeal aspiration
MBA	motor bicycle accident	N/S	normal saline
MCA	motor car accident	NTG	nitroglycerine (see GTN)
MEAC	mean effect anaesthetic concentration	NSAID	non-steriodal anti-inflammatory drugs
mcg	microgram	NYO	not yet ordered
Mg^{2+}	magnesium ion	N_2O	nitrous oxide
mg	milligram	O	oral
MH	malignant hyperthermia	O_2	oxygen
MI	myocardial infarction	O/A	on admission
MIC	minimum inhibitory concentration	O/call	on call
min	minute	OD	overdose
mm	millimetre	OPD	out-patients department
mmHg	millimetre of mercury pressure	OR	operating room
mmol	millimol	Ortho	orthopaedics
mosmol	milli osmol	OSA	obstructive sleep apnoea
ms	millisecond	OT	operating theatre
MS	multiple sclerosis	OXI	pulse oximetery
MSOF	multisystem organ failure	P	partial pressure as in PO_2
MRSA	multiple resistant Staphylococcus aureus	$PaCO_2$	partial pressure of carbon dioxide in the arterial blood
MTBF	mean time between failures	PACU	post-anaesthetic care unit
mV	millivolt	Paed	paediatrics
MVA	motor vehicle accident	PaO_2	partial pressure of oxygen in the arterial blood
MVPS	mitral valve prolapse syndrome	PA	pulmonary artery
Na^+	sodium ion	PAP	pulmonary artery pressure
NAD	nothing abnormal detected	PAT	paroxysmal atrial tachycardia
NBP	non-invasive blood pressure	PAWP	pulmonary artery wedge pressure
NIBP	non-invasive blood pressure		
Neg	negative	P.C.	after meals
NFO	no further orders	PCA	patient controlled analgesia
NFR	not for resuscitation	PCEA	patient controlled epidural analgesia
N/G	nasogastric		
NIDDM	non-insulin dependent diabetes mellitus	PCTA	percutaneous transluminal angioplasty
NMBD	neuromuscular blocking drugs	PD	peritoneal dialysis
NMDA	N-methyl-D-aspartic acid	PDE	phosphodiesterase
NMS	Neuroleptic malignant syndrome	PDQ	pretty damn quick
		PEA	pre-emptive analgesia

PEEP	positive end-expiratory pressure
PERLA	pupils equal and reacting to light and accommodation
pH	inverse logarithm of the hydrogen ion activity
PHx	past history
p.m.	after midday
PM	post-mortem
PND	paroxysmal nocturnal dyspnoea
PONV	post operative nausea and vomiting
PORC	postoperative residual curarization
POP	plaster of Paris
Pos	positive
PORC	post-operative residual curarization
PPF	plasma protein fraction
ppm	parts per million
PR	per rectum
PRBC	packed red blood cells
premed	premedication
PRN	when necessary (pro re nata)
PT	prothrombin time (also see INR)
PTH	post transfusion hepatitis
PTSD	post traumatic stress disorder
PTTK	activated partial thromplastin time (see APPT)
PUO	pyrexia of unknown origin
PV	per vagina
PVB	premature ventricular beat
PVC	polyvinyl chloride
PVC	premature ventricular contraction
PVR	pulmonary vascular resistance
QD	once daily (use of this is discouraged)
QID	four times daily
®	registered name
RBBB	right bundle branch block
RBF	renal blood flow

resps	respiration
RIA	radio-immuno assay
RIB	rest in bed
RIF	right iliac fossa
ROP	retinopathy of prematurity
RPAO	routine post anaesthetic orders
RUQ	right upper quarrant
RVF	right ventricular failure
SA node	sino-atrial node
SAP	systemic arterial pressure
S/B	seen by
SBE	subacute bacterial endocarditis
sec	seconds
S/C	subcutaneous
SG	specific gravity
SIADH	syndrome of inappropriate antidiuretic hormone secretion
SLE	systemic lupus erythematosus
SMR	submucosal resection
SNP	sodium nitroprusside
SOF	shaft of femur
SOOB	sit out of bed
Sp/A	spinal anaesthesia
SR	sinus rhthym
SSG	split skin graft
Stat	statum (immediately)
STD	sexually transmitted disease
STOP	suction termination of pregnancy
STP	sodium thiopentone
STP	standard temperature and pressure
Sux	suxamethonium chloride
SVR	systemic vascular resistance
SVT	supraventricular tachycardia
SWMA	systolic wall movement abnormality
tabs	tablets
TAH	total abdominal hysterectomy
TB	tuberculosis
TCP	transcutaneous pacemaker
tds	three times a day

TENS	transcutaneous nerve stimulation	#	fracture
THR	total hip replacement	#	number
TIA	transient ischaemic attack	5-HT	5 hydroxytryptamine (also called serotonin)
TMOA	too many obscure abbreviations	$[Na^+]$	concentration of sodium ion
TOF	train-of-four with a nerve stimulator	$[X]$	concentration of X
		<	less than
TOP	termination of pregnancy	>	greater than
TPN	total parenteral nutrition	«	much less than
TPR	temperature, pulse and respiration	»	much greater than
		/	per or each (breaths/min)
TRLI	transfusion related lung injury	%	per cent
Ts&A	tonsillectomy and adenoidectomy	@	at
		°C	degree centigrade
TTN	transient tachypnea of the newborn	°F	degree fahrenheit
TURP	transurethral resection of prostate	®	registered name
		©	copyright
T_3	tri-iodothyronine	™	trade mark
T6	sixth thoracic vertebra	α	greek letter, alpha
U&E	urea and electrolytes	β	greek letter, beta (pronounce bee-ta)
URTI	upper respiratory tract infection	γ	greek letter, gamma
UTT	up to toilet	δ	greek letter, delta
UWSD	under-water sealed drainage	Δ	greek letter upper case delta used to describe differences
V	volt	ε	greek letter, epsilon
VC	vital capacity	μ	greek letter, mu (pronounced mew)
VEs	ventricular extrasystoles		
VF	ventricular fibrillation	π	greek letter, pi (pronounced pie)
VO_2	oxygen consumption		
VPBs	ventricular premature beats		
VT	ventricular tachycardia		
VVs	varicose veins		
WEL	weekend leave		
WHO	World Health Organization		
WNL	within normal limits		
WPW	Wolff–Parkinson–White syndrome		
WYSWYG	What you see is what you get (a computer term)		
X-match	cross-match blood		
XDP	fibrin d-dimer		

INDEX